OXFORD MEDICAL PUBLICATIONS

Epidemiology of anencephalus and spina bifida

Epidemiology of anencephalus and spina bifida

J. MARK ELWOOD

Head of the Division of Epidemiology
Cancer Control Agency of British Columbia

AND

J. HAROLD ELWOOD

Professor of Social and Preventive Medicine
Department of Community Medicine
The Queen's University of Belfast

OXFORD
OXFORD UNIVERSITY PRESS
NEW YORK TORONTO
1980

Oxford University Press, Walton Street, Oxford OX2 6DP
OXFORD LONDON GLASGOW
NEW YORK TORONTO MELBOURNE WELLINGTON
KUALA LUMPUR SINGAPORE JAKARTA HONG KONG TOKYO
DELHI BOMBAY CALCUTTA MADRAS KARACHI
IBADAN NAIROBI DAR ES SALAAM CAPE TOWN

British Library Cataloguing in Publication Data

Elwood, J Mark
Epidemiology of anencephalus and spina bifida.
1. Spina bifida 2. Epidemiology 3. Anencephalus
I. Title II. Elwood, J Harold
614.5′97′3043 RJ496.S74 79-40890

ISBN 0-19-261220-4

Phototypeset by Western Printing Services Ltd, Bristol
Printed in Great Britain
at the University Press, Oxford
by Eric Buckley
Printer to the University

Preface

We describe in this book the epidemiology of two of the most common major congenital malformations of the central nervous system occurring in developed countries at the present time. Anencephalus and spina bifida not only comprise a significant health problem in early life but also illustrate many aspects of the wider phenomenon of the occurrence of congenital malformations in man. We therefore discuss some aspects of the role of epidemiology in attempting to elucidate the aetiology of birth defects.

Epidemiological methods can be applied in many fields and our studies may be of interest to all medical and allied personnel involved with the problems associated with infants having anencephalus or spina bifida. In addition to epidemiologists, the contents may be relevant to the work of community physicians, geneticists, neurologists, obstetricians, paediatricians, and teratologists. We do not aim at providing a comprehensive text on all aspects of neurological malformations as this undertaking would require a large team of contributors. Additional aspects relating to clinical observations of these infants and their management, particularly with respect to spina bifida, are contained in several recent books and journals. For this reason we have not included data on technical procedures, specialized investigations such as ultrasonography, amniography, amniocentesis and foetoscopy, and statistical methods. We also omit a review of early literature from the nineteenth century and before and our illustrative material is restricted to simple maps, graphs, and line diagrams. As these topics are covered elsewhere we present some findings from our own studies of the epidemiology of anencephalus and spina bifida in Canada and Ireland. These observations are compared with reports by other authors from various countries. We describe how the epidemiological approach may be used to investigate the problem of birth defects and appendices outlining some statistical methods adopted in our work are included.

Conclusive demonstration of the cause of anencephalus and spina bifida with recommendations for implementing an effective and efficient programme of primary prevention would be a logical end to our study. However, as with many conditions in medicine, an understanding of the aetiological factors involved has not yet been achieved. While some degree of primary and secondary prevention is possible, serious ethical, legal, and medical issues are associated with introducing these methods on a national scale. This book brings together material from many sources, presents some original data, and we hope, adds to knowledge regarding these malformations which may be of interest to the reader.

Vancouver J. M. E.
and J. H. E.
Belfast
March 1979

Acknowledgements

WE wish to acknowledge the many individuals in North America and the British Isles who provided assistance at various stages of this study.

The Canadian work was greatly helped by the encouragement of Dr John M. Last, University of Ottawa; valuable advice was given by Drs Stephen Walter, S. Raman, and Luciano Neri and Mr Giles Mousseau, University of Ottawa, Drs Brian MacMahon, Olli Miettienen, Kenneth Rothman, and Stella Yen of the Harvard School of Public Health, and by Mr Andrew Coldman, Cancer Control Agency of British Columbia. We also express our thanks to Dr Gerry Hill, Mr Norman Tompkins, and Mr John Silins and the staff of Statistics Canada for access to unpublished data and to Dr Philip Banister, Health and Welfare Canada, for access to data from the Congenital Anomalies Surveillance System. Studies based on the British Columbia Health Surveillance Registry were conducted with assistance from Mr Guy Renwick, Department of Vital Statistics, Province of British Columbia, Dr James Miller, Mrs Mary McBride and Dr Muriel Harris, Department of Medical Genetics, Dr Elizabeth Poland, Department of Obstetrics and Gynaecology, and Dr Cortlandt MacKenzie, Department of Health Care and Epidemiology, University of British Columbia. The British work was conducted with valuable advice from Professor John Pemberton, Professor Peter Froggatt, Dr Roger Blaney, Dr Maureen Scott, Mr Gilbert MacKenzie and Mr Maurice O'Flaherty, Department of Community Medicine, Dr Gordon Cran, Department of Physics and Applied Mathematics, Emeritus Professor E. A. Cheeseman, Department of Medical Statistics, Professor J. E. Morison, Department of Pathology, and Professor Norman Nevin, Department of Medical Genetics, The Queen's University of Belfast. We are grateful for comments from numerous individuals including Dwight Janerich, Albany, Irvin Emanuel, Seattle, Stanley Martin, Vancouver, Stephen Rogers, Rugby, Ian Leck, Manchester, and Professor R. G. Record and Professor George Knox, Birmingham. Considerable help was provided by research assistants and secretaries including Janice Rogers, Kathy Bell, Joan Camus, Kenneth Johnston, and Maxine Werner in Canada and Iris Hay, Margaret Bowker, Jennifer Clifton, Jean Ritchie, Emily McGurk, Phyllis Dorris, and Joseph Clint in Northern Ireland. Mr W. D. Linton, Miss A. H. P. McKeown and staff, Medical Library, Queen's University, Belfast, traced much published literature on our behalf and the illustrations were prepared by Elizabeth Rodgers and Helen McIlhenny, Medical Photographic Unit, Royal Victoria Hospital, Belfast.

This work could not have been completed without generous financial support to Dr Mark Elwood from Health and Welfare Canada (grants 606–1038–29, 606–1220–43 and 606–1119–43) and to Dr Harold Elwood from the Medical Research Council of the United Kingdom (Project Grants

G 972/919/c and G 977/1004/N). Dr Mark Elwood also was supported by a training Fellowship from the Physicians Services Incorporated Foundation, Ontario, a Health and Welfare Canada Fellowship and a Health and Welfare Scholar's Award.

Contents

I

Introduction

UNTIL recently congenital malformations were studied mainly as anatomical and pathological curiosities. At the beginning of this century diseases of early life presenting for medical care were predominantly infections. Analysis of the cause of death in the first 200 children dying and coming to autopsy at the Hospital for Sick children in Great Ormond Street, London in 1914 showed some 68 per cent due to tuberculosis, pneumonia, gastroenteritis, and other environmental conditions (Carter 1956). Out of a total of 1403 infant deaths in Belfast during 1915, only 43, some 3.1 per cent, were attributed to congenital malformations and the proportion in Dublin, 2.3 per cent, was even less (Elwood, J. H. 1973). With the decline of infectious diseases, congenital malformations are now more important and account for around 20 per cent or more of all mortality during the first year of life. Within this wide spectrum, two specific neural tube defects, anencephalus and spina bifida, are particularly common in Caucasian populations. The highest frequencies in the world so far reported occur in Ireland where these two defects alone account for 15 per cent of all perinatal and 10 per cent of all postperinatal mortality in Belfast (Elwood, J. H., MacKenzie, and Cran 1974). Prevalence rates for anencephalus and spina bifida in Dublin are similar (Coffey 1970, 1974). These malformations comprise an important part of early mortality at the present time (Table 1.1). For these reasons and because of the development of more effective surgical treatment for infants with spina bifida lesions, there is much current interest in these malformations and their possible causation. A sketch of the historical background gives a brief introduction to the present debate.

TABLE 1.1 *Proportions of early mortality attributed to anencephalus and spina bifida in Canada and the United Kingdom based on official statistics 1973*

Country	Total births (number)	Stillbirths and infant deaths (number)	Due to congenital anomalies (per cent)†	Anencephalus (per cent)‡	Due to spina bifida (per cent)‡	Both defects (per cent)‡
Canada	346 239	8205	17	28	7	35
Northern Ireland	29 589	999	23	34	19	53
Scotland	75 265	2285	30	26	16	42
England and Wales	683 889	19 343	36	17	15	32

† Per cent of all stillbirths of 28 or more weeks' gestation plus infant deaths.
‡ Per cent of stillbirths and infant deaths attributed to congenital anomalies.

1

Historical note

It would be incorrect to assume that anencephalus and spina bifida are recently observed conditions. A mummified anencephalic human foetus discovered in a sarcophagus at Hermopolis on the Nile was described and demonstrated at a meeting of the Academy of Sciences in Paris by Saint-Hilaire (1826). It was found in the catacombs of that city in the area where sacred animals, the ape and ibis, normally were buried according to the religious beliefs of ancient Egypt (Fig. 1.1). Brothwell and Powers (1968) note that the embalmer followed the usual methods of mummification attempting to remove the brain via an opening made through from the nose and apparently the significance of the deformities in the head and neck region posteriorly were not noticed. This specimen was acquired by the King of Prussia and formed part of the collection of the Berlin Museum which was later destroyed during the Second World War (Powers 1978). The earliest post-Renaissance description of an anencephalic is probably that by Lycosthenes (1557) and another is included in the register prepared by Ambrosinus (1642) of a collection of specimens of monstrosity assembled by Aldrovandus. Taruffi (1891) wrote that the term 'anencephaly' was used by Schlegal in 1812 and after this date the term 'anencephalus' became more widely adopted. Further details of various historical aspects are given by Warkany (1959, 1971, 1977) and Lemire, Beckwith, and Warkany (1978). Examples of spina bifida occulta have been reported in prehistoric human skeletons excavated in North America (Ferembach 1963) and well defined cases of spina bifida cystica were found in skeletons from the prehistoric, Roman, Anglo-Saxon, and Medieval periods in England (Brothwell and Powers 1968). Stewart (1931, 1953) noted neural-arch defects in ancient bony remains collected from Eskimo graves in Alaska and in the areas of the Yukon River, Point Hope, Norton Bay, and Bristol Bay and Bennett (1972) described a high frequency in skeletal remains of around 30 Modoc Indians found in Siskiyou County, California in 1967.

An extensive source of information on congenital malformations in the past are the teratological records of Chaldea (Ballantyne 1894). These consist of approximately one hundred clay tablets, many now stored in the British Museum, which have been variously interpreted by a number of scholars, the first being Oppert (1871), the second Lenormant (1875), and the latest Leichty (1970). These tablets covered with cuneiform script were found in the great mound of Koyunjik near the River Tigris in the nineteenth century by the archeologists Layard and Smith. They were part of the Royal

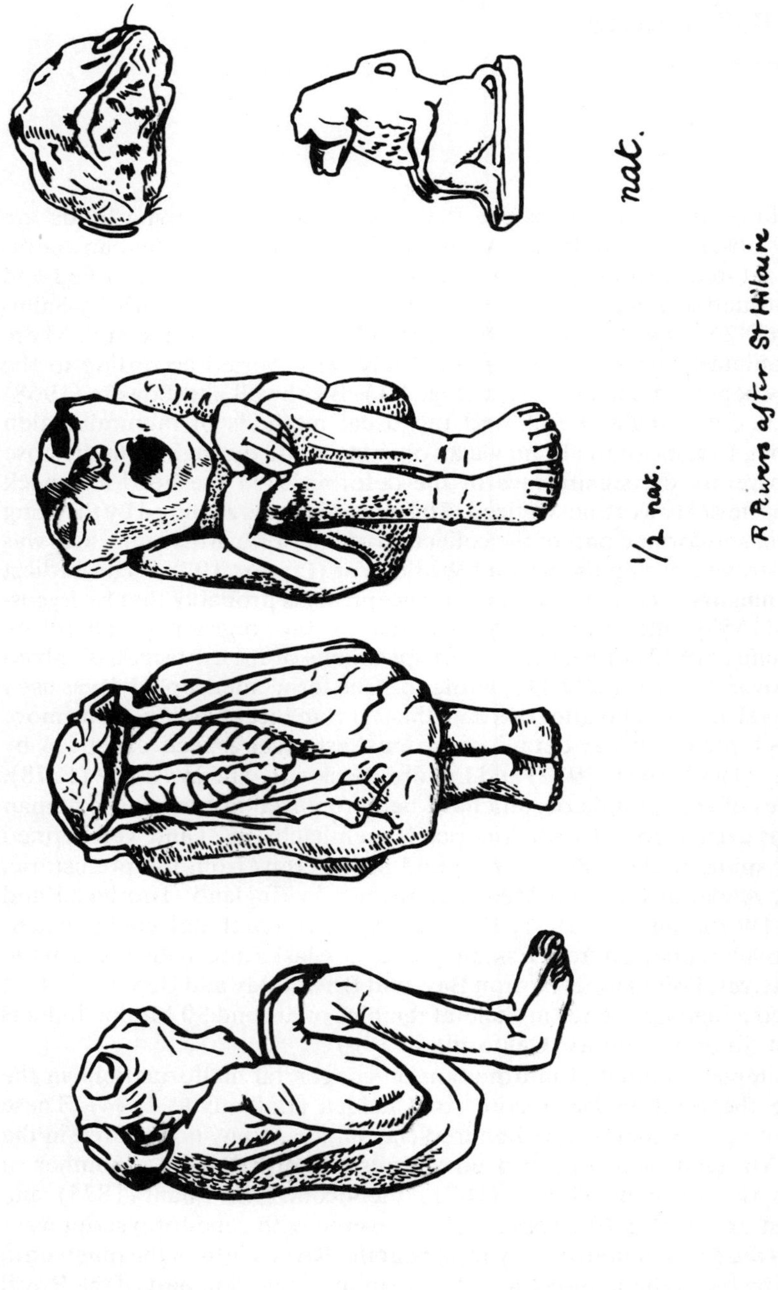

FIG. 1.1. The anencephalic mummy from Hermopolis. (Drawing by Powers 1978 after Saint-Hilaire 1826.)

Library of Nineveh assembled by Assurbanipal, King of Assyria from 668 to 626 BC. The tablets were arranged on shelves and if a work extended over several tablets an index listing first lines was provided while others, hanging down on straws like bookmarkers, gave the general title of each work. There were two libraries, one in the temple of Nabu and the other in the Royal palace. The records are written in Assyrian but may be copies of even older Babylonian texts dating from 2000 BC and were kept for the purpose of foretelling the future. This method of divination became established in many ancient civilizations and the Chaldean tablets include descriptions of several different types of human malformations although anencephalus is not mentioned.

Both in Egypt and India, the belief that union between members of different species could be fertile and produce monstrous offspring was widely held. The centaur of Greek mythology is one example and transmigration of souls from man to animal at death and vice versa as accepted by Hindus is another. This theory of causation was termed hybridization by Ballantyne (1904). Another explanation of malformed births was the theory of maternal impression. Similarity between monkeys and anencephalic infants gave rise to the belief that it was dangerous for a pregnant woman to look at monkeys whilst carrying a child *in utero*. Warkany (1971) quotes methods considered effective by the Spartans whose laws ordered pregnant women to look at statues of Castor and Pollux so that their children might be healthy and strong at birth. A less attractive side of ancient Greece and Rome was the widespread practice of infanticide both of malformed and normal children. The practice was carried out when there were too many infants born or if the infants were considered inferior or deformed. The Spartans accomplished this positive eugenic policy by throwing rejected offspring into a deep chasm on Mount Taygetus whilst the Romans preferred drowning unwanted infants in the River Tiber. Not that infanticide was limited to pre-Christian and non-Christian societies. Studies by Trexler (1973) of ecclesiastical records in Florence, Italy, and Helmholz (1974) of data for the Province of Canterbury, England, during the fifteenth century have shown such practices were widespread throughout medieval Europe. Kellum (1974) points out that despite the absence of demographic and historical records of infanticide much literary and church evidence exists. Imbalance of the sex ratio suggesting elimination of female infants is seen in the analyses of the heirs listed in 'Inquisition post mortem' from AD 1250 to 1348 and AD 1430 to 1545 by Russell (1948). These records show a ratio of male to female children of 1:1 but this later changes to 4:3. In another example from England, a list of serfs and their families on the lands of John F. Hastings from AD 1391–2 recorded 78 male and 46 female children, a ratio of 1.7:1. Specific synodal legislation against infanticide is included in the Decretals of Pope Gregory IX (AD 1234) and as early as AD 600 Columban defined the penance for overlaying one's child as one year on bread and water and two more years without wine or flesh. As in the ancient world the drowning of infants, often in a ditch or pond, was a common method of infanticide in England. Christianity, however, added one new feature as an unbaptized child was regarded as something evil and could do even more damage if laid to rest unbaptized. Some were buried with a stake through their heart to prevent the infant arising and injuring others (McNeil and Gamer 1938). Primitive folklore understood the newborn to be in great danger of being carried off by fairies and replaced by a changeling who would demand human milk (Gregor 1881). One method of getting rid of a changeling was to place the child in a basket and hang it over the fire and if it screamed, as it would, the diagnosis was confirmed and the changeling disposed of accordingly.

During medieval times the occurrence of malformed children was regarded as a portent of future disasters indicative of Divine wrath. This was especially so in Mosaic and Christian laws and the more extraordinary the abnormal birth the greater the disaster. Most of these examples today would be classified as monsters, a category (ICD No. 759.2) included in the *International Classification of Diseases* (World Health Organization 1967). One of the most famous, the birth of the Biddenden Maids at the village of Biddenden, near Staplehurst in Kent, about AD 1100 was associated in the same year with the death of William Rufus, King of England, who was found dead in the New Forest with the arrow of a hunter or possibly an assassin, in his chest. These sisters were twins conjoined at the shoulders and hips; they died six hours apart in 1134 and are buried in the churchyard of their native village. Their memory is preserved because of a curious will in which they bequeathed to

> the church-wardens of the parish of Biddenden and their successors, twenty acres of land, the annual revenue from which was to be spent in the distribution of cakes bearing the impression of their images, to be given away on each Easter Sunday to all strangers in Biddenden, also 270 quartern loaves, with cheese in proportion, to all the poor in the said parish.

This practice was discontinued at the beginning of this century owing to rowdy scrummages associated with the distribution of some 600 such cakes each Easter (Thompson 1930). There is a reference to similar conjoined twins in the Irish manuscript, Annals of the Four Masters (AD 1103), which may relate to the Biddenden Maids (Shrewsbury 1949). Paré, in his book, *Of monsters and prodigies* (1678), tabulates eleven causes accepted at that time as explanations for monstrosity and was of the opinion that single malformations and conjoined twinning arose due to the effects of the same aetiological factors (Guttmacher and Nichols 1967). The basic defect, according to Zimmermann (1967) who considered the Bayamon conjoined twins (Pantaléon-Mena, Díaz, Justiniano, Rudolph, and Nichols 1967) and the Port Lavaca conjoined twins (Griffin, Matthes, Hazlewood, and Nichols 1967) in detail, is an incomplete fusion occurring prior to the third week of ovulation age.

Often the doctrines of hybridity and maternal impression led to barbarous acts reminiscent of the hanging of witches in Salem, Massachusetts in 1692.

Mothers of these abnormal infants sometimes were put to death together with their offspring. By the end of the seventeenth century, London was a centre for exhibiting every variety of human form. They were displayed like circus animals in an area of West Smithfield and comprised part of an annual event known as the Bartholomew Fair. Handbills were printed describing each exhibit who, together with a manager, often toured Europe and the New World accumulating fortunes in the process. Well-known examples are the original Siamese conjoined twins, two brothers Eng and Chang who were born in 1811 at Maklong some 60 miles from Bangkok, and Charles Stratton, popularly known as General Tom Thumb who was 25 inches tall and came from Bridgeport, Connecticut. Tom Thumb's tour of Scotland and Ireland in 1846 is reputed to have grossed £150,000. Eng and Chang settled in North Carolina and were married at age 44 years to two sisters of English birth. There were 11 children in Eng's family and 10 in Chang's; the birth of one of the latter in 1868 was certified by Simpson of Edinburgh (Simpson and Barth 1869). Some 273 descendants comprising six generations of Eng–Chang families have been verified to date (Callahan and Mitchell 1970).

The first detailed descriptions of spina bifida are attributed to Nicholas Tulp who, in 1637 in Amsterdam, published an illustrated book recording observations based on six cases (Brocklehurst 1976). Tulp, a successful surgeon, held a post of anatomy demonstrator for 24 years and is depicted in Rembrandt's painting *The anatomy lesson.* This artist may have been the medical illustrator for Tulp's book (Rickman 1963). Later Morgagni (1761) examined several specimens of spina bifida with hydrocephalus and anencephalus with spina bifida and von Recklinghausen (1886) published observations on the dissection of 32 cases of spina bifida. Further anatomical and pathological studies were made by Cleland (1883), Humphry (1885), Arnold (1894), and Chiari (1891, 1896). Cleland's paper describes in great detail dissections of a full-term spina bifida infant with a lesion extending from the sixth thoracic vertebra to the first sacral vertebra and includes an account of the deformity now known eponymously as the Arnold–Chiari malformation. Chiari (1891) originally was of the opinion that there were three different types of deformity of the cerebellum as a result of hydrocephalus. Type I is associated with prolongation of the cerebellar tonsils and the medial part of the inferior lobe of the cerebellum and is sometimes called chronic tonsillar herniation. The second type, associated with extensive spina bifida, exhibits prolongation of the cerebellar vermis and inferior prolongation of the fourth ventricle into the cervical spinal canal causing displacement of the medulla oblongata. Type III is a severe defect having a dilated fourth ventricle and cerebellum present within the sac of a cervical encephalocele. Chiari's work, published in 1896 contains fourteen examples of the Type I deformity, seven of Type II, one example of Type III and also adds a fourth type characterized by cerebellar hypoplasia. Arnold's work and that of his pupils, Schwalbe and Gredig (1906) stressed the presence of cerebellar malformation to some degree in most spina bifida cases. They reviewed previous work, including the ideas of Morgagni, von Recklinghausen, and the Committee nominated by the Clinical Society of London on 10 November 1882 to investigate spina bifida and its treatment by the injection of Dr Morton's iodoglycerine solution (Marsh, Gould, Clutton, and Parker 1885). A fifth group of cerebellar abnormalities was added by Schwalbe and Gredig (1906) to the four already classified and these authors thought spina bifida occurred as a result of disturbance of the normal development of the neural tube at a time when the neural crests fold over. The descriptions of hindbrain deformities as Chiari Type I, Chiari Type II, etc. malformations may be of less value today than in the past. Variend and Emery (1976) suggest recording the precise lobular composition of the displaced segment of cerebellum.

The great interest in teratology during the late nineteenth and early twentieth centuries was based not only on ordinary curiosity but also stemmed from the publication on 24 November 1859 of Darwin's book, *The origin of species*. Previous observations such as Galileo's astronomy had produced fierce arguments between church, state, and scientist. However, these debates had taken place within the establishment, at that time a minority elite of probably less than ten per cent of the whole population who governed a largely illiterate peasant majority. Darwin's hypothesis was put forward during the period of the Industrial Revolution in England when a much greater proportion of the population could read and write. Moreover, unlike earlier scientific work during the Renaissance, it could be tested using fairly simple observational methods. Sophisticated apparatus, such as the telescope invented by Galileo, were not required. Because Darwin's book produced a powerful synthesis, explaining the great diversity of life as seen in plants, animals, and man, it was not long before others attempted to examine the theory directly by measuring natural biological variation. Congenital malformations and monsters, being unnatural, required explanation and therefore were studied with renewed interest. Books of that era dealing specifically with malformations include works by Ballantyne (1902, 1904) and the journal, *Teratologia*, which Ballantyne founded and edited, German texts by Förster (1865) and Ahlfeld (1880–2), and an eight-volume Italian treatise by Taruffi (1881–94).

This period of discovery up to about 1925 was characterized by a profusion of scientific observations and also severe and sometimes violent criticism of Darwinism. Proponents of the French naturalist, Lamarck, viewed natural variation and selection as too materialistic and not giving sufficient emphasis to the force of will and effort. The rediscovery in 1900 of Mendel's work (Gasking 1959) added fuel to this debate and produced a bitter controversy between two rival schools of thought in England, the Mendelians led by Bateson and the ancestrians led by Pearson and Weldon (Froggatt and Nevin 1971). The Mendelians soon discovered genetic units with large effect such as albinism; mutation was thought mainly responsible for positive evolutionary change whilst natural selection produced a negative function of getting rid of harmful variants by the process of biological competition and survival of the fittest. The ancestrians considered that an attribute of the phenotype was dependent on the manifestation of the same attribute in the ancestry, namely parent, grandparent, etc. Both groups were influenced by biometric data and particularly the work of Galton and his 'Law of Ancestral Heredity'. This is summarized in one of his articles (Galton 1865) as follows:

> The father transmits, on average, one-half of his nature, the grandfather one-fourth, the great-grandfather one-eighth; the share decreasing step-by-step in a geometrical ratio with great rapidity.

In order to test this law Galton assembled biological data and developed regression and correlation analysis for measuring degrees of resemblance in quantitative characteristics. His data on stature showing the mean height of offspring to be closer to the generation mean compared with the difference between mean parental height and its generation mean is well known (Pearson 1930). Pearson later expressed what he called 'Galton's Law of Ancestral Heredity' as a multiple regression equation. Early volumes of the journal *Biometrika* founded by Galton and Pearson in 1901, contain several articles on the measurement of natural variation. These were criticized at the time as denying the importance of Mendelism and as we now know, confused inherited genetic variation with nonheritable variation produced by changes in the common environment. Darwin, in fact, accepted the principle of the inheritance of acquired characteristics and elaborated this view in his hypothesis of pangenesis (Darwin 1868). A great number of disciplines have taken part in the case for and against Lamarckism. Brown-Séquard, the neurologist born in Mauritius of an Irish–American father and French mother, carried out numerous experiments in which local or sometimes general injury to the brain or peripheral nerves, particularly the sciatic, of guinea pigs caused epilepsy in the offspring (Olmsted 1946). This observation was first announced in Paris in 1859 (Brown-Séquard 1859) and was quoted by Darwin (1868) in the first edition of *The variation of plants and animals under domestication*. Few physiologists, however, could confirm this work. For example, Romanes (1895) initially accepted these findings, visited Brown-Séquard's animal laboratory in Paris, observed the experimental work, but had no success in his own later attempts to replicate the results. As a postscript to this study of inherited experimentally induced epilepsy, Stewart (1946) suggests these symptoms were produced by neurotoxins resulting from parasitic infections of the guinea pigs by lice. Delousing these animals abolishes the epileptogenic zone and puts an end to the fits (Pagniez and Plichet 1934). McDougall, the physiologist, organized a series of experiments with rats. Young rats were plunged into a tank of water having a choice of two escape routes. One route was illuminated but if chosen the animal received an electric shock; the second route was dimly lit but was not associated with any shock. The rats in time learned to take the latter escape route. Offspring of these rats received the same training and McDougall (1927, 1930) concluded that the time taken by rats to learn to take the escape route giving no electric shock gradually decreased in successive generations. Crew (1932) repeated this same experiment and found no improvement in eighteen successive generations and Agar, Drummon, and Tiegs (1935) also published negative results.

Advances in genetics and biometry enabled Fisher (1918) to lay the foundation of neo-Darwinism. A major difficulty of Darwin's theory was that attributes and the genes determining them were mixed together into a single blend when crossed; any new attribute therefore, would be progressively diluted by crossing in each generation. However if the genetic mechanism were particulate and most mutants recessive then new mutants may be stored indefinitely within the genetic constitution of a species. These then would become manifest when conditions are favourable (Huxley 1962). Fisher showed that natural selection resulted in the differential survival of variants and even small advantages, of a fraction of 1 per cent or less, could have significant long-term evolutionary effects. Many of these concepts are relevant to our study of the epidemiology of anencephalus and spina bifida.

II

Nature of Anencephalus and Spina Bifida

2

Anatomy, embryology, and classification

ANENCEPHALUS is a striking abnormality in which there is virtual absence of the forebrain and the skull vault. There are several anatomical variations of the defect which in the form when the brain is completely absent, is termed holo-anencephalus. These manifestations are described by Warkany (1971). Most infants are stillborn, although as the brain stem including the respiratory centres may be intact, liveborn infants may survive for short periods of time of the order of a few days or so. An exceptional case surviving 32 days was recorded by De Morsier and Bamatter (1952). Anencephalus often occurs in association with spina bifida; some 6.6 per cent of such infants out of a total of 360 infants having anencephalus or spina bifida in Belfast were observed during a five-year period (Elwood, J. H. and Nevin 1973). Other malformations sometimes noted in association include exomphalos, congenital heart disease, hare lip and cleft palate, and other types of defects (Record and McKeown 1949). Roberts and Powell (1975) analysed interrelationships of the common congenital malformations in a population of 90 921 singleton births in South Wales and found 9 per cent of anencephalics and 15 per cent of spina bifidas had defects of other organ systems. A necropsy series of 294 anencephalics and 50 cases of iniencephalus reported 41 per cent as having other defects outside the nervous system (David and Nixon 1976). The most frequent single malformations were hydronephrosis, cleft palate, diaphragmatic hernia, exomphalos, hare lip, and horseshoe kidney whose percentages in associations with anencephalus were, eight, five, five, four, and four respectively. Associated defects were more common in cases of anencephalus with spina bifida (occurring in 50 per cent of cases) than in those having anencephalus without spina bifida (31 per cent). Some 84 per cent of iniencephalics had other anomalies; urinary tract defects were the most common and occurred in 19 per cent of cases. Anencephalus is an abnormality affecting structures derived from or associated with the cephalic end of the neural tube. Other conditions lead to herniation of brain tissues through a defect in the skull—these include cranial meningocoele and cranium bifidum, encephalocoele, and hydrencephalocoele, containing respectively meninges only, meninges and brain tissue, or meninges, brain tissue, and part of the ventricular system. It is possible that cranial meningocoele and encephalocoele are part of the same disordered growth process although they are much rarer than and often clinically distant from anencephalus (Ingraham 1944). Lesions at the caudal end of the neural tube include rachischisis or myelocoele; spinal meningocoeles and meningomyelocoeles which represent herniation of meninges or meninges and spinal cord tissue through a defect in the vertebral arches. If a dorsal defect in the vertebral column exists with no herniation, the condition is called spina bifida occulta. Both cephalic and caudal development may be abnormal, yielding craniorachischisis in the most extreme case and combinations of anencephalus and spina bifida otherwise. Spina bifida is frequently associated with an Arnold–Chiari malformation and hydrocephalus. Scott's (1975) survey of malformations observed in 41 925 total births in Belfast during the quinquennium 1964–8 found only 21.6 per cent of spina bifida infants had no additional major defect; some 50.6 per cent had hydrocephalus, and clubfoot was the next most frequently noted malformation occurring in 20.8 per cent of cases.

Anencephalus was described in considerable detail by von Recklinghausen (1886) who suggested that it was caused by failure of closure of the neural tube. In the human anencephalic infant, there is usually virtually complete absence of the forebrain and of the skull (Morison 1970). In the place of the forebrain there is a mass of haemorrhagic fibrovascular tissue containing some neural elements, referred to as the area cerebrovasculosa. There are no recognizable anatomical structures, but the brain stem is present, and there are usually normal eyes and optic nerves which end blindly at the base of the skull. The midbrain and cerebellum may be intact and normally developed, or may be absent. Marin-Padilla (1970) has emphasized the constancy of the skeletal abnormalities in anencephalus where the nervous system anomalies may vary considerably. The bones of the base of the skull are abnormally shaped, especially the sphenoid and petrous temporal bones. The cranial vault bones, namely the parietal, frontal, the squamae of the temporal bones, and the occipital bone, are present only as rudimentary fragments. The facial bones are more nearly normal, but are deformed due to their articulation with the abnormal skull base, being rotated posteriorly leading to the characteristic appearance of an elevated and pointed nose, a short and elevated maxilla, and a protruding tongue. In addition to skeletal abnormalities many other body systems exhibit patterns of disordered growth (Nañagas 1925).

The term cranioschisis is often used in animal studies as being equivalent to anencephalus. If the open lesion extends through the cranium and spine, the condition is called craniorachischisis; this occurs although rarely, in humans (Warkany 1971). The cranial defects are similar to those described above, and in addition the vertebral bodies are abnormal in shape and irregularly ossified. The vertebral column is thus rudimentary and lacks a proper spinal cavity. In craniorachischisis the proximal exposed portions of the spinal nerves are destroyed; the peripheral nerves are normal in position but consist only of afferent elements, the efferent nerves degenerating after destruction of their nuclei of origin. The spinal ganglia are usually intact (Marin-Padilla 1970). Other features noted regularly are a reduction in size or absence of the neurophypophysis, and the presence of very small adrenal glands which lack the normal foetal zone. The lack of adrenal secretion leads to abnormally low levels of maternal urinary oestriol which have been used as the basis for a diagnostic test.

Exencephaly

In animal experiments, the condition of exencephaly has been known for many years. In this condition there is an overgrowth of the cerebral hemispheres accompanied by normally developing cranial nerves, eyes, midbrain, and hindbrain structures. The overgrowing material expands from the cranial base, the cranial vault being open in the midline, and the cerebral material is everted, the ventricular surface being exposed. In animals such as rats and hamsters it is established that exencephaly is followed by degeneration of the exposed neural tissues and replacement by fibrovascular tissue giving the area cerebrovasculosa typical of anencephalus. This development of everted brain material followed by destruction of the exposed tissue accounts for the finding in anencephalus of normal structures such as the eyes, cranial nerves, spinal ganglia, and peripheral spinal nerves. The foetal adrenals in exencephaly are normal with a foetal zone present but degeneration occurs later following replacement of the diencephalon by cerebrovasculosa tissue.

Exencephaly is seen frequently in animals because the time spent *in utero* after this stage is short. In humans, destruction of the everted tissue to produce anencephalus is likely to occur by 8 weeks of gestation and so only a few early human embryos with exencephaly have been observed (Dekaban 1963; Stevenson 1960; Warkany 1971).

Embryology

The brain and spinal cord develop from the neural tube which is formed by dorsal folding of the neural plate. Two basic concepts of the origin of anencephalus and spina bifida were expressed initially and continue to be debated; either the neural tube fails to close normally (von Recklinghausen 1886) or it closes but later opens (Morgagni 1761). Most investigators currently favour primary non-closure as the likely mechanism and we now describe a concept of normal neural tube development and of the formation of exencephaly and anencephalus based on the views of Källén (1968), Marin-Padilla (1970, 1970*a*), and Warkany (1971) (Fig 2.1) and on an embryological timetable for man by Shepard (1976). These times calculated from work conducted by several embryologists, as Shepard explains, are two- to three-days greater than in Streeter's (1942, 1945, and 1948) data because he estimated timing in man by extrapolating from observations on comparable stages in the monkey (Table 2.1). The University of Washington material (Iffy, Shepard, Jakobovits, Lemire, and Kerner 1967) agrees quite well with the Japanese reports (Nishimura, Takano, Tanimura, and Yasuda 1968; Nishimura, Tanimura, Semba, and Uwabe 1974).

The first stage in the formation of the central nervous system is thickening of the outer germ layer. This ectodermal material constitutes the neural plate, the epithelium changing from cuboidal to pseudostratified; the epithel-

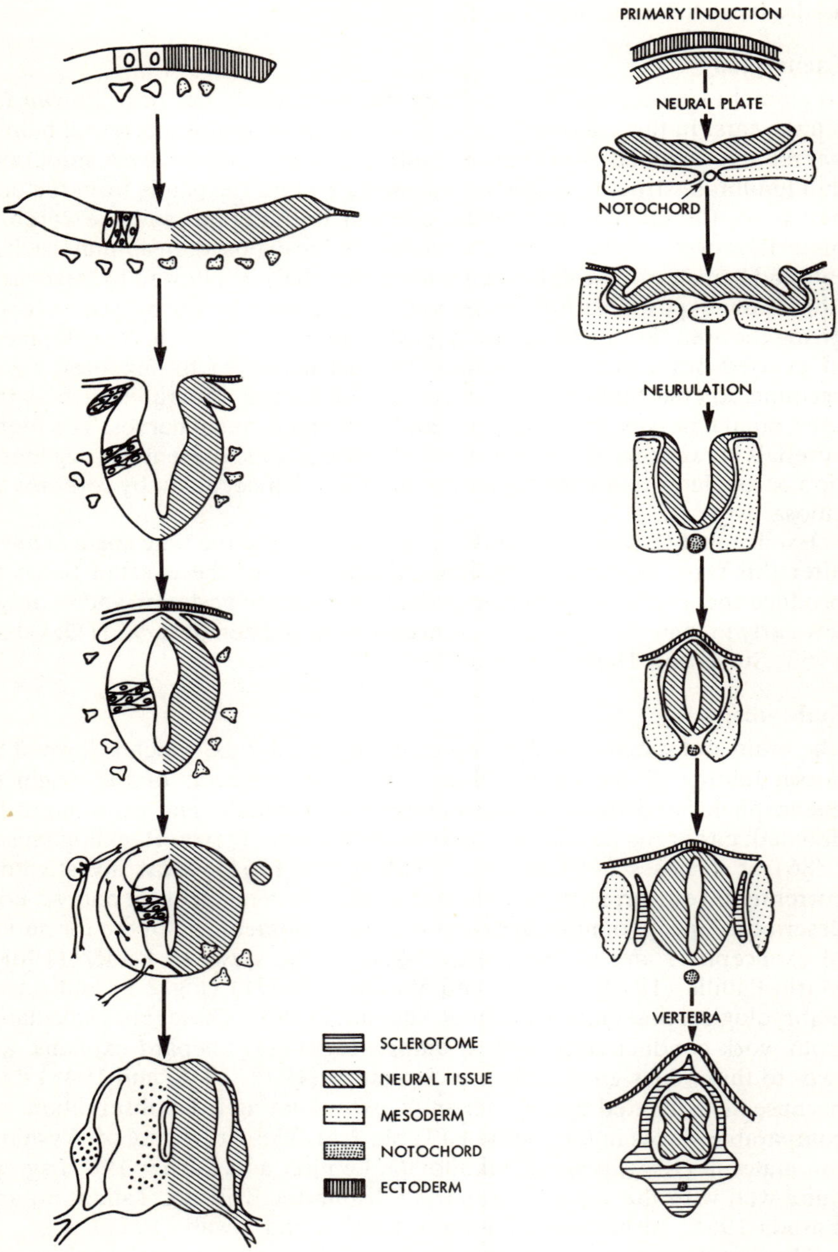

FIG. 2.1. Embryology of the central nervous system. (After Källén 1970 and courtesy of *Developmental Medicine and Child Neurology.)*

ial cells will later give rise to neurons and most neurological cells. This process is induced by the underlying mesoderm via at least two diffusible factors, of which one activates neural plate formation and the other influences differentiation to more caudal levels namely to spinal cord rather than to brain formation. Experimental transfer of the mesoderm to underlie a different area of ectoderm leads to neural plate formation at the new site.

TABLE 2.1 *Embryological timetable in man*

Age in completed days		Embryological event
–		Last menstrual period
0		Ovulation
4–6		Blastula stage
7	1 week	Implantation
14		Primitive streak
18–20		Neural plate forms
21	3 weeks	Early somites
22		Heart first beats
22		Pronephros
24		Oral Plate perforation
24–5		Anterior neuropore closed
25		Mesonephros
25–6		10 Somite stage
26–7		Posterior neuropore closed
27–8		Upper limb bud appears
27–8	4 weeks	20 Somite stage
29–30		Crown rump length 5 mm
37		Crown rump length 10 mm
40–3	6 weeks	Ossification begins
56–8	8 weeks	Palate closed completely
267		Total gestation time (from ovulation to birth)
280 (267 + 13)	40 weeks	Total gestation time (from date of last menstrual period to birth)

After Shepard (1976) and courtesy of The Johns Hopkins University Press.

The inducing factor can cross a millipore membrane and is presumably a chemical. There is a feedback interaction from the developed neural cells themselves. The neural plate then folds dorsally and commences to fuse in the thoracic region at the six-somite stage; fusion proceeds in cranial and caudal directions and is normally complete at 15 and 20 somites respectively. The 20-somite stage is reached approximately four weeks after conception. This folding of the plate (neurulation) is accompanied by increased mitotic activity, and there is probably active contraction of the apical (dorsal) surfaces of the cells. The nuclei migrate towards the ventral surface of the plate (Glaser 1916); this may be either a cause or a consequence of the apical contraction. An isolated neural plate will undergo folding and tube formation. Jacobson (1962) has shown that cell streaming in a median direction occurs in both the neural plate and in the underlying mesoderm, and if the plate is removed, this streaming still occurs in each tissue showing that both have inherent actions. If the plate is removed and replaced upside down, normal neurulation occurs showing that the mesodermal control is dominant. Jacobson suggests that the folding of the plate is basically due to increased adhesiveness of the cuboidal epithelial cells, associated with contraction of the adjacent mesoderm, rather than to active contraction of the neural plate cells.

Marin-Padilla (1970*a*), studying hamsters, has stressed the role of the neural folds which are the lateral extremities of the neural plate containing neural tissue, future neural-crest cells (which will form the lateral ganglia) and ectoderm; these folds are elevated by accumulation of mesodermal cells and lack of these will prevent apposition and fusion. Early changes seen when anencephalus is produced by excess vitamin A include reduction in the size and the number of mesodermal cells (Marin-Padilla 1966) which may be a basic mechanism of non-closure. However, in amphibian embryos neurulation may occur after removal of the lateral parts of the neural plate (Jacobson 1962). Successful neurulation leads to a closed neural tube with pseudostratified epithelium. Further development into mature neurons occurs by waves of mitotic activity during which the nuclei migrate to the ventricular surface of the tube causing bulgings called neuromeres; after mitosis the daughter cells move back into the epithelium and the neuromere disappears. The mitotic activity appears to be regulated by an inductive influence from the substratum, which at this stage of embryogenesis comprises prechordal plate, the notochord, and the surrounding mesoderm. If the prechordal plate is removed from an amphibian embryo, there is no development of paired structures such as eyebulbs or hemispheres (Adelmann 1937); so normal bilateral development requires mesodermal influence and the lack or malfunction of this may cause cyclopian malformations. The interaction of neural tissues and mesoderm is reciprocal, the diameter of the spinal canal being controlled by the size of the neural tube, and the formation of cartilaginous vertebrae is induced by the neural tube and the notochord.

Pathogenesis

Only a small number of early human embryos with neural-tube defects have been described in the literature.

Lemire, Shepherd, and Alvord (1965) reported a 5.5-mm embryo with spina bifida cystica of the lumbo-sacral region and thought that the lesion originated before the neural tube closed. Other specimens have been described by Patten (1953), Wrete (1959), and Gruenwald (1941). One of the youngest anencephalic embryos was of size 2.75 mm, 14-somite stage at 24±1 days of gestation, having total dysraphism (Dekaban 1963) and other embryos of less than 10 mm have been described by Bremer (1906), Politzer (1952, 1955), and Sternberg (1929). These show definite abnormalities present at developmental stages before full closure is expected and suggest that anencephalus is due to failure of closure rather than later reopening of the tube. At the site of the defect, the neural-plate cells are more randomly arranged than is normal and fusion may occur at the ends of the neural tube leaving a central defect. Overgrowth of neural tissue around the defect has been seen (Patten 1953), and in chick embryos experimental operative opening of the neural tube roof is followed by hyperplasia in 25 per cent of cases suggesting that the closure defect is the primary lesion (Fowler 1953). Giroud (1960) demonstrated the formation of excencephaly, followed by anencephalus after degeneration of the hyperplasic tissue, in rats given excess vitamin A. However, similar hyperplasia may be produced without a closure defect by removal of the tip of the notochord or by disturbance of the floor of the spinal cord neural groove at another site (Källén 1970). In chick embryos, cutting the spinal cord with a glass needle after normal fusion may produce a normal embryo after secondary closure, or a myeloschistic condition, or else the neural tissue develops normally but mesodermal closure and normal vertebral development does not occur; this gives a possible model for spina bifida cystica.

The production of exencephaly and anencephalus by excess vitamin A in foetal rats has been studied in detail at the cellular level. An abnormal accumulation of mitoses in the neuroepithelium was observed by Langman and Welch (1967) who suggested that vitamin A may act by prolonging the cell cycle. The cell nuclei accumulate at the dorsal rather than the ventral surface of the neural plate and the plate tends to evert rather than form a tube, allowing exencephaly to develop. Marin-Padilla (1966) suggests vitamin A excess in hamsters acts primarily by retarding mesodermal development, and points out that the deformity produced in the base of the skull, particularly the sphenoid bone, is similar to that seen in humans with various degrees of neural tube defect. He suggests the constancy of the mesodermal abnormalities indicates a primarily mesodermal cause of non-closure of the neural tube. Currently many researchers favour primary non-closure of the neural tube as the most likely mechanism producing anencephalus and spina bifida, although whether the basic lesion is in the ectodermal-neural tissue or the surrounding mesoderm is not clear.

A different hypothesis postulated by Vogel and McClenahan (1952) suggests the primary cause may be maldevelopment of the internal carotid arteries as the adjacent parts served by the ophthalmic and vertebral arteries (eyes, hindbrain, cervical cord) are normal. Vogel (1961) states there is a failure of formation of a normal anastomosis between cerebrovascular and systemic vessels at about 6 to 7 weeks of gestation; however, about 40 human cases of anencephalus have been described before this gestation time (Hanaway and Welch 1970), and ligation of the carotid arteries experimentally produces only dysgenesis and retardation of development, not anencephalus (Myers 1969). Also, vascular abnormalities are not always found in human anencephalics (Epstein and Kolker 1965). A further hypothesis by Keen (1962) postulates excess cerebrospinal fluid pressure in the foetal ventricles leads to rupture of the dorsal surface of the brain. This concept is similar to that expressed originally by Morgagni in 1761. Jelinek (1960) has demonstrated the production of anencephalus in the chick by mechanical reopening of a closed neural tube and Wilson, Jordan, and Brent (1954) concluded radiation-induced anencephalus is due to rupture of a necrotic area of the closed tube. Although the reopening mechanism is favoured by several authors (Gardner 1973, Padget 1968), there is evidence against this hypothesis because abnormalities are seen in early embryos before the time of normal closure (Dekaban 1963). The deformity produced by a mechanical reopening after normal closure may not represent naturally occurring anencephalus, and in particular, abnormalities of mesodermal structures such as the vertebral bodies and the base of the skull are not found (Marin-Padilla 1970). To produce anencephalus by an insult such as vitamin A excess or irradiation the agent must be given before the time of normal neural-tube closure (Hicks and D'Amato 1966).

Animal teratology

Anencephalus or exencephaly have been produced in various laboratory animals by a great variety of procedures, which we have arbitrarily classified into genetic mechanisms, operative procedures, and exogenous agents (Table 2.2). Anencephalus has been described in an inbred mouse population where it follows a Mendelian recessive genetic pattern (Bonnevie 1936) and also has been produced by X-radiation leading to chromosomal translocation (Snell 1935). A great variety of exogenous agents including physical insults such as X-rays, freezing, heat stress, and deficiencies or excesses of nutrients, vitamins, drugs, metals, or other substances are known to cause anencephalus in animals. Most of these agents also produce other abnormalities and the relevance of these observations to human studies is difficult to assess. Observations concerning the time of action of these teratogens, however, are particularly relevant to man. In the production of anencephalus in rats, excess vitamin A has a maximal teratogenic action if administered between the 8th and 10th days of gestation (Giroud and Martinet 1957). Some teratogenic activity is seen after earlier administration, which may be due to retention of the vitamin A in the tissues. In rats neural tube closure occurs on the 10th or 11th day, so the critical time appears to be at or just before the time of normal closure which supports the hypothesis of primary non-closure. The equivalent stage in humans is the 24th day (Warkany 1971). Other teratogens such as pteroylglutamic acid, anoxia, trypan blue, and X-rays also appear to be most effective at the 8th to 10th days in rats (Giroud 1960).

Congenital anomalies of the lower spine are known to occur naturally in tail-less cats. These cats are widespread throughout the world but probably the best known is the Manx. This occurs in two forms, the 'stumpy' possessing a very short tail and the 'rumpy' which has no visible tail (James, Lassman, and Tomlinson 1969). Many exhibit severe physical disabilities and they have a high early mortality. The Government of The Isle of Man has set up an experimental cat farm to safeguard the decreasing numbers of

TABLE 2.2 *Agents (excluding infectious organisms) producing anencephalus or exencephaly in laboratory animals*

Method	Animal	Reference
Genetic		
Recessive gene in certain strains	Mouse	Bonnevie 1936
Chromosomal translocation after X-ray	Mouse	Snell 1935
Operative		
Surgical reopening of neural tube	Chick	Jelinek 1960
Exogenous agents		
X-rays	Mouse	Hicks 1953; Rugh and Grupp 1959
	Rat	Wilson and Karr 1951
Heat stress	Chick	Alsop 1919
	Rat	Škreb and Frank 1963
Freezing	Hamster	Smith 1957
Short wave diathermy	Rat	Hofmann and Dietzel 1966
Ultrasound	Chick	Lutz and Lutz-Ostertag 1958
Starvation	Mouse	Runner 1959
Anoxia	Mouse	Ingalls, Curley, and Prindle 1950
	Bird	Gallera 1951
Excess CO_2	Bird	Gallera 1951
Actinomycin	Rat	Tuchmann-Duplessis *et al.* 1959*a*
Insulin	Mouse	Smithberg, Sanchez, and Runner 1956
Salicylate excess	Rat	Warkany and Takacs 1959
Streptonigrin	Rat	Warkany and Takacs 1965
Sulphonamides	Rat	Tuchmann-Duplessis *et al.* 1959*b*
Vitamin A excess	Rat	Cohlan 1954, Giroud 1960
Vitamin E deficiency	Rat	Cheng, Chang, and Bairnson 1957
Folate deficiency	Rat	Tuchmann-Duplessis *et al.* 1957
Pantothenic acid deficiency	Rat	Lefebvres 1951, Giroud 1952
Pteroylglutamic acid deficiency	Rat	Nelson *et al.* 1955
Riboflavine deficiency	Rat	Nelson *et al.* 1956
Thiamine deficiency	Rat	De Watteville, Jürgens, and Pfatz 1954
Trypaflavine	Bird	Ancel 1955
Trypan blue	Rat	Wilson 1955
	Hamster	Ferm 1958
Hydrourea	Rat	Chaube & Murphy 1966
Mercury and Cadmium	Hamster	Gale 1973
Nitrogen mustard	Mouse	Danforth and Center 1954
Prochlorpemazine	Rat	Roux 1959
Retinoic acid	Hamster	Shenefelt 1972
Zinc deficiency	Rat	Hurley and Swenerton 1966
	Rat	Warkany and Petering 1972
Zinc and Cadmium	Hamster	Ferm & Carpenter 1968
5-bromodeoxyuridine	Chick	Lee *et al.* 1976

these animals. Lesions similar to human spina bifida have been noted (James *et al.* 1969, Clark and Carlisle 1975), as also has syringomyelia associated with spina bifida occulta (Martin 1971).

From studies of several human embryos having anencephalus, Lemire, Beckwith and Warkany (1978) emphasize the range of variability in the morphology of cranioschisis and craniorachischisis and consider there are experimental observations supporting both the non-closure and the reopening hypotheses. Most evidence, however, favours initial non-closure of the neural tube as the basis for these defects although it is possible that some lesions may be caused by reopening of a previously closed neural tube.

Classification

There is no ideal or generally agreed classification of neural-tube defects. Consideration of their embryology and anatomy as described indicates a great variety of manifestation while more recent chromosomal and genetic studies point towards some degree of aetiological heterogeneity (Holmes, Driscoll, and Atkins 1976). The conventional clinical classification includes in the category anencephalus the many anatomical variations outlined by Nañagas (1925) and Warkany (1971) (Fig. 2.2); the much rarer anomalies of exencephaly and iniencephalus should be considered separately as they may not be aetiologically similar to anencephalus. Spina bifida is a general term describing the many varieties of lesions due to midline separation of the vertebrae. The great majority of lesions are of the dorsal elements but spina ventralis bifida lesions do occur. Cases of combined anterior and posterior spina bifida are very rare especially if those associated with anencephalus are excluded; Saunders (1943) collected only 37 such reports from the literature. Spina bifida aperta describes the open lesions seen in the newborn where there is exposed neural tissue, an open spinal canal, and no skin cover; if skin cover is present, the lesion often becomes cystic and is described as spina bifida cystica. Clinically, defects having no skin cover are more liable to infection than those having some membrane present. Spina bifida occulta implies that the lesion is covered by epithelialized skin and may not be obvious clinically. The overlying skin may be pigmented, dimpled, or have an abnormal tuft of hair but X-rays of the spine will reveal the underlying bony defects in the vertebrae. The terms meningomyelocele, syringomyelocele, myelomeningocele, myelocystocele, and hydromyelocele imply basically spina bifida aperta lesions. The South Wales survey recorded around 90 per cent of cases of spina bifida cystica as open myeloceles while approximately 5 per cent were true meningoceles which carry a good prognosis of physical and mental normality provided the sac is removed surgically, and around 3 per cent were skin covered myeloceles (Laurence 1964, 1976). In the Edinburgh series of 200 consecutive myelomeningoceles reported by Stark (1977), there were only 19 closed lesions of which one was situated in the thoracic area, 6 in the lumbar area, and 12 in the lumbo-sacral area.

In many clinical and most epidemiological studies the rubric spina bifida

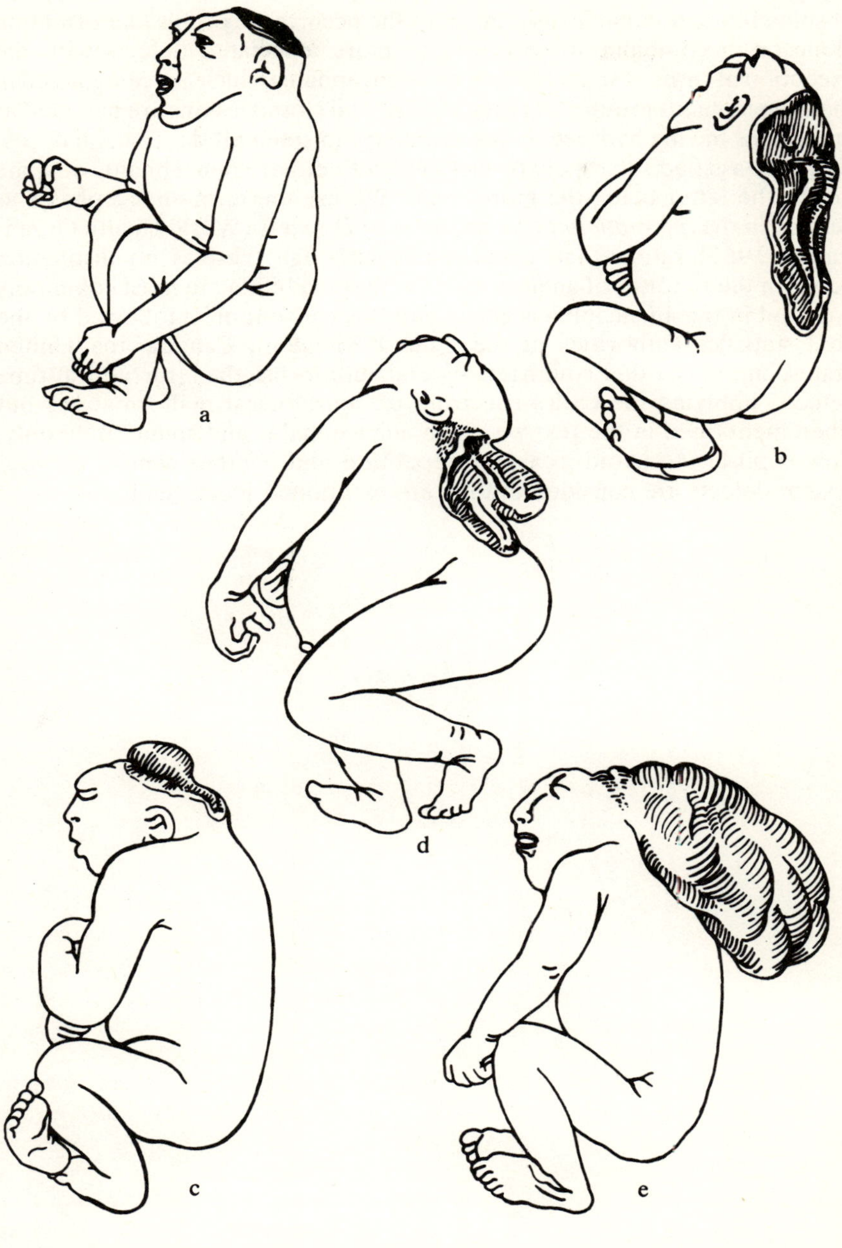

FIG. 2.2. Five anatomical types of anencephalus: (a) anencephalic acranius; (b) anencephalic craniorachischisis; (c) microcephalic acranius; (d) microcephalic craniorachischisis; (e) exocephalic acranius. (After Nañagas 1925 and courtesy of the *American Journal of Anatomy.)*

comprises the manifestations of this lesion just outlined with the exception of spina bifida occulta. Thus it includes the occurrence of this malformation alone or in combination with one or more associated defects with the exception of cases of spina bifida with anencephalus which are categorized in the anencephalus group. All types of open and closed lesions are included as are infants having hydrocephalus secondary to spina bifida. Encephalocele may be classified separately or included with either anencephalus or spina bifida, the latter being the more usual. We use the term anencephalus as defined in the *International Classification of Diseases* (World Health Organization 1967) rather than anencephaly although there is no distinction between them. Cases of anencephalus with spina bifida are most commonly included in the anencephalus group and this convention is followed by the vital statistics authorities of the United Kingdom, Canada, the United States, and most other countries. Several authors use the term 'neural-tube defects' implying the entire spectrum of neurological malformations but when mentioned in the text we mean anencephalus and spina bifida only. This is purely to avoid excessive repetition and if other central nervous system defects are considered, they are mentioned individually.

III

Role of epidemiology

3

Epidemiological approach to the problem of birth defects

THIS book is written from an epidemiological perspective but as the issues discussed are relevant to many other disciplines, we now outline an epidemiological approach to the problem of birth defects so that the remainder of the text may be more easily understood. Epidemiology has been defined as 'the study of the distribution and determinants of disease frequency in man' (MacMahon and Pugh 1970). Thus the approach of the epidemiologist to the question of the causation of anencephalus and spina bifida is primarily based on observations of the frequency of these defects in human populations. Knowledge of the causes of these defects will increase as hypotheses are formulated and tested. Many disciplines have contributed to our current understanding, including epidemiology, genetics, clinical medicine, the laboratory sciences such as pathology and biochemistry, and experimental teratology. Often a hypothesis arising from one of these sciences is best tested by another discipline.

To many, the process of scientific research is most clearly exemplified by the animal experiment. Here the hypothesis that a particular agent causes a certain condition is tested by forming two groups of similar animals, applying the postulated causal agent to one group and perhaps a placebo to the other, keeping all other conditions the same for both groups, and observing the outcome, for example the frequency of malformed offspring born to exposed and control animals. If the outcome is more frequent in the group to which the agent has been applied, the hypothesis is supported; if not, it is rejected, a new hypothesis formulated, and the process is repeated. However, not all science adopts this approach. Epidemiology uses the human population and therefore the researcher rarely controls the conditions to which the experimental groups are exposed; instead he observes natural occurrences. To compensate for the inability to produce the artificial simplicity of the animal experiment, the epidemiologist uses a range of other techniques which have been designed to deal with the special properties of his type of research. Unfortunately, practitioners of one type of scientific method may fail to appreciate the contributions of another discipline because of an incomplete understanding of their complementary roles.

For example, let us consider the hypothesis that neural-tube defects in humans are caused by exposure to influenza in early pregnancy. The epidemiologist may interview several thousand mothers in early pregnancy and evaluate their exposure to influenza by means of a symptom questionnaire, supplemented perhaps by serial serum antibody measurements. Then he follows all mothers throughout their pregnancy and ascertains the frequency of neural-tube defects in the infants. The teratologist may use a group of mice, randomly allocate them to receive influenza virus or a placebo, and then evaluate the occurrence of neural-tube defects in their subsequent offspring, or may directly infect embryos such as those of chicks. These two approaches differ in their strengths and weaknesses. The major differences are due to contrasting qualities in terms of internal and external validity.

Let us assume each study found that the risk of anencephalus is twice as high if the mother (human or animal) is exposed to influenza during early pregnancy. We first ask if we can accept this result as indicating the true state in the experimental situation namely, in those particular women or particular animals who were studied. Here the teratological experiment, if well performed, is much easier to interpret because it possesses high internal validity. In other words, it should be relatively easy to state with assurance that the association between influenza and the occurrence of anencephalus in the animals studied is due to a causal relationship. This is because the experiment will be conducted on selected, genetically similar, animals in whom all other known conditions are as far as possible specifically set the same for infected and for control animals, and unknown factors are arranged to be equally distributed between the two groups by the statistical technique of randomization. If the number of animals studied is large enough to ensure that the findings are unlikely to occur purely by chance, we are able to have confidence in the result as it applies to those animals. In contrast, the epidemiologist has a much more difficult job convincing us that the association which he has observed is indeed causal. The two groups of women, infected and uninfected with respect to influenza, are not derived from a common population by randomization, and we have no assurance that they are similar in relation to other characteristics which may be relevant to the occurrence of anencephalus. In fact, from our knowledge of the epidemiology of influenza we would predict many differences in terms perhaps of social class, family size, immune response, and so on. Nor can we assume that the exposure under test (influenza) is not accompanied by other differences between the groups of mothers in the conditions in early pregnancy as again differences with respect to many factors such as the frequency of physician visits and drug usage might be present.

However, the epidemiologist's disadvantage in terms of internal validity is accompanied by a much higher degree of external validity, by which we mean the accuracy in extrapolating any observed findings to the relevant community which always will be a human population. Extrapolation of the experimentalist's results involves not only the difficulties of species differences, but also questions of equivalent dosages, of the relationship between the animal defects and the human defects, and of possible interactions of the exposure (influenza) with other factors in the human situation. Clearly it is not particularly fruitful to consider issues of whether one or other of these approaches is more valid or more 'scientific'; the two are complementary and where possible an hypothesis should be tested using both methods.

Practical issues also demonstrate contrasts between these two approaches to the same problem. Frequently, an experimental study may be adequately performed quickly and cheaply. The teratologist, therefore, may follow the familiar scientific pathway of hypothesis formulation, testing, revision, and re-testing. Epidemiological studies usually take longer and the number of potential subjects namely, affected individuals, is often limited. Thus in one project the epidemiologist must attempt the equivalent of a series of related experimental studies. Often, it is wasteful to perform an epidemiological study in which only one hypothesis is tested; any opportunity to simultaneously test other hypotheses, or to gather descriptive data relating to another question, should be used. Sometimes epidemiological studies are more expensive than experimental work but this is not always the case. Studies which can be based on already existing information, for example by record linkage techniques, may provide valuable information at little additional cost. Although both the teratologist and the epidemiologist must adhere to ethical and legal standards, clearly the scope of the epidemiologist is much more limited. While the laboratory investigator can determine which animals are exposed to the postulated causal agent, the epidemiologist in most instances may observe only the results of exposure. In the event that an intervention can be postulated to have a high probability of a beneficial effect and a low risk of major detrimental effects, the best method of investigation is a randomized prospective trial on a human population, which combines the strengths of both the experimental and the epidemiological approach.

Terminology

An important quantitative index used in epidemiology is the incidence rate, defined as the number of new occurrences of disease per unit of population during a specified period of time. One of the major limitations in our understanding of birth defects is that this quantity has never yet been validly measured in a human population. Given that anencephalus and spina bifida probably occur at approximately 4 weeks of gestation, the incidence rate of these defects is the number of new cases occurring divided by the number of conceptions surviving to this age, in a defined population of mothers over a given time. To measure this we need to know the fate of all conceptions surviving beyond four weeks of gestation. Those that are lost before four weeks are unimportant as they are not at risk of neural-tube defects (if our timing hypothesis is correct) and so contribute neither to the numerator nor to the denominator of the incidence rate.

The prevalence rate of a disease is the number of cases of disease per unit population at a specified time. Most studies of birth defects give the number of affected births and the total number of births, defined as livebirths or total births (live and still) from a specified gestational age, usually 28 or 20 weeks. The ratio of these quantities is the 'prevalence rate at birth' of the malformation, although some earlier literature refers to this index as an incidence rate. Clearly, this prevalence rate depends on both the true incidence rate of the condition and on the rates of early foetal losses of both affected and unaffected conceptuses.

A mortality rate is the number of deaths, from all causes or from a specified cause, in a given time per unit population. The infant mortality rate is defined as the number of deaths in infants aged under one year, occurring in a given time period (usually one year), divided by the number of live births occurring over the same time period. This formula has been used for many years largely because it can be directly applied to data collected in the traditional manner. It does not produce a true 'rate' as the criterion for this is not fulfilled, namely that the denominator should be a count of all persons who if affected would be included in the numerator. If we followed all live-born infants delivered during one year until death or their first birthday we would measure the true death rate at ages under one year in that group. However, differences between these two estimates usually will be very small unless either the birth rate or the mortality rate changes rapidly over a short interval.

The neonatal mortality rate is defined as the number of deaths within 28 days of birth divided by the total number of live births, and the perinatal mortality rate is the ratio of the number of still births plus first week deaths to the total number of births (live and still) occurring in a given time (usually one year).

4

Types of epidemiological study

As epidemiology is a relatively new discipline there is no universally accepted terminology to describe the several major types of study which are commonly conducted. If little is known about the occurrence of a disease, the first approach often is to examine data already available through routine sources and to describe the major features which characterize the occurrence of the disease. Most epidemiological studies of neural-tube defects are of this 'descriptive' type and describe the frequency (usually prevalence at birth) of anencephalus or spina bifida in a particular community and how this frequency varies by geographical area, year or month of birth, or with maternal characteristics such as age and parity. The aim is to understand some of the features of the disease and so generate aetiological hypotheses. This type of study is usually based on information available from existing sources such as birth certificates, death certificates, or hospital records. The validity of such a study will be maximal where the disease can be simply and accurately diagnosed by any medical practitioner, without special tests, and where the condition is unlikely not to be recorded by the sources of ascertainment selected. As anencephalus is easily recognizable and always fatal, it is one of the few congenital anomalies which may be ascertained fairly completely from stillbirth and death records. Death registrations do not give as complete data for spina bifida because many cases are not fatal, the primary cause of death may not be recorded as the defect itself but as a condition such as meningitis, and also the diagnosis of some types of spina bifida is not straightforward. Clearly the usefulness of such descriptive studies will depend on the completeness and accuracy of the data and the nature of the information recorded.

We shall illustrate various aspects of the epidemiological approach to the problem of birth defects by considering several studies which have examined the relationship between anencephalus and spina bifida and influenza exposure during early pregnancy.

Routine data sources may be used to test specific hypotheses. For example, Leck (1963) analysed available data to see if there was any trend in anencephalus prevalence rates which could be linked to influenza epidemics in the same population, and Elwood, J. M. (1976) used Canadian vital statistics to test the foetus-foetus interaction hypothesis which predicts a number of relationships between the prevalence and sex distribution of anencephalus and the twinning rate in a population. Such studies are sometimes classified as descriptive, for example by MacMahon and Pugh (1970), as they may not require specific data collection, but in terms of their hypothesis-testing aim and their methodological sophistication they may also be regarded as analytical studies. Leck (1977) gives them the distinctive title of 'correlative studies of groups'. Some other types of study are similar in that they apply complex methods to already available data as shown by the examination of time–space clustering of births with neural-tube defects in Quebec (Siemiatycki and McDonald 1972), the separation of secular trends and maternal age effects in New York State (Janerich 1972*a*), and the investigation of a very large number of dietary factors in relation to anencephalus mortality in England and Wales in which analytical techniques were used to minimize the likelihood of reporting chance associations (Knox 1972).

The two most frequently used types of investigation in which special groups of people are selected for study are case-control and cohort studies. Often these are called analytical studies (MacMahon and Pugh 1970), although Leck's (1977) title of 'correlative studies of individuals' is perhaps a more precise term. In a cohort study, a group of persons (mothers in our context) is defined as an 'exposed cohort' by virtue of having the characteristic under investigation at some defined time prior to the incidence of the disease. This cohort, and one or more comparison cohorts which differ with respect to the exposure, are followed in time and the prevalence at birth of the defects observed in each group. Thus to assess the association between events in early pregnancy and the subsequent occurrence of infants having congenital defects, McDonald (1961) interviewed women during their first attendance for prenatal care at hospital and public health clinics in Watford and St Albans, England. To examine febrile illness in pregnancy, we can define in her study two cohorts on the basis of clinical history. The results show that 9 of 148 infants born to mothers with febrile illnesses had severe ('type A') defects compared to 81 of 3103 infants whose mothers had no such history (Table 4.1).

In a case–control study, two or more groups of mothers are defined in terms of pregancy outcome. Coffey and Jessop (1957) surveyed all births over a two-year period in the three largest maternity hospitals in Dublin. They identified 137 anencephalic births, and interviewed these mothers together with 192 mothers of normal infants, asking about, amongst other factors, illnesses during the first three months of pregnancy. Their findings show that 21 'case' mothers and 7 'control' mothers reported such illness (Table 4.2). The prevalence rates of anencephalus amongst exposed and unexposed infants cannot be calculated from these results but the difference between the exposure rates in the case and control groups demonstrates an association.

The relationship between the time when the epidemiological investigation is carried out and the time period to which the data refer may also be used to classify the study. The commonest designs are those described above. In McDonald's cohort study, the cohorts were defined at the beginning of the investigation and followed forward in time giving a prospective design. In the case control study by Coffey and Jessop, cases and controls were identified at a point in time and information about past events obtained, thus using a retrospective design. However, Coffey and Jessop's study also reported on the blood-group distributions of the case and control mothers. In this instance, the data refer to the situation at the time of the study and there is no retrospective component; this is a cross-sectional case–control design. Walker and McKee (1959) performed laboratory tests and interviews on mothers after delivery to define cohorts on the basis of influenza exposure in early pregnancy; in its design and therefore in regard to the appropriate methods of analysis this is a cohort study, but is not prospective—all data used refer to events completed when the study is performed. It can be classified as a retrospective cohort study.

Measures of association

The cohort study may seem more simple in concept because the process of recording the exposure and subsequently observing the outcome is the same as that used in animal experiments and clinical trials. The results yield the prevalence rates in each exposure group. From these rates two comparative indices are often obtained—the relative risk, or risk ratio, being the ratio of the prevalence rate in the exposed to that in the unexposed group; and the risk difference, or attributable risk, being the difference between these two rates. Thus the findings from McDonald's study yield a relative risk of 6.1/2.6 or 2.3 and an attributable risk of 6.1 minus 2.6 or 3.5 per cent (Table 4.1). The 'aetiological fraction', defined as the proportion of disease which is associated with the exposure, represents the amount of disease due to the exposure if we assume the results reflect causation. It may be calculated for either the exposed sample or the total study group. For the exposed sample the aetiological fraction is (6.1–2.6)/6.1 or 57 per cent. Thus 57 per cent of

TABLE 4.1 *Cohort study: distribution of total number of births (live and still) and number having major ('type A') congenital defects by maternal health status in early pregnancy in Watford 1952–5 (after McDonald 1961)*

Maternal health in early pregnancy (exposure category)	Numbers of births: Malformed infants	Total infants	Malformation prevalence rate (per cent)
Exposed (Febrile illness)	9	148	6.1
Unexposed (No febrile illness)	81	3103	2.6
Total	90	3251	2.8

Groups defined by exposure and followed up.
Relative risk = 6.1/2.6 = 2.3
Attributable risk = 6.1 − 2.6 = 3.5 per cent
Aetiological fraction in exposed = (6.1 − 2.6)/6.1 = 57 per cent
Aetiological fraction in population = (2.8 − 2.6)/2.8 = 7 per cent

disease in the exposed mothers is related to being exposed to influenza in early pregnancy. The aetiological fraction for the whole study group is (2.8–2.6)/2.8 or 7 per cent.

A case–control study does not provide estimates of the prevalence rate in each exposed group, so the attributable risk and aetiologic fraction cannot be directly determined. However, the relative risk will be closely approximated by the cross-products ratio or odds ratio which may be calculated from the data (Table 4.2). This ratio is (21 × 185)/(7 × 116) or 4.8. The approximation to the relative risk is good so long as the disease is a fairly rare event as usually is the case with congenital defects. However, a special situation obtains in a case–control study where the sampling fractions of cases and controls are known. An example is the study of anencephalus in 14 Canadian cities. The data applying to the 'exposure' of a previous stillbirth yield a relative risk of 4.1 (Table 4.3). Here the cases comprise all stillbirths and deaths attributed to anencephalus in a defined population and the controls are a random sample of the 1 193 000 births occurring in that same population. Thus the total numbers of unaffected births in the exposed and unexposed categories may be estimated (with some sampling error) and the prevalence rates and attributable risks calculated.

TABLE 4.2 *Case–control study: distribution of cases of anencephalus and control births (live and still) by maternal health status in early pregnancy at three Dublin Maternity Hospitals 1953–5 (after Coffey and Jessop 1957)*

Maternal health in early pregnancy (exposure category)	Cases (anencephalus) number	Controls non-malformed (live and still) births
Exposed (Illness in first trimester)	21	7
Unexposed (No illness)	116	185
Total	137	192

Groups defined by birth outcome and information on exposure obtained retrospectively by interview.
Odds ratio = (21 × 185)/(7 × 116) = 4.8.

Attributes of cohort and case–control studies

Cohort and case–control studies vary greatly in terms of size and cost. If the outcome of interest is uncommon, cohort studies must be very large to be effective. Consider an investigation which is to have a high chance (90 per cent) of detecting a threefold increase in the prevalence at birth of anencephalus in the study compared with the comparison group, and this result will be accepted only if demonstrated at a significant level of 5 per cent, using a one-sided test. In a cohort study we would need to follow up about 10 000 exposed and 10 000 unexposed women (Walter 1977). The size of a

TABLE 4.3 *Case–control study: distribution of cases (total series of anencephalics) and a random sample of control livebirths by exposure status defined as history of one or more previous stillbirths—Canadian 14-city study*

Exposure status	Cases (anencephalus) number	Controls (livebirths) number	Estimated total number of livebirths in population	Prevalence of anencephalus per 1000 births
Exposed (One or more previous stillbirths)	141	133	31 734	4.44
Unexposed (No previous stillbirth)	1250	4867	1 161 266	1.08
Total	1391	5000	1 193 000	1.17

Relative odds = (141 × 4867)/(133 × 1250) = 4.1
Attributable risk = 4.44 − 1.08 = 3.36 per thousand
Aetiological fraction in exposed = 4.44 − 1.08/4.44 = 75.7 per cent
Aetiological fraction in population = 1.17 − 1.08/1.17 = 7.7 per cent

case–control study of similar power will depend on the proportion of control mothers exposed. If this were 10 per cent, a study including 100 mothers of anencephalics and 100 control mothers would have a similar chance of detecting the association. The difference in time required for those two types of studies will not be great for most studies of congenital defects as a cohort study requires follow-up for only nine months or so, However, consider an hypothesis such as that of Baird (1974) postulating that the occurrence of anencephalus is related to chronic malnutrition during the early childhood of the mother. Here a case–control study may be conducted using interviews, but a prospective cohort study would require a 20- to 30-year follow-up period. In these circumstances a retrospective cohort approach may be very valuable. Within a population, it might be possible to identify adult women who by reason of place and time of birth or other circumstances will have been inadequately nourished during early childhood and to compare the prevalence rates of congenital defects in infants born to these women with the rates in infants born to one or more control groups of mothers without such exposure.

The major considerations in both cohort and case–control studies are those regarding the completeness and quality of the information used and the validity of the control groups selected. There are many possible sources of error and of bias in either design. In a prospective cohort design, information concerning exposure should be of high quality as interviews will apply to current or very recent events and special investigations, for example blood tests, can be used if necessary. Thus several prospective studies of influenza used serial antibody estimates. The choice of a control group will pose problems. In our example, women with no clinical or laboratory evidence of infection may be suitable, although we may wish to match the controls on factors such as social class. Matching is discussed more fully below. Controls need not always be totally 'unexposed' women, Doll, Hill, and Sakula (1960) studied only women who reported having had influenza, and defined the exposed group as those with influenza during pregnancy, using as controls women who had influenza before they became pregnant and women whose symptoms were regarded as not likely to be due to influenza. The most critical part of a cohort study is to ensure that all women initially entered are followed, and that assessment of the outcome is unbiased. Often some women are lost to follow-up, for example they may move out of the study area or may deliver at a hospital not included in the study. If such losses are random, namely within each exposure cohort the prevalence rate of affected infants is the same in those lost to follow-up as in those retained, the results will not be biased. Usually it is impossible to check this and experience suggests that the pattern of losses is unlikely to be random. Even loss rates of 5 or 10 per cent may compromise the validity of the results. Certainly a cohort study such as that of Wilson, Heins, Imagawa, and Adams (1959) in which 377 women entered the survey on the basis of influenza antibody tests and the outcome was ascertained on only 126, provides little useful information. In a cohort design it is important to guard against bias in the assessment of outcome. When this assessment is somewhat subjective the assessor may show conscious or subconscious bias if he is aware of the mother's exposure category. Such bias may be avoided if the assessor is unaware of the exposure information, and this precaution is advisable if there is any possibility of variations in ascertainment or recording of outcome as for example with respect to minor degrees of spina bifida or the diagnosis of even major defects in stillbirths. As a cohort study is defined by exposure, it allows assessment of multiple outcomes in relation to that exposure; thus in studying influenza, even if the main objective is to assess the association with neural-tube defects, the study should include all other outcomes such as abortions, prematurity, and other defects.

Owing to the large numbers of subjects and the long period for follow-up required by cohort studies, case control studies have been performed much more frequently. Careful attention must be given to the definitions adopted for both case and control groups. The case group is best selected as a total series of affected cases in a defined population and time period, but restrictions may be accepted if the implications of these are understood. For example, in Coffey and Jessop's study the case group consisted of all anencephalic births in three Dublin maternity hospitals (Table 4.2). If the control series had been chosen from all births in Dublin, some characteristics might have appeared to be associated with anencephalus when in fact they were related to referral to the hospitals used in the survey. The controls, therefore, were chosen from the same hospitals. The problem, however, is not quite solved. Let us assume there was a population group, defined on some social or ethnic basis or by place or residence, which tended not to use these particular three hospitals. Mothers from this group would form a small proportion of the control series. But if such women had had previous abnormal births or had hydramnios or premature labour, they might be referred to these hospitals and so be over-represented in the case series leading to a spurious association. The likelihood of such a bias in the Dublin study is small because the hospitals surveyed cared for 80 per cent of the births in the city. Restrictions applied to the case series, if reflected by similar restrictions to the controls, should not produce bias. There is no requirement that the case or control series are 'representative' of their respective total populations. Thus in a case control study of anencephalus, both cases and controls may be restricted to women in a certain age, racial, or social group but the findings of course may only apply to this group and not to anencephalus in the total population. The choice of controls is important. They should be taken from the same source as the cases (same hospital or same area of residence) and often a simple scheme such as using the next-born normal infant, as was selected in the Dublin study, is adequate. Use of a random sample of the total unaffected population, as was used in the Canadian studies, has certain advantages as previously described.

Most case–control studies depend on retrospective information about exposure and this is the most common reason for inaccuracy. Many surveys are based on postpartum interviews which ask about infections, diet, or drugs taken during pregnancy. Two problems, random error and systemic bias, should be distinguished. Obviously retrospective data will have some inaccuracies, but if these are similar between cases and controls the only effect will be to reduce the estimated relative risk towards the null value of one. Systematic bias, however, may produce a reduction or an increase in the estimated relative risk. Mothers of cases may remember or report events differently than mothers of controls perhaps due to having different educational standards or different reactions to the interview situation. Most importantly, mothers who have had an abnormal child will clearly react to questioning about previous events in a different manner to mothers who have had a healthy infant. The direction of the bias rarely can be predicted. More complete reporting or even over-reporting of ill health by mothers who have had malformed infants seems likely to occur, and this bias may have occurred in the case control study described above. Several strategies may help to recognize and overcome this bias. Information recorded before the birth by medical records may be useful although there may even here be differences in recording as case mothers may be treated differently to controls, perhaps because of previous pregnancy losses or defects. A retrospective interview may include some questions about events unlikely to be associated with the condition under study and similar reporting of these makes the presence of bias less likely. Mothers of infants having other handicaps or illnesses may be used as an additional control group as their reactions to interview should be comparable to mothers of infants having the defects being studied. Ideally, the interviewers should be unaware of the case or control status of the mother being interviewed.

The remaining type of epidemiological study is the intervention trial. This is a cohort study where the 'exposure' of a group of subjects is intentionally changed by the investigator and the outcomes compared to those of a comparison group. Such trials are ethical only if there is strong evidence that the proposed intervention may be potentially beneficial, without any major concomitant risks. No valid intervention trials of primary prevention of neural-tube defects have ever been carried out. Nevin and Merrett (1975) attempted to test Renwick's (1972) hypothesis that anencephalus and spina bifida are usually preventable by avoidance of potatoes during early pregnancy. They advised all mothers who had had an infant with a neural-tube defect to avoid eating potatoes as soon as they decided on another pregnancy. Amongst those who had a subsequent term pregnancy there were 27 mothers who stated they had avoided potatoes and 61 who stated that they had eaten a normal diet which included potatoes. Amongst the 24 stillborn or liveborn infants born to the potato avoiders, two (8.3) per cent) had anencephalus or spina bifida, while of 57 infants born to non-potato avoiders, two (3.5 per cent) were so affected: thus there was no evidence that the avoidance of potatoes decreased the risk. This prospective study is however not an intervention trial as exposure to potatoes was decided by the mothers and not by the investigators, and therefore there are the same difficulties in judging whether the difference in outcome is causally related to the one difference between the two groups of mothers which was of greatest interest to the investigators. Another aspect of this study which illustrates a frequent limitation is that it tested a somewhat different hypothesis than the one proposed, by studying the effects of potato avoidance on the recurrence risk of neural-tube defects, rather than on the risk of a first affected child. The chief advantage of intervention trials is that the investigator, by controlling the amount of exposure, may be able to ensure that the two cohorts are similar with regard to certain factors related to the outcome. The best method of assuring this is by allocating the exposure randomly, and here the study becomes similar in design to an animal experiment or a clinical trial. However, no randomized trials of factors postulated to cause or prevent neural-tube defects have been conducted although they would be considered if a specific and apparently safe preventive measure were suggested.

5

Association and causation

THE objective of any epidemiological approaches, whether descriptive or analytic studies, or intervention trials, is to demonstrate an association between exposure and outcome. Then the investigator must assess if the association is likely to reflect a causal relationship. The epidemiologist's concept of causation is that of a link, but not necessarily a one-to-one relationship, between exposure and outcome. Thus such a change (qualitative or quantitative) in the exposure to the causal agent is followed by a change in the outcome, provided all other conditions remain the same. The mechanism or the immediacy of the cause is not a prime issue. Snow (1855) reduced the incidence of cholera in London in 1854 by closing one water-supply point and demonstrated that the water supply was clearly a cause of this disease even though the mechanism by which it acted was unknown. Before interpreting an association as a causal relationship, we must first consider and exclude other explanations for the observed association and also search for other evidence supporting a causative mechanism. An association between exposure and outcome may be due to any of four mechanisms: observation bias, confounding, chance, and causation. The three non-causal explanations require different methods of evaluation.

Observation bias

Observation bias refers to systematic, as opposed to random, errors in the validity of the study data. A positive association between a history of infectious disease and an abnormal birth derived from a case–control study may be due to mothers of abnormal infants reporting more infections even if they did not actually have more such illnesses. As mentioned, case–control studies are particularly prone to bias in historical data and cohort studies to bias in the information relating to outcome. Such errors may be minimized by high response rates or high rates of successful follow-up, and by the use of multiple sources of information. Estimates of the presence of such biases may be based on comparisons between several data sources, use of multiple comparison groups, additional questionnaires or interviews, and other methods specific to the study. The decision as to whether an observed association is wholly or partially due to observation bias, or is obscured by such, will rarely be based entirely on objective evidence but will involve some subjective judgement.

Confounding

Confounding is a central issue in epidemiology, and a large amount of epidemiological methodology has been developed to permit examination of this problem. Despite this, the term has no widely accepted definition. We define a confounding factor as one which alters the measured association between an exposure and an outcome, by virtue of its association with both these factors (Miettinen 1970). For example, the prevalence rate of Down's syndrome increases with increasing maternal age but is not influenced by birth order. Examination of prevalence rates by maternal age and birth order demonstrates that the rate changes little with birth order within each age group, but varies greatly with maternal age within each birth-order category (Table 5.1). However, let us consider the relationship when birth order only is examined. The prevalence rates increase with increasing birth order and this relationship is due to a third factor, maternal age, which is associated both with the prevalence of Down's syndrome and with birth order. In this instance, maternal age is acting as a confounding factor.

TABLE 5.1 *Prevalence rates at birth of Down's syndrome per 1000 livebirths by maternal age and birth order, Lower Michigan 1950–64*

	Birth order						
						Total	
Maternal age	1	2	3	4	5+	Crude	Adjusted
<20	46.9	36.0	(20.7)	(45.3)	(00.0)	43.2	31.3
20–4	42.6	47.1	40.2	39.3	23.7	42.8	39.9
25–9	53.3	51.3	51.7	48.6	51.3	51.2	51.6
30–4	102.6	101.1	84.1	87.7	75.5	86.6	92.4
35–9	270.5	299.2	242.2	242.2	246.5	263.8	272.1
40+	850.9	753.6	864.6	940.1	851.7	858.9	839.9
Total							
Crude	56.7	68.5	81.4	114.4	165.6	89.1	
Adjusted	93.2	92.9	83.7	92.4	74.4		

Rates in parentheses are based on fewer than 10 cases.
From Stark and Mantel (1966).

The relationship between an exposure and an outcome may be distorted by a factor which has independent associations with both exposure and outcome. This distortion may increase or decrease the observed association in relation to the real situation. Any factor which is associated with the true causal agent will for that reason show an association with the outcome; however, it will not be confounding if that is its only association with the outcome. To produce confounding the factor must show independent associations with the exposure and the outcome (Miettinen 1970, 1974). If such independent associations exist, the confounding factor will be associated with the exposure even in the absence of the outcome, for example within the control group in a case–control study, and will be associated with the outcome in the unexposed group. Furthermore, both these associations must hold within the data set under examination. Consider again a case–control study where mothers of malformed infants and mothers of normal infants are compared with respect to influenza exposure. Maternal age will be confounding if two conditions are fulfilled: firstly, the maternal age distributions differ between cases and controls, and secondly the maternal age distributions of mothers with and without histories of influenza are different. It may be that in the particular sample set the ages of case and control mothers are similar, even if the prevalence of the defect varies with maternal age in the population. If this is so, no confounding will result. The amount of confounding will depend on the strength of the associations. If influenza exposure and the malformation rate change greatly with maternal age, even a small difference in the age distributions may lead to a large degree of confounding. Thus the demonstration that the difference between mean maternal ages of cases and controls is not statistically significant is not a sufficient reason to rule out confounding.

Control of confounding

There are a number of techniques used to control confounding: restriction, matching, randomization, stratification, and the use of mathematical models. Restriction means exclusion from the study of groups of subjects; thus the possible confounding effects of a family history of a birth defect may be avoided if all women with such a history are excluded. Such restriction must of course be made for the whole study—cases and controls, exposed and unexposed.

Matching involves choosing controls, for either a cohort or case–control design, who are similar to the exposed or the case group with respect to the potentially confounding factors. In practice, two types of matched study are common. In a fully matched design, the intention is to match the two series with respect to all relevant confounding factors, and then the analysis is based on the matched groups, for example pairs or triplets. In a matched-pair situation the final analysis is simple, the relative risk being derived as the ratio of the number of pairs in which only the exposed is affected to the number in which only the unexposed is affected. However, while the analysis is attractive, simple and powerful, this type of study is difficult to design. Choosing controls matched for more than a very few factors is usually difficult and expensive, and if a confounding factor is not anticipated and used as a matching factor, it is difficult to adjust for its effect in any subsequent analysis as the original matching must be preserved. Also, the associations with the disease risk of the matching factors themselves cannot be assessed in the study. Fully matched designs are most practical if the matched controls can be chosen from a large number of potential controls. For example, in a prospective cohort study of smoking, Hammond (1964) had information on 422 094 subjects and was able to match smokers and nonsmokers on sixteen potentially confounding factors, producing 36 975 matched pairs.

If the number of study subjects, diseased or exposed, is very small, full matching is useful because of its high statistical power, meaning the ability to detect a significant difference in a small sample. This is seen in the case–control study of adolescent vaginal cancer which demonstrated trans-placental exposure to diethylstilboestrol as a causative factor; only eight cases were available for study and for each, four controls were matched with respect to three factors (Herbst, Ulfelder, and Poskanzer 1971). Although few epidemiological studies employ fully matched designs, almost all have some matching if only for administrative reasons such as the selection of cases and controls from the same hospital population. Where matching has been carried out only on one or two factors such as place of residence and age, and other confounding factors have to be controlled in the analysis, there is little value in preserving the original matching. Instead, stratification or multivariate methods may be used which ignore any initial matching. The matching factors should be included in the analysis, as although matching by age will ensure no age confounding when the total study group is examined, if this group is partitioned the age distributions within each subgroup may be dissimilar and confounding by age may still be present.

Randomization is the method of controlling confounding most familiar to experimentalists but it can be used only in intervention trials. The use of randomization to divide subjects into two or more groups ensures that the groups will be similar with respect to all factors. If each group is very large, the similarity will be close. In practice the numbers of subjects may be fairly small and therefore the major potential confounding factors should still be examined, because there may be substantial differences in their distributions between groups despite the randomization. Often the major potential confounding variables are specified in advance and randomization is carried out within the groups defined by these factors. Thus randomization does not replace the need for collecting information on other factors and assessing their confounding effects. However, unlike the other methods discussed, it does provide some assurance of control for factors not assessed because of ignorance of their effects or inability to collect the relevant data.

Stratification is a widely used method of controlling confounding and consists of measuring the association between a risk factor and outcome within groups or 'strata' defined in terms of the confounding factor. An example has been given already where the apparent association of prevalence of Down's syndrome with birth order disappears when examined within strata of maternal age (Table 5.1). As the number of subjects within one stratum may be small, it is useful to calculate summary indices of risk recombining the data over all strata. In cohort designs direct and indirect standardization are applicable methods (Hill 1966). For each group defined by exposure, the data are stratified and a standardized rate computed as a weighted average of the stratum specific rates, the same weighting factors being used for each exposure category. For case control designs, several summary estimates of risk ratio after controlling confounding, and appropriate significance tests have been proposed for situations where exposure and outcome are dichotomous (for example, Mantel and Haenszel 1959; Gart 1970; and Miettinen 1972) or where either or both are polychotomous (Mantel 1963).

Mathematical modelling controls confounding by applying an equation in which the outcome of interest is the dependent variable and both the exposure and the confounding factors are included as independent variables. A simple example is the assessment of the effects of maternal weight on birth weight taking into account the influence of maternal age: a regression model expressed as:

$$\text{(birth weight)} = \text{(constant)} + \beta_1 \text{(maternal weight)} + \beta_2 \text{(maternal age)}$$

may be used and appropriate statistical techniques are applied to estimate the size and statistical significance of the regression coefficients β_1 and β_2. If the data are continuous, methods such as multiple least-squares may be used to solve this equation taking into account any underlying mathematical assumptions. The parameter b_1 estimates the effect of maternal weight after controlling for maternal age; if confounding is present b_1 will differ from the value obtained when maternal age is excluded from the model. In many epidemiological studies, the relevant variables are not all continuous but are often dichotomous (absent or present, male or female) or have a number of unordered categories such as ethnic origin or social class. Rather more complex methods be used to examine this type of mixed data. Further treatment is not appropriate here, but an example of a multivariate model applied to continuous data is given is Section 19 and the use of models for discrete data is discussed in Appendix A.3.

Confounding effects therefore may be controlled either in the study design, by restriction, matching, or randomization, or in the analysis, by stratification or mathematical modelling. A combination of methods may be used. It is evident that in any study potential confounding factors should be anticipated as far as possible and relevant data collected. In this regard the necessary attributes of independent associations with outcome and with exposure provide valuable guidance. Actual confounding, however, must be assessed within the data set and frequently a factor considered as a potential confounding variable will be found not to be so in practice. This assessment is best made by comparing measures of association between exposure and outcome calculated with and without control for confounding.

Use of statistics

If an association between an exposure and an outcome seems not to be due to observer bias or to confounding, we then estimate the likelihood of this result being due to chance. In epidemiological studies all measures to control confounding should first be performed and then appropriate statistical tests applied to the unconfounded measures of association. The results are usually expressed in terms of probability values (*P* values) or as confidence limits. Confidence limits are particularly useful if no significant association is shown. For example, expressing a result as a risk ratio of 1.1 with a statement that this is not statistically significant is less informative than reporting the confidence limits. If these are for example 0.9 to 1.3 (95 per cent, two-sided) this makes it unlikely that the true risk-ratio is substantially different from one. A smaller study may yield limits of 0.2 to 5.3 and their width clearly indicates that this study should not be interpreted as strongly suggesting no association. The asymmetry of the confidence intervals is due to the log–normal distribution of risk-ratio estimates.

The diagnosis of causation

We have discussed the interpretation of the results of individual studies and shown that if observation bias, confounding, and chance can be shown to be unlikely reasons for the observed association then a causal interpretation is favoured. To make further progress towards reaching a decision on the likelihood of causation, certain other features of the findings and information from other studies should be considered. The conclusion that the association is causal is reached as a reasoned judgement and cannot be totally based on any statistical or other procedure. Several characteristics indicative of causality can be described as more fully discussed by Hill (1966), MacMahon and Pugh (1970), Susser (1973), and others.

The time sequence of events must be consistent: the putative cause must precede the outcome. Thus an event occurring after four to eight weeks of gestation cannot cause neural-tube defects if our current understanding of their embryology is correct, although it could affect the prevalence at birth by influencing abortion rates. On the other hand, we may include as causal factors events before pregnancy if we suspect that they may affect a later conception. In prospective studies the timing of the exposure can often be well defined, but in retrospective studies this may pose considerable difficulty. The strength of the association, estimated after confounder control, is helpful, largely because the likelihood of a strong association being due to an unassessed confounding factor is usually small. Even very strong associations, however, may be produced by observation bias, or result if the postulated cause is closely associated with the true cause. Thus a strong association with a particular disease of the mother may be due to a causal association with the treatment given for that disease. Demonstration of a dose–response relationship is helpful; for example if a viral infection were causal, births to mothers having high antibody titres would be expected to have a higher prevalence rate of defects than births to mothers having lower titres. If the association is specific, a particular exposure being associated with neural-tube defects but with no other types of abnormalities, this supports a causal mechanism, partially by making observation bias a less likely explanation. Obviously there is no biological requirement that the relationship be totally specific, and in fact any major teratogen may be expected to cause more than one type of malformation. The cell-rest hypothesis was first visualized as specific to neural-tube defects (Clarke,

Hobson, McKendrick, Rogers, and Sheppard 1975), but subsequently modified to include other midline defects (Gardiner, Clarke, Cowen, Finn, and McKendrick 1978). However, as neural-tube defects show many epidemiological features which are not shared by other major abnormalities, an hypothesis requiring an exposure to account for most cases of neural-tube defects should be able to explain these differences.

These aspects of causation may be assessed within one study. Then the question must be widened and other relevant information evaluated to assist the interpretation. Results of other epidemiological studies must be assessed, searching for consistency in demonstrating the observed association, and if possible consistency in strength– and dose–response characteristics. Care must be taken to make a fair evaluation of other work, and a single well-performed study may outweigh a large number of inadequate investigations. A study should not be dismissed because of some methodological inadequacy unless it can be shown that this is likely to produce substantial bias in the results. Frequently, a study demonstrating an association is criticized because of errors in the assessing of outcome, exposure or both, and yet a spurious association can only arise if such errors are systematically different between the groups being compared; random errors will bias the result towards the null hypothesis making them conservative. On the other hand, studies showing no association are better assessed in terms of the confidence limits of the results; if they are small studies, even if adequately conducted, they may provide little evidence against the presence of an association. Any hypothesis should explain the descriptive epidemiology of the malformations under investigation and should be tested if possible by both case–control and cohort studies. Intervention trials are a much more powerful tool because they are direct tests of the causal mechanism, and demonstrate if a change in exposure results in a change in outcome; if randomization is used in a trial of adequate size confounding should be minimal.

Less direct support for an hypothesis may be given by observations made by other disciplines, for example the putative exposure may be shown to produce neural-tube defects in experimental animals. Thus, an hypothesis derived from epidemiology should be tested using animal models and vice versa. However, the absence of such interdisciplinary support, especially if it has not been strenuously sought, is not critical. Viable hypotheses for human congenital abnormalities are too rare to be discarded solely on the grounds of insufficient support from other disciplines. The final decision about causation depends on reasoned judgement together with some degree of subjectivity. Intervention trials on human populations will provide the nearest thing to scientific proof.

IV

Clinical presentation

WE consider in this section the diagnosis and complications of pregnancy associated with a foetus *in utero* having anencephalus or spina bifida. Each aspect is examined according to the time sequence presented by the mother to her doctor except for the question of prenatal diagnosis by measuring levels of alpha-foetoprotein and other markers in amniotic fluid and maternal blood which is discussed in Chapter XII.

If the uterus is too small or too large for the duration of gestation and the length of pregnancy is not in doubt, foetal abnormality should be suspected. Although sometimes a small-for-dates pregnancy may be observed, a more common finding when a foetus has some type of neurological malformation is a fundal height larger than the dates would suggest. This is most often due to hydramnios.

6

Diagnosis and complications of pregnancy

THE traditional diagnostic methods of clinical history and physical examination are of most value after 20 weeks of gestation and to evaluate pregnancies of less than this gestation time special investigations such as ultrasonography and amniocentesis in order to measure various biochemical markers are required (Section 28). An accurate history of previous reproductive experience is important as up to 5 per cent of mothers of infants with anencephalus or spina bifida previously will have had one or more affected infants, or there may be a history of neural-tube defects in the more distant family. Also, mothers of anencephalic or spina bifida infants report significantly more spontaneous abortions, stillbirths, and child deaths, irrespective of cause than do mothers of normal infants (Section 21).

Biochemical tests

Foetal adrenal hypoplasia in anencephalus is associated with very low levels of maternal urinary oestriol excretion (Frandsen and Stakemann 1961, 1964) and this forms the basis of a diagnostic test. Using this screening method, Macafee, C. A. J. (1973) reported a prevalence of foetal abnormality three times that of a control group having normal levels of maternal oestriol excretion. This test is not specific for neural-tube defects and subnormal oestriol levels may occur in relation to hydrocephalus, mongolism, congenital heart disease, the Potter syndrome, and abnormalities of foeto-placental function (MacLeod, Brown, Beischer, and Smith 1967; Macafee, C. A. J., Beischer, Brown, and Fortune 1972; Macafee, C. A. J., Beischer, and Fortune 1973; Beischer, Ratten, Fortune, and Macafee, C. A. J., 1973). Generally the lowest levels are found when the foetus is anencephalic and Dean, Abell, and Beischer (1977) suggest routine screening by urinary oestriol assay, with foetal radiography when values are below 20.8 μmol/24 hours, as the most reliable method of detecting anencephalus before birth. The genesis of oestrogen in four patients pregnant with an anencephalic foetus studied by MacDonald and Siiteri (1965) indicated that at least 50 per cent of this hormone was derived from placental utilization of dehydroisoandrosterone sulphate (DS) circulating in the maternal blood. Steroidal precursor substances are supplied from both maternal and foetal circulations and in the case of anencephalus with absence of the foetal zone of the adrenal cortex, the amount of DS contributed is very small. This chemical, detectable in the circulation of normal foetuses, was absent in the cord blood of anencephalics examined by Nichols, Lescure, and Migeon (1958).

Amniography and X-rays

Radiology, a widely used diagnostic aid in obstetrics, became less acceptable after reports of possible hazards of leukaemia and other cancers if the foetus was X-rayed during early pregnancy (Stewart, Webb, Giles, and Hewitt 1956). The recently developed computerized tomography probably would detect foetal abnormality *in utero*, but this procedure also is associated with a radiation hazard (Horsley and Peters 1976). An early estimate of the order of 1.0 rad per scan for computerized axial tomography (Perry and Bridges 1973) probably is too low as most patients irrespective of diagnosis require multiple scans. A plain X-ray of the foetal skeleton at 16 weeks of gestation will demonstrate anencephalus. Spina bifida defects, unlikely to be seen using plain film, may be detected prior to 20 weeks of gestation by amniography and foetography (Frigoletto and Griscom 1974; Mennuti, Moranz, Schwarz, and Mellman 1977). Amniography uses a water-soluble contrast medium to visualize the amniotic sac and the foetus while a fat-soluble contrast medium is used for foetography. About 20 ml of amniotic fluid are removed and around 10 ml of contrast medium injected via the amniocentesis needle. X-ray pictures are then taken some 24 hours later. These procedures have certain complications such as damage to the uterus, placenta, and maternal internal organs and irritation of the pregnancy which may produce bleeding, abortion, or premature labour.

Foetoscopy

Foetoscopy is a technique using a fibre-optic telescope which is introduced into the uterus via an incision made in the anterior abdominal wall. This likewise is associated with serious complications in a fair proportion of cases. Scrimgeour (1974) examined 28 patients by this method and thought the best results were obtained if the investigation was made at 18 weeks of gestation. Thirteen foetoscopies were carried out in Cardiff in women whose pregnancies were between 14 and 20 weeks of gestation (Laurence, Pearson, Prosser, Richards, and Rocker 1974). Twelve were followed by immediate hysterotomy or hysterectomy and one was followed by a normal liveborn male delivered by elective lower-segment caesarean section at the 35th week. This patient, whose foetoscopy was performed at 18 weeks, was readmitted at 26 weeks due to leakage of amniotic liquor; at 28 weeks she came into hospital again due to intermittent loss of blood-stained liquor and remained there until delivery which was precipitated by more severe bleeding. Valenti (1978) has described various uses of a foetoscope or endoscope using a transcervical or transabdominal approach. Further experiences have been reported by Scrimgeour (1976), Aladjem (1976), Hobbins and Mahoney (1976), Levine, McNeil, Kaback, Frazer, Okada, and Hobel (1976), Alter, Modell, Fairweather, Hobbins, Mahoney, Frigoletto, Sherman, and Nathan (1976) and Wheeless (1976). The cervical route seems inadvisable owing to the likelihood of interrupting the pregnancy. Also, the placenta requires careful localization by ultrasonography and among the complications encountered are amnionitis, foetal haemorrhage, and foetal death due to injury of the umbilical cord by the foetoscope, foetal death from injury to the foetus and spontaneous abortion subsequent to the diagnostic procedure. In Valenti's report based on 59 cases studied in San Francisco and Cagliari, Italy, the frequency of serious foetal complications was 11 per cent.

These techniques are now largely replaced by the use of ultrasonography and amniocentesis. Sonar scanning, apart from plain X-rays is the only non-invasive technique permitting direct visualization of the foetus. Anencephalus may be detected as early as 12 weeks of pregnancy (MacVicar 1976) and Campbell, Pryse-Davies, Coltart, Seller, and Singer (1975) diagnosed a large dorso-lumbar myelomeningocele at 19 weeks of gestation. In one series of 329 patients scanned between 17 and 20 weeks of gestation for the early detection of neural-tube defects, 81 per cent had been referred because they had had a previous foetus with a neural-tube defect (Campbell 1977). These new diagnostic aids will increase the likelihood of detecting anencephalus and spina bifida prior to labour and consequently reduce the need for radiography in obstetrics. In Oxford less than 10 per cent of the foetuses are now radiographed (Fletcher 1978) and introduction of an ultrasound service at Northwick Park Hospital, Harrow, was associated with a 55 per cent decrease in obstetric referrals for abdominal radiography (Meire, Farrant, and Wilkins 1978).

Complications of pregnancy

Several complications of pregnancy have been studied in relation to congenital malformation and some are reported to occur more frequently if the foetus has anencephalus or spina bifida. Record and McKeown (1949) found a small excess of threatened abortion in mothers of anencephalics compared to controls and an excess of placenta praevia, 1 per cent in contrast to 0.1 per cent of all births. Some 8.9 per cent of mothers of anencephalics in Southampton had some vaginal bleeding in early pregnancy but Williamson (1965) concluded there was no real excess of threatened abortion. However, Smithells, Chinn, and Franklin (1964) reported 3.4 per cent of 180 mothers of anencephalics had a threatened abortion and 5.7 per cent an antepartum haemorrhage, the frequency of these two signs being significantly increased compared with findings in a control group of 366 mothers of normal infants.

Hydramnios

The most frequent complication of pregnancy associated with anencephalus or spina bifida is hydramnios which also may occur in relation to many other types of congenital defects, twins, and other causes. Clinical diagnosis of excess amniotic fluid is unreliable unless large quantities of 3000 ml or over are present. A dye dilution test whereby a dye is introduced into the amniotic cavity by amniocentesis and the fluid then sampled a few hours later by a second amniocentesis, is necessary to estimate accurately amniotic-fluid volume (Fuchs 1966; Whitfield, Neely, and Telford 1968). The amount of amniotic fluid present is calculated from the amount of dilution of a known concentration of dye added to the amniotic fluid at the time of the test amniocentesis. Early studies used X-rays to confirm the diagnosis of hydramnios (Macafee, C. H. G. 1950) but this is no longer acceptable owing to the radiation hazard. Estimates of the frequency of hydramnios vary greatly. Stevenson (1960) reviewed the incidence in all pregnancies and found reported rates were from 0.1 per cent to 3.2 per cent with the highest frequencies being in areas of high anencephalus prevalence. It is clear that hydramnios is a common sign of foetal malformation and occurs in between one-quarter and two-thirds of such pregnancies (Table 6.1). The particular birth defect most likely to be present in association with

TABLE 6.1 *Frequency of hydramnios in selected series of hospital deliveries and proportions of pregnancies having hydramnios associated with malformed births of all types (after Stevenson 1960)*

		Pregnancies having hydramnios					
		Deliveries			Malformed		
Area	Deliveries total number	number	per cent	Births number	number	per cent	Reference
Northern Ireland	12 021	147	1.2	172	79	45.9	Macafee, C. H. G. 1950
Belfast	15 449	494	3.2	523	123	23.5	Stevenson 1960
Republic of Ireland	13 194	213	1.6	231	159	63.8	Barry 1958
Oxford	15 967	194	1.2	217	89	41.0	Stevenson 1960
United States	34 272	204	0.6	219	78	35.6	Yordan and D'Esopo 1955
Holland	19 816	260	1.3	292	79	27.0	Van der Velden 1957
Total	110 719	1512	1.4	1654	607	36.7	—

this excess of amniotic fluid appears to be anencephalus where hydramnios occurs in between 48 per cent and 93 per cent of cases. It is also a fairly frequent concomitant of pregnancies associated with spina bifida and hydrocephalus (Table 6.2) and several other birth defects as described in detail by Stevenson (1960). It may be more common when the anencephalic is female (Macafee, C. H. G. 1950); Guha-Ray (1975) reported hydramnios in 65 per cent of female and 28 per cent of male anencephalic pregnancies. Normal amniotic fluid and that in hydramnios are identical in composition and the association with anencephalus may be because the anencephalus foetus swallows less amniotic fluid than a normal foetus (Pritchard 1965). Other hypotheses are increased urine output due to lack of antidiuretic hormone (Naeye, Milic, and Blanc 1970) or by secretion of cerebrospinal fluid into the amniotic cavity (Warkany 1971). Hydramnios probably is a major cause of premature labour because pregnancies with anencephalus but no hydramnios frequently have delayed onset of labour possibly due to lack of normal foetus pituitary–adrenal function (Anderson, Laurence, and Turnbull 1969). There are not many recent studies of hydramnios in relation to foetal malformation due to the inaccuracy of clinical diagnosis and the hazards associated with X-rays.

TABLE 6.2 *Frequency of hydramnios in pregnancies associated with neural-tube defects observed in hospital births*

Centre	Malformation	Total observed number	Hydramnios present number	Hydramnios present per cent	Reference
Belfast	Anencephalus with and without spina bifida and other defects	270	142	53	Stevenson 1960
Belfast	Spina bifida alone	73	10	14	Stevenson 1960
Belfast	Spina bifida with and without hydrocephalus and other defects	162	18	11	Stevenson 1960
Dublin	Anencephalus	150	135	90	Comerford 1965
Birmingham	Anencephalus	262	182	69	MacMahon and McKeown 1952
Liverpool	Anencephalus	180	90	50	Smithells *et al.* 1964
Liverpool	Spina bifida	258	39	15	Smithells and Chinn 1965
Liverpool	Anencephalus	76	71	93	Edwards and Balfour 1976
	Spina bifida	2	1	50	Edwards and Balfour 1976
	Hydrocephalus	20	7	35	Edwards and Balfour 1976
Oxford	Anencephalus	177	76	43	Fedrick 1976
Viipuri and Helsinki	Anencephalus	39	27	69	Hiilesmaa 1945
Malmo and Lund	Anencephalus	67	33	49	Böök and Rayner 1950
Beirut	Anencephalus	16	9	56	Mufarrij and Kilejian 1963
Pittsburgh	Anencephalus	60	27	45	Guha-Ray 1975
Johannesburg	Anencephalus	12	9	75	Glietenberg 1967

Length of gestation

The hormone imbalances together with the absence or presence of hydramnios just described are related to and influence the length of gestation of anencephalic pregnancies. A series of 66 anencephalic infants born at the Columbia-Presbyterian Medical Center between 1942 and 1967 exhibited two patterns (Milic and Adamsons 1969). Some 22 pregnancies were significantly prolonged averaging 311 days and 44 pregnancies were significantly shortened, averaging 253 days, compared with a mean of 270 days for a control group of 6052 deliveries. Of the 44 short-gestation pregnancies, 34 were associated with hydramnios, some 30 came into labour spontaneously and had normal deliveries, six had Caesarean sections and the remainder were induced. There were no failed inductions.

We have examined the distributions of 457 anencephalics and a random sample of 4052 livebirths by gestational age at the time of delivery; these represent a consecutive series of anencephalics together with a sample of all livebirths delivered to women resident in several selected urban locations across Canada during the years from 1968 to 1972 (Fig. 6.1). The mean periods of gestation for the anencephalics (36.13 weeks; S.E. 4.53) and the livebirths (39.37 weeks; S.E. 2.17) are significantly different but there is no difference between the mean gestation times for the 158 male anencephalics (36.54 weeks; S.E. 4.64) compared with the 299 female anencephalics (35.91 weeks; S.E. 4.46). These data show a similar pattern to the hospital study by Milic and Adamsons (1969) whereby a proportion of anencephalics are delivered at early gestation times probably related to the presence of increasing hydramnios and another group spend a longer than average time *in utero* and are born at 42 or more weeks of gestation. There is little information on the gestation times of pregnancies associated with spina bifida but because hydramnios occurs less frequently the pattern may well be different from that described with respect to anencephalus.

Mode of delivery

The more widespread use of ultrasonography and other special investigations should ensure that a greater proportion of foetal malformations are diagnosed prior to the onset of labour than in previous years. For example, over the period 1959–73 during which 90 000 deliveries occurred at Magee Women's Hospital, Pittsburgh, 68 per cent of anencephalics remained undiagnosed until the onset of labour (Guha-Ray 1975). In this series of 60 anencephalics, 69 per cent were vertex, 19 per cent face, and 10 per cent breech presentations compared with 96 per cent, 9 per cent, and 3 per cent in a control group having normal infants respectively. Spina bifida infants are particularly prone to birth injury associated with breech delivery, the mode of birth of around 25 per cent of all such infants. Ralis (1975) dissected the locomotor system of 49 fatal cases of spina bifida born by normal delivery and 15 born by breech. Muscle damage, nerve damage and tendon haemorrhage were more common and severe in the latter infants possibly due to forcible extraction and manipulation. Rupture of the myelomeningocele was noted by Stark (1977) in 10 out of 130 consecutive infants studied in Edinburgh. Failure to commence labour spontaneously may occur in relation to anencephalus hence postmaturity is associated with the presence of this abnormality as also are retained placenta and postpartum haemorrhage. Some obstetricians favour Caesarian section as the mode of delivery if there is rapidly developing hydramnios, previous uterine scars or pelvic dispro-

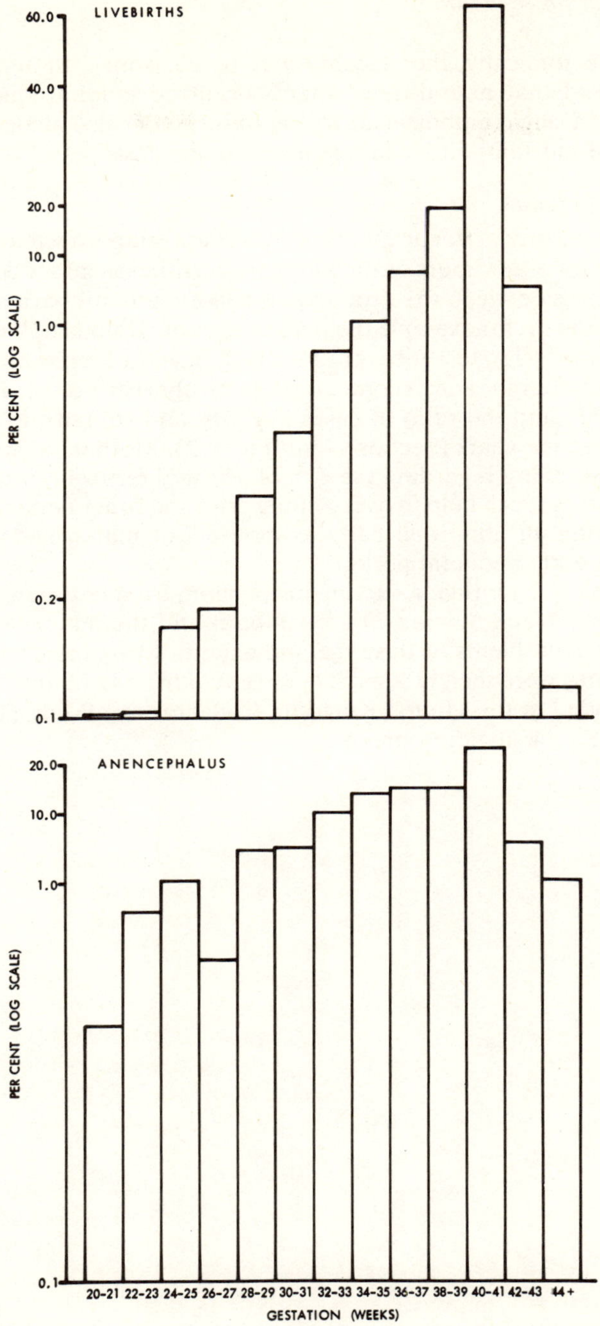

FIG. 6.1. Distribution of 457 cases of anencephalus and a random sample of 4052 livebirths by gestation time at delivery in urban areas with populations of 10 000 persons or over—Canada 1968–72.

portion. Anatomically, the placenta may be abnormal; Bryan and Kohler (1974) found that neural-tube defects occurred more frequently in the presence of a single umbilical artery, an observation also made in the study of perinatal mortality in Ireland (Cahalane and Jessop 1970).

Pregnancy outcome

The great majority of anencephalic foetuses are stillborn while the remainder survive for a few hours or days and are certified as infant deaths. There are differences between the proportions reported as stillborn and liveborn from area to area; for example the percentages of all anencephalics liveborn over the period 1956 to 1966 were 19, 10, 7, 5, and 1.5 in Belfast, Glasgow, Dundee, Edinburgh, and Aberdeen respectively (Elwood, J. H. and MacKenzie 1971) and the ratio of cases liveborn and stillborn in Canada has changed over the years (Section 8 and Fig. 8.2). Mothers of anencephalics require counselling regarding the risk of affected births in future pregnancies and also as much help in overcoming grief and other personal problems due to having an abnormal baby as mothers of malformed infants who survive the early neonatal period.

Regarding spina bifida, a varying proportion, from between 16 to 26 per cent (Table 7.1 and Section 7) are stillborn and the majority present the many serious problems of this type and extent of treatment to be offered. Closed lesions were seen in some 24 per cent of the 142 infants having spina bifida included in the United Kingdom Collaborative Study (1977) which screened 18 684 singleton pregnancies.

7

Spina bifida and results of treatment

TREATMENT is not an issue with regard to anencephalus because the great majority are stillborn and the remainder die at or around the time of birth. The situation in the case of spina bifida, however, is quite different because a varying proportion survive and pose serious problems of treatment and management. Clinical aspects have been described in several monographs (Ingraham 1944; Menelaus 1971; James and Lassman 1972; American Academy of Orthopaedic Surgeons 1972; Brocklehurst 1976; Stark 1977). Also, Allum (1975) discusses social problems based on her interviews of spina bifida children and their parents living in South Wales.

Attempts to treat spina bifida date back many years and in Morgagni's text of 1761 there is a note of such a patient dying at operation during crude surgery without anaesthetic (Cooke 1822). In the last century, Morton (1877) of Glasgow popularized a method in which the spina bifida lesion was injected with a solution of iodine in glycerine. A committee appointed by the Clinical Society of London investigated this therapy (Marsh *et al.* 1885) and in addition collected data on 60 cases not subjected to any operative interference. They concluded that about 1 per cent of liveborn spina bifida individuals survived at that time without treatment. A smaller number underwent spontaneous cure due to gradual shrinking of the sac and injection of from half a drachm to two drachms of Morton's fluid was recommended in preference to puncture or incision of the tumour, treatment by ligature, excision, or plastic surgery. Even in the last century it was recognized that selection of cases for surgery was important. Bayer (1892, 1897), reporting a 59 per cent mortality based on 17 patients treated, stated he would only operate in future if three clinical conditions were fulfilled namely, when there was no marked hydrocephalus, no paralysis, and no complications to be expected in the sac. Hildebrand (1893) also thought operation inadvisable if severe paralysis or irreparable deformities were evident and Sachtleben (1903) obtained five 'permanent' cures out of 30 cases, all five having simple meningoceles. Robson (1895) described a 30 per cent mortality in twenty operations carried out in the United States. Moore (1905) collected from the literature 385 cases treated by excision and advised not operating on newborns, patients with progressively growing lesions, hydrocephalus, paralysis, or deformities. Ingraham's (1944) series of 546 infants seen over two decades at The Children's Hospital, Boston, had an overall mortality of 49 per cent for 462 patients with spina bifida and 37 per cent for 84 patients with cranium bifidum (encephalocele).

After this period and until Nulsen and Spitz (1951) devised their valve for controlling advancing hydrocephalus there was little enthusiasm among surgeons for operative surgery in spina bifida infants. Many surgeons refused to do anything at all about these cases and advised a policy of conservative management. This however had one major limitation in that the children in question did not always die (Rickman 1976). They were admitted to paediatric units in large numbers, occupied a significant proportion of hospital beds, and presented multiple clinical problems. Further work by Holter, who in 1957 constructed a silicone rubber valve, provided a means of controlling hydrocephalus and closure of open myelomeningoceles as early as possible became an active policy. Lister, Zachary and Brereton (1977) describe that in 1965 some 134 spina bifida infants were admitted to the neonatal surgical unit at the Children's Hospital, Sheffield, but by 1968 the number attending their follow-up clinic was approaching 1000 with up to 20 per cent of all paediatric beds in the hospital occupied by spina bifida children.

Owing to the observation that expected deaths of untreated patients did not always occur and that it did not appear possible to accurately predict prognosis, resulting in around one-third of these children surviving in a state of paraplegia, hydrocephalus with mental retardation, incontinence, and severe recurrent renal infections, an era of active management was initiated. The object was for as many patients as possible to survive with a minimum of disability. This involved a multi-disciplinary approach combining several clinical specialities, social work and education, rehabilitation, and community care. Survival rates improved, the quality of some survivors undoubtedly increased and further work in Sheffield (Sharrard, Zachary, Lorber, and Bruce 1963) demonstrated early closure of the sac within 24 hours preserved muscle innovation and appeared to result in improved muscle function in groups previously paralysed.

Laurence and Tew (1971) described the survival of 425 cases of mainly untreated spina bifida children observed in a total population of 800 000 persons ascertained between 1956 and 1962 in the mining valleys of South Wales, excluding large towns. Some 110 (26 per cent) were stillborn, 239 (56 per cent) had died during infancy and 76 (18 per cent) were alive at one year. Robards, Thomas, and Rosenbloom (1975) reported that of the infants with spina bifida referred to their neonatal surgical unit in Liverpool over a three-year period and denied early closure, a significant proportion survived long enough to require drainage of hydrocephalus. Some 30 per cent of these infants denied early closure survived at least one year, a proportion quite different from Oxford where 92 out of 99 infants with unoperated myeloceles died before their first birthday (Hide, Williams, and Ellis 1972). Hide *et al.* (1972) also noted a higher mortality for children placed in institutions and given custodial care only instead of being cared for at home by their parents. Studies from other centres demonstrate indirectly the effects of treatment as illustrated by a 24 per cent survival rate at one year in Birmingham, 36 per cent in Liverpool, and 43 per cent in Belfast

(Table 7.1). The survival rate of the 185 Belfast infants was better for males (45 per cent) than for females (34 per cent). Apart from the objective measurement of mortality, Reid (1977) has emphasized the suffering non-selection imposes on these unfortunate children. Barden, Meyer, and Stelling (1975) described the fate of 143 spina bifida patients treated between 1928 and 1951 in Greenville, South Carolina, and followed up for 20 years or more; one-third of these survivors were self-supporting at ages ranging from 20 to 43 years although all had some degree of disability.

TABLE 7.1 *Survival rates in four series of spina bifida infants in the United Kingdom*

	Spina bifida infants		Stillborn		Died (0–364 days)		Alive at first birthday	
Place	total number	per cent	number	per cent	number	per cent	number	per cent
Belfast 1964–8 (Elwood, J. H. and Nevin 1973)	185	(100)	30	(16)	75	(41)	80	(43)
Birmingham 1960–2 (Knox 1967)	132	(100)	29	(22)	71	(54)	32	(24)
Liverpool 1960–2 (Rickham and Mawdsley 1966)	203	(100)	46	(23)	84	(41)	73	(36)
South Wales 1956–62 (Laurence and Tew 1971)†	425	(100)	110	(26)	239	(56)	76	(18)

† Majority of this series were untreated, other series include treated and untreated cases.

This period of active surgical management has been assessed by Lorber (1971, 1972). Around 35 per cent of the infants referred to the Sheffield unit from all areas of Great Britain were treated: the remainder were given only supportive care and feeding on demand. Lorber describes his aim as 'to add life to their years rather than years to their life'. This experience demonstrated that a high mortality and severe disability are related to the level of the lesion, thoracic lesions having a worse prognosis than lesions at the lumbar or sacral level. A poor prognosis was also associated with a degree of hydrocephalus having a head circumference exceeding the 90th percentile by 2 cm or more at birth, gross physical deformity, or other major associated defects. Of the several criteria to be considered for and against treatment (Lorber 1977) one which can be assessed at birth and which greatly affects the chance of survival is the level and extent of the spina bifida lesion. In their ten-year review of 200 consecutive closures of open myelomeningoceles, Lister, Zachary, and Brereton (1977) found a better survival rate in infants having lesions limited to the sacral area compared with infants having lesions at higher levels (Fig. 7.1). Intermediate and long-term survival as well as the prognosis regarding the quality of life is very much dependent on the management of hydrocephalus and other conditions. Poor social circumstances also increased mortality. Many of these infants are unlikely to earn a living and they will live severely restricted lives.

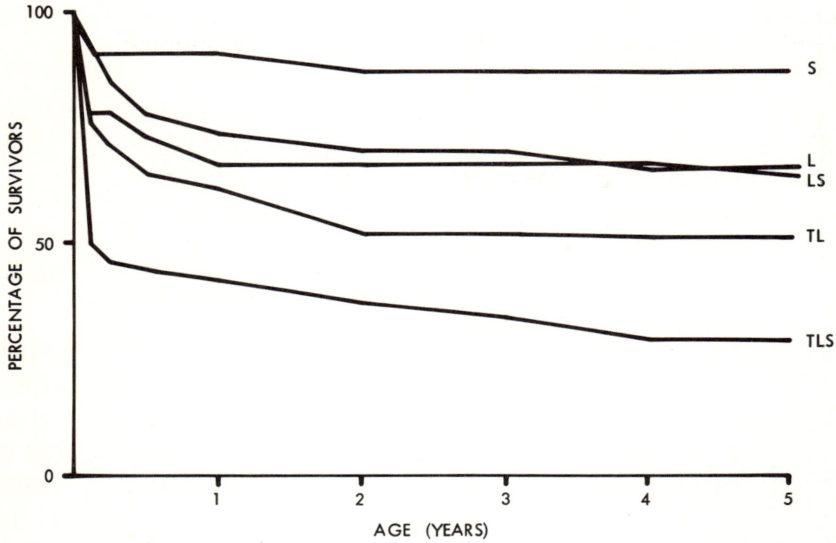

FIG. 7.1. Distribution of 200 consecutive liveborn infants with spina bifida by anatomical level of the lesion and survival time. (After Lister *et al.* 1977 and courtesy of *Progress in Pediatric Surgery*.)

If a comparison is made of the degree of the handicap in the 475 treated cases followed up in Sheffield (Lorber 1971) with the 426 mainly untreated cases followed up in South Wales (Laurence and Tew 1971) it is evident that the increased proportion of survivors aged four to eight years in Sheffield (45 per cent) compared with South Wales (21 per cent) is virtually all accounted for by an increase in the proportion of children having physical or physical and mental handicap (Table 7.2). The proportion of survivors having no handicap is virtually the same being 7 per cent in the South Wales series and 5 per cent in the Sheffield series. Furthermore, of the 288 Sheffield infants with myelomeningocele and hydrocephalus only one survived without handicap. Illingworth (1974) has summarized the Sheffield experience as follows:

The suffering which these children have to tolerate is immense. They have prolonged and repeated stays in the hospital. They suffer numerous operations and it is not surprising that some older children live in dread of further operations and admissions to hospital. Forty-one children with paralysed legs had a total of 500 operations by the age of 8 to 12 years. One nine year old girl with normal intelligence had had 18 major operations. Of 200 cases over an eight year period, 97 died, having had 203 operations, and having spent 898 weeks in the Children's Hospital, Sheffield (from whence they were discharged as soon as possible to regional hospitals. We do not know how long they were in-patients in these hospitals). Of the 200 cases, 103 survived; they had a total of 885 operations and spent 2796 weeks in the Children's Hospital, Sheffield. In other words to produce 103 survivors, a total of 1088 operations were performed, and a total of 3694 weeks were spent in this one hospital. Valve replacements averaging about one per 18 months, were one cause for hospital admission. Fractures of the femur or other bones are common; many children had had eight or more fractures. Dislocation of the hip is common. Almost all those with paralyzed legs have serious urinary tract infections, often with hydronephrosis. Of those with meningomyelocele and hydrocephalus, 83 per cent are incontinent of urine and faeces. Most of the boys will be impotent.

TABLE 7.2 *Degree of handicap observed at follow-up of 901 liveborn spina bifida infants in the United Kingdom (after Illingworth 1974)*

Degree of Handicap	Cardiff (untreated cases)	Sheffield (treated cases)
	Rates per 100 affected liveborn infants	
None	7	5
Physical only	2	25
Physical and mental	12	15
Total (proportion surviving at ages from 4 to 8 years)	21†	45
Total number of infants followed up	426	475

† Includes some infants with meningoceles which were excluded in the Sheffield series.

How accurate are methods of selecting children for surgical treatment? Experience at the Royal Children's Hospital, Melbourne, based on 318 patients, shows no active surgical treatment was offered in one-third and 93 per cent of these infants died indicating that prediction was accurate in all but 7 per cent of cases (Medical Journal of Australia 1971). Only some 2 per cent of 79 untreated cases lived for two years. Problems relating to selecting infants for treatment have been discussed by Freeman (1974) in the United States, Cooperman (1977) in Canada and others. Katzen (1975), at the Transvaal Memorial Hospital, Johannesburg, studied 61 children with myelomeningocele over the period 1970 to 1975 of which 39 were actively treated surgically with a mortality of 33 per cent. Some 22 were 'selected out' and nine having severe defects died within two weeks. The remaining 13 were not treated but survived for periods of time varying from 3 weeks to 9 months. Some eight children had lesions at the level of the third lumbar vertebra or above and three of these died from infection within 3 weeks while the lesions in the other five children epithelialized over within 2½ months. Although these children developed progressive hydrocephalus, the parents insisted that they receive treatment which Katzen carried out by inserting ventriculo-peritoneal shunts. Two children subsequently died, one of septicaemia from a urinary infection at 3 months and the other of pneumonia at 9 months, and three were alive at age 8 months, 13 months (mentally retarded), and 5 years. This description illustrates some of the problems facing the clinician and Katzen also emphasizes the difficulties of arranging home care for these spina bifida infants and of non-treatment being interpreted by some parents as medical malpractice.

Guiney, Fitzgerald, Mehigan, Puri, and Sundar (1977) described 127 open-myelomeningocele patients, 77 of whom were operated upon and 50 received no operations, at Our Lady's Hospital for Sick Children, Dublin. Of the 50 patients treated non-surgically only five (10 per cent) were alive 15 months later whilst 65 (84 per cent) of the operated group were alive. In another report from the same unit, Fitzgerald and Healey (1974) consider surgery has increased the proportion of survivors from 27 per cent in 1963 to 67 per cent in 1968. A communication from the Richmond Hospital, Dublin, by Archer and Pate (1975) based on 469 children treated between 1967 and 1973 gives an overall survival rate of 50 per cent. The survival rates according to the type of lesion were 80 per cent for meningocele in which a simple sac with no nerve involvement was present; for closed myelomeningoceles in which the sac contained nerves or a lump of neural tissue the survival rate was 88 per cent and for open myelomeningoceles with exposed neural tissue the survival rate was 38 per cent. Laurence, Evans, Weeks, Thomas, Frazer, and Tew (1976) formally compared the reliability of prediction of outcome on spina bifida. Clinical findings relating to 85 affected infants were given to two neurosurgeons and two paediatricians who were asked to use the data to predict the length and quality of survival. Out of 170 choices made by the assessment team regarding survival or death relating to these 85 infants the surgeons were more pessimistic than the paediatricians and made 100 compared with 36 incorrect predictions respectively. Surgeons predicted shorter survival times and paediatricians longer survival times than in fact were observed. Estimates of the quality of survival with regard to intellect, locomotion and continence were fairly good although prediction of the level of intellect was unreliable due to the inability to anticipate complications of infection and valve failure. Pertinent to this debate is the prospective randomized controlled trial of immediate and delayed closure of myelomeningocele which was conducted by Smyth, Piggot, Forsythe, and Merrett (1974) to determine if immediate closure prevented or minimized muscle paralysis. Their results based on 99 infants treated in Belfast did not show any significant difference in mortality or alteration of muscle power between the two groups and they concluded that closure of the lesion may be delayed for 48 hours after birth or longer to allow detailed clinical assessment of the infant.

Lorber's policy of selective treatment has considerably influenced the active management of spina bifida and there is evidence that mortality in recent years has increased. The first-year mortality of spina bifida infants in

Northern Ireland was 54 per cent in 1964, but 73 per cent in 1972 (Elwood, J. H. 1976). A similar trend is seen in data for spina bifida children in England and Wales (Weatherall 1976; Weatherall and White 1976) where survival rates improved annually up to 1969. After this date infant mortality rates for children born with spina bifida increase and survival rates decrease for each year up to 1972 (Fig. 7.2). This rise in mortality has occurred concomitantly with a fall in the number of operations performed on children having spina bifida, hydrocephalus, or both spina bifida and hydrocephalus.

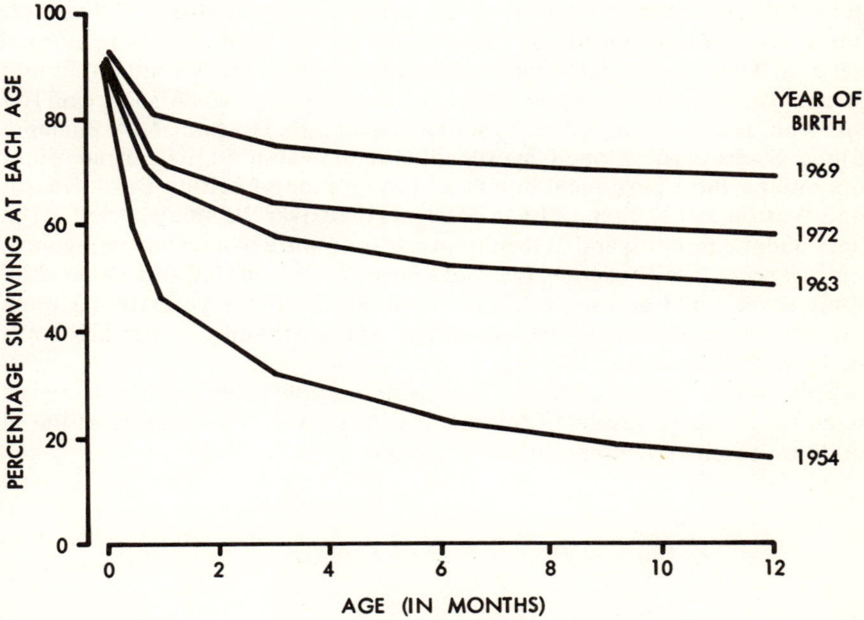

FIG. 7.2. Distribution of children born alive with spina bifida, hydrocephalus, or both by year of birth and survival time in England and Wales for various years from 1954 to 1972. (After Weatherall and White 1976 and Crown Copyright.)

Despite the influences of modern medical and surgical treatment (Eckstein and MacNab 1966) there is serious concern about the quality of survival of spina bifida children. They now comprise a sizeable cohort who are reaching adulthood, some of whose parents are either dead, elderly or in a large number of instances separated or divorced (Tew, Laurence, Payne, and Rawnsley 1977). They are further faced with the social problems of earning a living, travel, accommodation, and being an independent individual as well as the personal problems of physical and mental health (Illingworth 1974, British Medical Journal 1978). There are no good estimates of the true prevalence of spina bifida children and adults in the United Kingdom or elsewhere; as we emphasize, the work which we examine in this book is based mainly on prevalence at birth data as an approximation for the estimates of incidence (Chapter III). No valid estimates of prevalence rates in the community are available although they are essential for health-care planning in terms of institutional care, hospital beds, and medical and social services. Attempts to assess costs point to large amounts of money being needed (Lightowler 1971). Of the 117 spina bifida children who had open myelomeningoceles at birth and were assessed at their fifth birthday by Lister and colleagues (1977) some 80 (68 per cent) out of the 117 children examined had normal intelligence quotients (Stanford Binet test), 36 (31 per cent) were educationally subnormal, and one child was profoundly retarded. At the time of a ten-year follow-up 106 of the 117 five-year survivors were reviewed; of these 27 per cent were attending normal schools. The authors state that an assessment of the child's ability to fit into society can be made fairly accurately at five years of age. A survey of 107 spina bifida children cared for by staff at Wellington Hospital, New Zealand, found 89 cases developed hydrocephalus of whom 61 had atrial shunt operations, three peritoneal shunts, and 25 no shunts (Arthur, Bush, Guard, and Weston 1972). Some 41 (38 per cent) died over the study period, 27 at ages under 6 months, and of the 66 survivors 43 were of normal intelligence, nine were retarded but educable, and four severely retarded and ineducable. Only seven children out of 22 survivors aged from 4 years to 10 years attended normal schools, virtually all the remainder being at special schools or in institutional care.

Spina bifida children, therefore, present multiple problems and there is a need for assessing results of treatment with regard to the quality of life in addition to objective measurements of mortality.

V

Ascertainment

8

Modes of ascertainment

In order to study the epidemiology of anencephalus and spina bifida in a population, it is essential to be able to identify or at least count all affected births occurring in the defined population during a given time period. Also, it must be possible to enumerate all births so that an estimate may be obtained of the population at risk. The methods available range from total reliance on routine records, such as stillbirths and death registrations, to special examination of all births by a committed individual or team. As Smithells (1971) has stated:

> The smaller the number of observers, the higher will be the standard of ascertainment, the highest standard being achieved by a single enthusiast. But the larger the population surveyed, the more information will be obtained. The one extreme will produce a negligible quantity of completely reliable data; the other will provide vast quantities of suspect information.

The best method of ascertainment will depend on the circumstances and objectives of the particular study. Virtually all publications on the epidemiology of anencephalus and spina bifida are based either on vital statistics, data from special registries or hospital records. We will now examine some of the issues relating to these sources of ascertainment.

Definitions of anencephalus and spina bifida

We mention other aspects of the important question regarding the definitions of 'anencephalus' and of 'spina bifida' (Section 2) but we emphasize here that the generally accepted definition of 'anencephalus' includes a proportion of cases having anencephalus with spina bifida, the definition 'spina bifida' includes a large proportion of cases having spina bifida with hydrocephalus, and both diagnostic categories contain infants having neural-tube defects together with congenital abnormalities of other body systems. A classification adopted and used by official vital statistics in many countries is the *International Classification of Diseases* (World Health Organization 1967) which, however, is revised and altered every ten years or so.

Hospital births

Perhaps the most common mode of ascertainment is from hospital records and particularly records of births in teaching hospitals associated with medical schools. As many doctors are hospital based and obstetric records easily accessible such a study is not difficult. If only one hospital is studied and the number of births delivered in this institution is fairly small relative to the total number of births occurring in the community served by that hospital, any findings may be biased by a substantial but unknown amount, owing to the hospital deliveries not being representative of all those in the community. Usually the rates in hospital births will be higher, as mothers with hydramnios will tend to be referred to hospital, as will mothers with other characteristics associated with a higher risk of neural-tube defects, such as a history of a prior affected child, stillbirth, or miscarriage or extremes of age and parity. Excluding mothers delivered in the hospital but referred from elsewhere usually because of complications of pregnancy may reduce this bias somewhat but again, results may not be relevant except to that one unit. That hospital rates are not the same as estimates of prevalence in the community is demonstrated by a survey of anencephalus in Belfast (Fig. 8.1, Elwood, J. H. 1970).

The prevalence rate of anencephalus in all births occurring between 1950 and 1966 to women resident in Belfast was 4.2 per 1000 (221 anencephalics, 52 452 total births). Deliveries at the two largest obstetric centres, the Royal

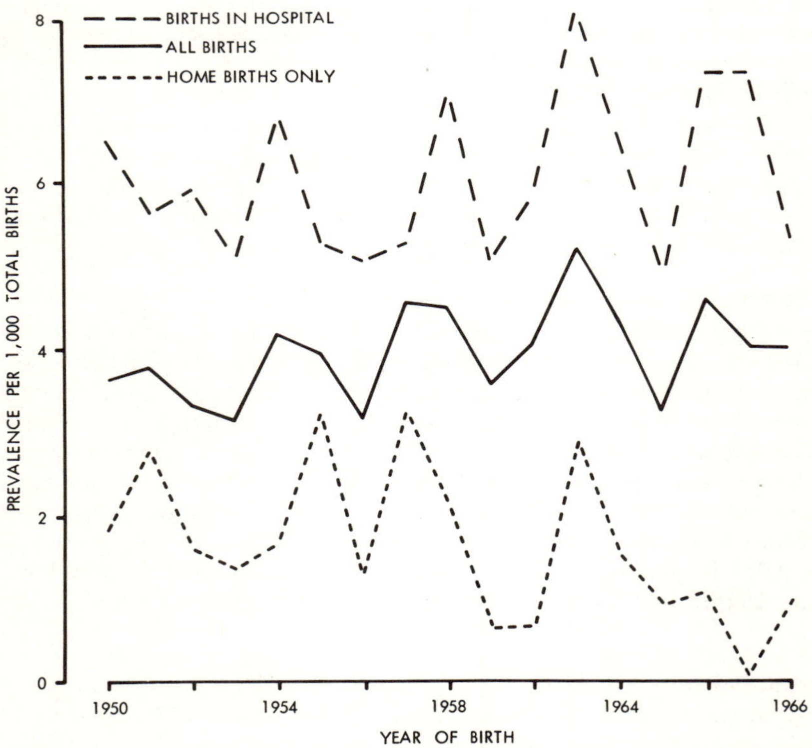

FIG. 8.1. Prevalence of anencephalus per 1000 total births ascertained from three sources for Belfast 1950–66. (Courtesy of the *British Journal of Preventive and Social Medicine*.)

Maternity and Jubilee Maternity Hospitals, included 81 per cent (179) of the anencephalics but only 54 per cent (28 365) of the total births, giving a prevalence rate of 6.3 per 1000 births. In contrast, amongst births occurring at home, delivered by family doctors, the rate was 1.4 per 1000 (17 cases, 11 967 births). The remaining 25 anencephalics and 12 140 total births occurred in smaller hospitals and lying-in units, showing an intermediate rate of 2.1 per 1000 births. Interpretation of hospital series, therefore, is not straightforward unless the proportion of births in the community delivered in the hospitals surveyed approaches 100 per cent. Even so, when hospital records alone are searched the number of cases expressed as a percentage of all known cases found using multiple sources of ascertainment may be low as indicated by the Hungarian figure of 52.6 per cent based on this one source of ascertainment (Czeizel and Révész 1970). Naggan (1976) has discussed these points with particular reference to international comparisons.

Birth-defect monitoring systems

There are a number of birth-defect registries, surveillance systems, or monitoring programmes operating in different countries (Miller 1977). Their essential common characteristics are that they relate to a defined population and are on-going from year to year but they differ with regard to completeness and accuracy of recording birth-defect events, speed of data processing and communication of any reports, and administration which may be by government departments, municipal health units, universities, hospitals, individuals, or any combination of these.

United Kingdom

Certain local birth registries have been set up in the United Kingdom for the purposes of examining numerous outcomes of pregnancy of which the occurrence of birth defects is one component. These usually are maintained on a prospective basis by mutual agreement between the municipal health department and a university and contain more detailed information on all births in a defined local population than is available from national vital statistics. Record and McKeown (1949) and later Leck *et al*. (1968) used the Birmingham registry (Charles 1951) for several surveys and a similar registry was initiated in 1957 in Belfast by Stevenson primarily for the study of population genetics (Stevenson and Warnock 1959). After the thalidomide tragedy in 1961 registers of voluntary notifications for congenital malformations were set up by the Registrars General for England and Wales (Rogers and Weatherall 1976; Weatherall and Haskey 1976) and Northern Ireland (Elwood, J. H. 1972, 1976). Data are available for each year beginning with 1964. No comparable system operates in Scotland. The notification forms are completed by a community physician, health visitor or other member of the maternal and child-health division of the area health authority based on examination of each stillborn and liveborn infant having a malformation noted within seven days of birth. Forms are forwarded to the General Register Office, now the Office of Population Censuses and Surveys, for data processing. No name is sent centrally but an identification number is used so that the record may be traced at local level if necessary. The information is analysed monthly hence short-term changes and epidemics are detectable. No systemic follow-up of these notifications is made at present and the diagnoses are not verified by clinical consultants. More specialized computer-based information systems also exist. Newcombe's (1967) work on the British Columbia population study laid the foundation for developing medical record linkage in Oxford (Acheson 1967), Scotland (Heasman 1968), and Northern Ireland (Cheeseman 1968) and some studies of birth defects have been conducted based on these sources.

A survey by Scott (1975) investigated the completeness of ascertainment of the voluntary notification system for Congenital Malformations in Northern Ireland as operated in Belfast compared with a number of other sources. If ascertainment is based on the Registrar General's notification system alone then all anencephalics (100 per cent) but only 74 per cent of known spina bifida cases would be ascertained. The degree of completeness of ascertainment was found to vary considerably according to source and type of defect. Weatherall (1969) measured the efficiency of reporting one defect, anencephalus, through the Congenital Malformation Notification System for England and Wales by matching 1233 anencephalic infants notified during 1966 against all the 1584 stillbirths and infant deaths registered from this cause during the same period. Some 1155 anencephalic deaths correctly matched against notifications, 429 infants certified at stillbirth or death to have anencephalus were never notified and the efficiency of notification varied greatly geographically with some local authority areas having 100 per cent and others less than 60 per cent notifications.

North America

A registry of handicapped children and adults, known as the British Columbia Health Surveillance Registry since 1974 (Miller 1976), has been maintained in this province of Canada since 1952 (Miller 1964; Lowry, Miller, Scott, and Renwick 1975; Miller and Lowry 1977). This system ascertains and cross checks birth-defect events from a number of sources and forms the basis of the Canadian medical record linkage project described by Newcombe (1967). Also, by agreement between the provincial governments and the federal department of Health and Welfare Canada, a central registry of congenital defects occurring in infants born in four provinces namely, New Brunswick, Manitoba, Alberta, and British Columbia commenced in 1966 and is referred to as the Congenital Anomalies Surveillance System (Banister 1971). A fifth province, Prince Edward Island, will be added in 1979. All stillbirths and death certificates and Physician's Notice of Birth Certificates are collected by the provincial registrars and copies sent to Statistics Canada, Ottawa. The Physician's Notice of Birth Certificate is a statutory document which must be completed within 24 hours or 48 hours of the birth by a physician who is either present at the delivery or else examines the infant shortly afterwards. These certificates are scrutinized and any mention of a congenital defect coded by a paediatrican. The coded data are then punched and computerized. Linkage of different documents referring to the same individual is carried out clerically as the forms come in and is checked using computer routines.

This system operated from 1966 to 1969. It gives the most accurate recording for defects which are fatal or else obvious at birth and a defect not diagnosed within 24 hours of delivery or one which does not contribute to death will be missed. From 1970, information from the Hospital Discharge Certificate is included in the system. This document, required under hospital by-laws in each province, is completed by the physician responsible for the infant's discharge from the hospital and contains all diagnoses made during the period of hospitalization. Inclusion of this information in the Congenital Anomalies Surveillance System has greatly improved the reporting of birth defects. No document corresponding to the Hospital Discharge Certificate is in use for home deliveries but these comprised only 1 per cent of all births in 1970. Stillbirths from 20 weeks of gestation are included and data relate to either the number of abnormalities or to the number of malformed infants. The large increase in the reporting of many abnormalities after Hospital Discharge data were included in 1970 shows the relative incompleteness of ascertainment of the 1966 to 1969 returns for many defects, but no abrupt change in the reported rates of anencephalus or spina bifida occurred (section 10). Even with these more recent data, comparisons of prevalence rates between provinces may be influenced by different standards of diagnosis and recording. These, however, are probably minor within one province over short time periods and do not affect analyses of such factors as seasonal variation. The Surveillance System is more complete for British Columbia and Alberta than for Manitoba or New Brunswick (National Academy of Sciences 1975).

There are no monitoring programmes for birth defects in the United States which exactly parallel the Canadian systems, mainly because of the differences in health care in these neighbouring countries, but there are two registries which have very similar aims. The Metropolitan Atlanta Congenital Defects Program began in 1967, monitors 130 categories of congenital birth defects and publishes regular reports. Around 23 000 births annually are scrutinized and the data have been used to test hypotheses relating to cleft lip and prenatal exposure to diazepam (Safra and Oakley 1975). Secondly, there is the Birth Defects Monitoring System set up in 1973 as a collaborative venture between government departments (The National Institute of Child Health and Human Development and the Center for Disease Control) and two voluntary bodies (Commission on Professional Hospital Activities and the National Foundation). The data are based on all births (live and still) delivered in over 1200 hospitals across the United States which represent about one million out of around three million births occurring in this country each year. The National Foundation (March of Dimes) also supports the International Clearinghouse for Birth Defects Monitoring Systems by which ten countries (Canada, Czechoslovakia,

England and Wales, Finland, France, Hungary, Israel, Norway, Sweden, and the United States) have agreed to a standardized format for reporting defects and exchanging information (Miller 1977).

Mortality data

The source of ascertainment in a large number of surveys is mortality data based on the causes of stillbirth and death as certified by registered medical practitioners and published in government vital statistics reports annually or at other time intervals. As anencephalus is a striking malformation incompatible with life, mortality statistics may provide acceptable information concerning the frequency of this defect. More specifically it is assumed that stillbirth and death registrations will give a valid estimate of the prevalence at birth of anencephalus in deliveries of 20 or 28 or more weeks' gestation. McKeown and Record (1949) found all of 366 anencephalics reported in Birmingham between 1940 and 1947 were stillborn or dead within 28 days. Gittelsohn and Milham (1965) reported on 2205 anencephalics ascertained in New York State from 1945 to 1959 of which 1430 were stillborn, 647 died within 24 hours of delivery, and 102 died between one and 27 days after birth. The length of survival of the remaining 26 cases casts doubt on the diagnosis. In our Canadian studies deaths attributed to anencephalus at ages over one year were excluded but there were only 13 such cases out of a total of 10 340 registered in the national mortality statistics during the period from 1950 to 1969. The likelihood of attributing mortality to anencephalus on a death certificate will depend on the accuracy of diagnosis and certification practice. For example, of the 36 neonatal deaths ascribed to anencephalus in the British Perinatal Mortality Survey, only 32 (89 per cent) were recorded as such on the death certificates while five other deaths (two from spina bifida and three from other abnormalities) were erroneously attributed to anencephalus (Fedrick and Butler 1972). In this situation comparison of the numbers of cases reported by official mortality records and by special study sources will give very similar results without showing that the diagnoses recorded are accurate.

Thus although more specific data are preferred for any study of individual cases of anencephalus, for studies of population groups routine mortality data are usually as accurate and may be more accurate than special systems of recording. A comparison of the numbers of cases of anencephalus reported by routine stillbirth and death notifications with the numbers reported by the Congenital Anomalies Surveillance System and other special studies in several areas of Canada shows that the total recorded by vital statistics was 98.4 per cent of the total reported by other systems (Elwood, J. M. 1974), although for any one area and time period the vital statistics total ranged from 84 to 116 per cent of the total from the other sources. In Iowa, Hay (1971) found that 94 per cent of anencephalics ascertained from multiple sources were recorded by vital statistics. Special surveys and ongoing registries in their initial years of operation are prone to errors due to both missing cases and to duplication of reports. As the British Columbia Registry is probably the most accurate in Canada, we compared the numbers of cases of anencephalus and spina bifida occurring in British Columbia as reported by vital records and by the Health Surveillance Registry (Table 8.1). For the years 1964 to 1970, death registrations reported 161 cases of anencephalus and the Registry reported 158. The discrepancy may be due to differences in diagnosis, in coding practices or in the date of reporting. We were unable to directly compare individual records because of confidentiality regulations. For spina bifida, the situation is quite different with 209

TABLE 8.1 *Numbers of anencephalics and spina bifidas ascertained from two sources in British Columbia, 1964–70*

	Anencephalus		Spina Bifida	
Year	B.C. registry	Vital statistics	B.C. registry	Vital statistics
1964	23	26	42	14
1965	20	21	28	11
1966	22	23	30	11
1967	29	28	27	10
1968	18	18	24	12
1969	22	21	30	5
1970	24	24	28	13
TOTAL	158	161	209	76

Registry includes stillborn, dead and live cases (unpublished data). Vital statistics includes registered stillbirths of 20 or more weeks of gestation plus deaths.

cases reported by the Registry and only 76 by mortality data. The discrepancy for spina bifida is expected as many affected infants survive well past the neonatal stage, and deaths may be certified as due to hydrocephalus, meningitis, or other causes rather than to spina bifida. The use of multiple sources of ascertainment is an important method of overcoming this problem especially as the proportion now surviving is markedly influenced by treatment (Lorber 1971). Examination of spina bifida mortality using death registrations and the *International Classification of Diseases* is confusing and much less valid than is the case with anencephalus. There have been frequent changes in coding procedures by the three Registrars General of the United Kingdom mainly in relation to classifying spina bifida and hydrocephalus. These problems of interpretation are amplified by Lorber (1968) and Elwood, J. H. (1976).

Although mortality data alone provide good estimates of the prevalence at birth of anencephalus, findings based on ascertainment from deaths occurring in livebirths only, that is excluding stillbirths, as in the study of anencephalus in West Virginia (Poole 1960), have little validity because they exclude up to 90 per cent of births having anencephalus. In the United Kingdom stillbirths are defined as deadborn infants of 28 or more weeks of gestation and are medically certified and registered by law. The Republic of Ireland has only a voluntary notification system for stillbirths and no statutory registration as yet while in the United States the gestational age defining the 'late fetal death period', synonymous with the period of stillbirth, is usually 20 weeks but this varies from state to state. The various provinces of Canada changed the minimum age for definition of a stillbirth from the 28th week to the 20th week between 1959 and 1964; however this produced no change in the prevalence at birth of anencephalus, as the prevalence in stillbirths of 20 to 27 weeks of gestation is similar to that in later stillbirths (Elwood, J. M. 1976*a*). A varying proportion of anencephalics are liveborn and later registered as infant deaths. In a survey comparing births from 1956 to 1966 in Belfast and in four Scottish cities, Glasgow, Dundee, Edinburgh, and Aberdeen, the percentages of cases of anencephalus reported as livebirths in each city were 19.2, 10.5, 6.6, 5.4, and 1.5 respectively (Elwood, J. H. and MacKenzie 1971). The Canadian national mortality data show a rise in the proportion of anencephalics registered as infant deaths rather than stillbirths from 11 per cent during 1943–9 to 42 per cent during 1965–9. Thus although the total mortality rate attributed to anencephalus has declined, the rate based only on liveborn cases has risen (Fig. 8.2).

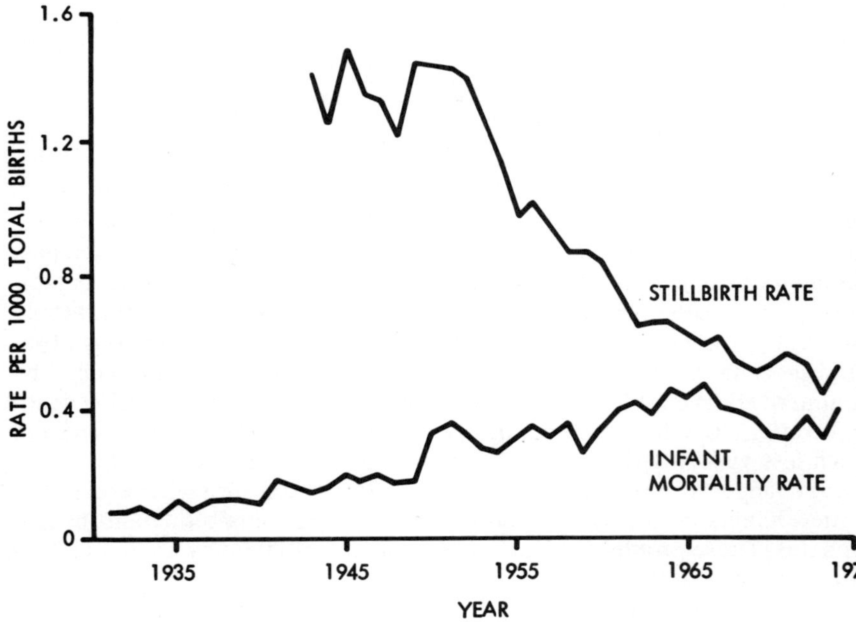

FIG. 8.2. Annual stillbirth rates attributed to anencephalus 1943–74 and annual infant mortality rates attributed to monstrosity 1931–68 and to anencephalus 1969–74 in Canada. Both rates are calculated per 1000 total births.

Monstrosity

To assess the validity of accepting the *International Classification of Diseases* (7th revision) category, monstrosity (ICD No. 750), as predominantly reflecting infant deaths due to an anencephalus at our request Statistics Canada staff examined the records of all infant deaths in Canada coded by this number for the years 1953, 1963, and 1968 (Table 8.2). From a total for the three years studied of 433 infant deaths, 395 (91 per cent) mentioned anencephalus. Of the remaining 38, specified in Table 8.3, eight were judged to probably represent anencephalus, 16 probably represented other defects, and for 14 no decision could be reached. Thus at least 93 per cent and possibly 96 per cent, of infant deaths recorded under this ICD code represent anencephalus. In more recent data, the problem does not arise as the Eighth Revision Classification of Diseases codes deaths due to anencephalus under ICD No. 740 and monstrosity is subdivided into six descriptive types distributed over three ICD numbers (740, 759.1, and 759.2). Only one type, acephalic monster, is coded as ICD No. 740.

Anencephalus is probably the only common congenital abnormality for which routine mortality records give a reasonable estimate of prevalence at birth. This fact has allowed us and other investigators to study the epidemiological features of anencephalus in very large birth populations, allowing useful assessments of geographical, secular, and other factors. Spina bifida, like most other congenital defects, can only be directly studied if special registries or survey systems are used.

TABLE 8.2 *Classifications of all infant deaths registered in Canada and coded as Monstrosity (ICD number 750) in 1953, 1963, and 1968*

Classification	1953 number	1963 number	1968 number	Total number	Cumulative percentage
Coded as ICD number 750	116	178	139	433	–
With mention of anencephalus	96	170	129	395	91
Other					
Probably anencephalus	6	2	0	8	93
Unknown	7	3	4	14	96
Probably not anencephalus	7	3	6	16	100

TABLE 8.3 *Listing of exact form of death certificate entries coded ICD number 750 in which anencephalus was not mentioned based on a search of all infant deaths registered in Canada for the years 1953, 1963, and 1968*

Group 1:	Considered as probably anencephalus	
1	1953	Premature monster—small head, brain out of the skull, harelip
2	1953	Monster—malformation of head, spina bifida, malformation of lower limbs
3	1953	Monstrosity, breech birth, harelip, polydactylism, spina bifida
4	1953	Premature, hydramnios, monster
5	1953	Spina bifida, monster
6	1953	Inanition, hydrocephalic, malformation of spine, monster
7	1963	Absence of skull (infectious hepatitis during pregnancy)
8	1963	Brain malformation, cyclops, arrhinencephaly
Group 2:	Considered as probably not anencephalus	
1	1953	Myocarditis, macrocephalic, hemiplegic, mental retardation
2	1953	Congenital malformation, cleft palate, harelip, one eye, one ear
3	1953	Rachitism, macrocephalic, idiotic
4	1953	Malformation of fetus, teratology
5	1953	Congenital hydrocephalic monster
6	1953	Fetal monstrosity, hydrocephalus, harelip, cleft palate, malformation of fingers
7	1953	Mongolian monstrosity, premature
8	1963	Monstrosity (mouth, feet and hands), hydramnios (age of mother 50 years)
9	1963	Monstrosity—malformation of abdominal organs
10	1963	Cyclops malformation
11	1968	Siamese twins (one heart, one liver, hemorrhage sub-cranial in largest twin)
12	1968	Microcephalic, club foot, pulmonary atelectasis
13	1968	Multiple deformities (congenital)
14	1968	Multiple deformities macrocephalic, hypocalcification, premature
15	1968	Epilepsy, microcephalic, subocclusion intestinal, cyclopia, tetralogy of Fallot
16	1968	Cyclops, multiple congenital abnormalities
Group 3:	Unknown: defined as 'monstrosity'	
1–6	1953	Monstrosity
7	1953	Fetal monster, mental deficiency
8	1963	Multiple fetal abnormalities (monster)
9	1963	Pneumonia—monstrosity birth
10	1963	Premature—deformed, cyclops, atresia faciale
11	1968	Bronchopneumonia, cachexia, microcephalic, mental retardation
12	1968	Epilepsy, encephalopathic chronique, monster, dehydration
13	1968	Terminal pneumonia, monster
14	1968	Multiple abnormalities (monster)

Entries are recorded in their exact original form.

VI

Present studies

9

Studies of anencephalus and spina bifida in Ireland and in Canada

WE discuss in this book several aspects of the epidemiology of anencephalus and spina bifida. When dealing with each major epidemiological feature we present a review of work by other investigators together with any relevant findings from our own research carried out in the British Isles and in Canada. We now briefly outline some of the studies we ourselves have performed.

The work in the British Isles is largely based on information from Northern Ireland where one of us (J. H. E.) is based. Anencephalus and spina bifida have the highest frequencies in the world reported to date in this area. Northern Ireland (1976 estimated population 1 538 100 persons) consists geographically of six out of the 32 counties of Ireland. Since 1921, Northern Ireland has been part of the United Kingdom, governed from Westminster but with its own regional parliament near Belfast which is the capital and largest city (1976 estimated population 363 000 persons). As in the rest of the United Kingdom, health care has been provided by the National Health Service since 1948. Some 31 per cent of the total population of Northern Ireland are Roman Catholic and 69 per cent are Protestant. To some extent Roman Catholic reflects a celtic origin and Protestant a Scots–Irish or Anglo–Irish origin but this distinction is oversimplistic (Evans 1973). We have carried out several surveys of neural-tube defects observed in the population of Belfast.

The Belfast birth register was set up in 1957 by Alan Stevenson who was the first Professor of Social and Preventive Medicine at The Queen's University. This register, similar to that in Birmingham, contains information on all livebirths and stillbirths of 28 or more weeks of gestation delivered annually to women resident in Belfast. The data are collected by arrangement between the municipal health department and the university and do not rely, at least for the earlier years, on official statistics. Stillbirths for example, were first registered in Northern Ireland in 1961. The unit of observation is a birth and for each, detailed biosocial data are available; they are identified by unique serial numbers with each year being numbered independently. This system operated from 1957 to 1969. From 1970 onwards the data are incorporated into the Northern Ireland medical record linkage project which covers all stillbirths of 28 or more weeks of gestation and livebirths (30 000 approximately) occurring in the province each year. The project is along the lines of the British Columbia population study (Newcombe 1967) but computer analysis and other aspects are not yet developed to the same degree. We have also used birth and death registrations maintained by the Northern Ireland General Register Office and also the voluntary notification system for congenital malformations in Northern Ireland which began in 1964 (Section 8). The Republic of Ireland, and particularly Dublin, have high prevalence rates for both anencephalus and spina bifida. We have examined official statistics and the voluntary notifications of late foetal deaths (that is, stillbirths of 28 or more weeks of gestation) in the Republic of Ireland. However, as there is known to be underascertainment of stillbirths by this system and because stillbirths are not legally registered in the Republic of Ireland, we examined reports on all deliveries in each of the three main Dublin maternity hospitals, the Rotunda Hospital, the Coombe Lying-In Hospital, and the National Maternity Hospital. These are large units, responsible for between 50 per cent and 80 per cent of all births to Dublin residents depending on which particular year is studied, and have made notable contributions to obstetrics and paediatrics. The oldest, the Rotunda Hospital, was founded in 1745 (Kirkpatrick 1913).

We have also conducted a number of epidemiological studies of anencephalus and spina bifida in Canada. Several of these are based on mortality data relating to anencephalus (stillbirths and infant deaths) made available through the generous cooperation of the staff of Statistics Canada in Ottawa. For the descriptive epidemiological work, the study population was defined as all births occurring from 1943 to 1974 in Canada, excluding Newfoundland, the Northwest Territories, and the Yukon. These areas were excluded as information on stillbirths by cause of death was only available in recent years, and even then, the risk of considerable underreporting was high; they include less than 3 per cent of all births in Canada. *The International Classification of Diseases* (7th and 8th revisions) codes used were for stillbirths, Y.38.0 (1943 to 1968) and p. 69 (1969–70) 'anencephalus', and for infant deaths, code 750 'monstrosity' (1943 to 1968) and 740 'anencephalus' (1969–70). The older infant death code 750 includes cases of conjoined twins and some other major abnormalities, but as we show (Section 8) it is likely that at least 93 per cent of these cases are in fact anencephalus. Stillbirths are notifiable from 28 weeks of gestation in the earlier years studied, but between 1959 and 1964 each province adopted a definition based on 20 weeks of gestation; this alteration was not accompanied by any abrupt change in the recorded mortality rate of anencephalus. Throughout the time period examined, infants with both anencephalus and spina bifida are coded as anencephalus. In most of our work, we present the results as mortality rates, defined as the number of anencephalics (stillbirths plus infant deaths) per 1000 total births (stillbirths plus livebirths). For the investigation of seasonal variation, information was obtained for the years 1954 to 1972. The statistical methods employed in our analyses of seasonal variation are described in Section 13 and in Appendix A.2.

Information from the Congenital Anomalies Surveillance System relating to the prevalence at birth of all congenital defects in the four provinces of New Brunswick, Manitoba, Alberta, and British Columbia for the years 1966 to 1971 was made available to us by Dr Philip Banister. We therefore were able to compare geographical and seasonal variations in anencephalus mortality rates with the variations in prevalence rates at birth of anencephalus, and the corresponding rates for spina bifida and other congenital abnormalities. With the assistance of Dr James Miller and Ms Mary McBride, we studied cases of anencephalus and spina bifida recorded by the British Columbia Health Surveillance Registry, which allows linkage of birth information into sibships using computerized medical record linkage techniques. This investigation further clarified the associations of these defects with maternal reproductive history (Section 21).

Some of the original work which we present is based on a case–control study of anencephalus in infants born between 1950 and 1969 to women resident in 14 major Canadian cities. The cities were selected to provide a large geographical range, although the two largest cities, Toronto and Montreal, could not be used owing to several major boundary changes with the recent creation of new administrative areas which invalidated comparisons of information over the study period. The cities chosen were Vancouver (British Columbia), Calgary and Edmonton (Alberta), Saskatoon and Regina (Saskatchewan), Winnipeg (Manitoba), Hamilton, Kitchener, London, Windsor, and Ottawa (Ontario), Quebec (Quebec), St John (New Brunswick), and Halifax (Nova Scotia)—Fig. 9.1. The case group comprised the 1391 stillbirths and infant deaths attributed to anencephalus or monstrosity observed in infants born to women resident in these 14 Canadian cities from 1950 to 1969. The control group was a sample of 5000 livebirths,

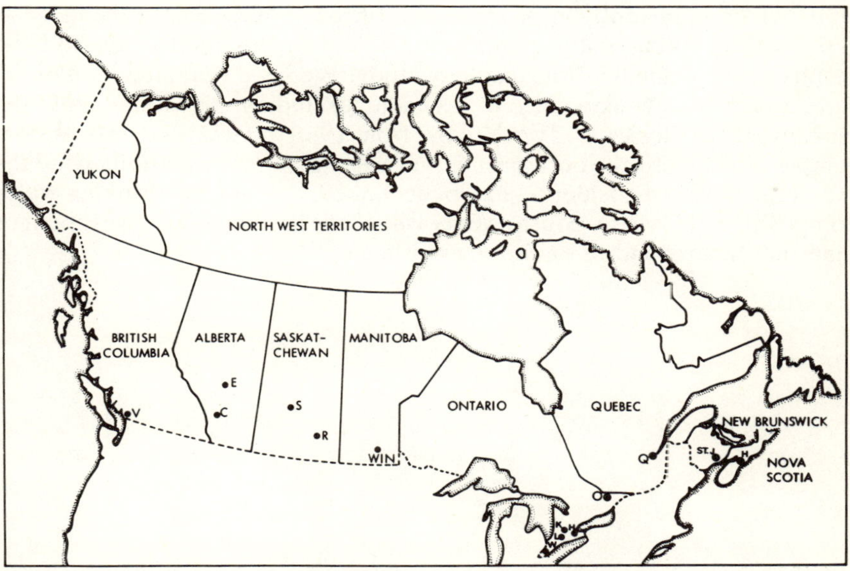

FIG. 9.1. The urban populations included in the Canadian 14-city study: V, Vancouver; E, Edmonton; C, Calgary; S, Saskatoon; R, Regina, WIN, Winnipeg; H, Hamilton; K, Kitchener; L, London, W, Windsor; O, Ottawa; Q, Quebec; ST.J, St. John; and H, Halifax.

chosen randomly from the 238 720 livebirths occurring to women resident in the selected 14 cities and registered in the years 1952, 1957, 1962, and 1967. Of the 1391 cases of anencephalus 73 per cent were stillborn and 27 per cent were liveborn. For the latter the infant death and birth records were linked manually, and the analysis was based on the data recorded on the stillbirth record or on the livebirth record. The main analysis examined eleven factors: city of residence, year of birth, month of birth, maternal age, the number of previous livebirths and the number of previous stillbirths occurring to the mother, the number of previous liveborn children who were deceased, maternal ethnic origin, plurality of birth (single or multiple), legitimacy, and place of birth (hospital or non-hospital). Multivariate statistical methods were used to assess the association between anencephalus risk and each of these factors after adjustment for effects of all the other factors. Further analyses dealt with interactions between certain of these factors, and interactions with the sex of the affected birth. Our methods are detailed in Appendix A.3.

We also have carried out a pilot study to assess if any association exists between the mortality rate from anencephalus and the composition of drinking water. We compared the mortality rates from anencephalus and from certain other causes in 36 large cities in Canada (populations over 50 000) and in the fourteen smaller towns in Ontario (populations 20 000 to 50 000) over the period 1950 to 1969 with information on the composition of drinking water obtained by special surveys conducted by Dr Luciano Neri and his colleagues at the University of Ottawa (Section 19). A case control study which is currently in progress will further evaluate both the associations with drinking water composition found in this pilot study and the results of the Canadian fourteen-city study. We have obtained data on all fatal cases of anencephalus in Canada, excluding Newfoundland, the Northwest Territories, and the Yukon, from 1968 to 1972, and on a random sample of all livebirths born during that period, and information giving the maternal place of residence has been linked to data on drinking-water composition. This case–control study will allow simultaneous assessment of maternal factors and of environmental factors.

VII

Descriptive epidemiology of anencephalus and spina bifida

10

Geographical variation

PREVALENCE rates at birth of anencephalus and spina bifida exhibit large geographical differences both between and within countries. We have summarized the relatively few studies including both anencephalus and spina bifida (Table 10.1) and also some 120 studies of the prevalence at birth or mortality from anencephalus (Appendix A.1). Any interpretation of this variation by place, however, must bear in mind the various modes of ascertainment used and the quality of data obtained by investigators working under many different conditions throughout the world. Ideally, all available records should be examined and special enquiries into all livebirths and stillbirths in the community made using standardized diagnostic criteria. This situation has rarely, if ever, been met. Several large studies have used multiple sources of ascertainment including stillbirth registrations, birth and death records, hospital records, birth defect notifications, and registers of abnormal births. As anencephalus is fairly easy to diagnose without specialized investigation, variability in diagnosis is not as large a problem as in studies of spina bifida or other abnormalities.

British Isles and Europe

The area which has been most studied is the British Isles where several surveys based on multiple sources of ascertainment are available. The highest prevalence rate for anencephalus reported by a community survey is 4.2 per 1000 births in Belfast, while hospital series in Dublin show rates up to 5.9 per 1000. Other areas with rates of above 3 per 1000 include county Galway, South Wales, Glasgow, Dundee, Liverpool, and Exeter. The lowest recorded rates of anencephalus are in South-east England. The prevalence of spina bifida shows a similar gradient from a maximum of 4.5 per 1000 in Belfast to a minimum of 1.5 in London. There is a pattern of decreasing prevalence rates for both defects from the northern and western areas to those in the south-east, the lowest rates being recorded in London, Northampton, and Oxford. The variation seen by comparing community studies is also apparent in studies of mortality from anencephalus, which has been estimated from official statistics for all areas of the British Isles (Elwood, J. H. 1970*a*, 1976 and Fig. 10.1). Considerable differences in prevalence are evident within Northern Ireland (Elwood, J. H. 1972), Scotland (Edwards 1958) and Wales (Laurence, Carter, and David 1967), and even within cities such as Glasgow (Wilson 1971). This gross geographical pattern suggests a high risk in people of Celtic (Welsh, Irish, Scottish) origin (Section 11) but

TABLE 10.1 *Selected studies of the prevalence of anencephalus and spina bifida per 1000 births in the same populations*

Area	Number of births	Anencephalus prevalence	Spina bifida prevalence	Ratio spina bifida/ anencephalus	Sources of Ascertainment	Reference
British Isles						
Birmingham	158 307	2.31	2.46†	–	H, M	Record and McKeown 1949
Birmingham	190 236	2.41	2.36	0.98	R	Leck, Record *et al.* 1968
Liverpool	91 176	3.14	3.36	1.07	R	Smithells 1968
London	409 466	1.41	1.54	1.09	H, M, B	Carter and Evans 1973
Southampton	14 094	1.95	3.22	1.65	H, M	Williamson 1965
South Wales	102 786	3.55	4.13	1.16	H, M, B	Laurence *et al.* 1968
South Wales	90 921	3.09	3.92	1.27	R	Richards and Lowe 1971
Glasgow	104 431	2.80	2.80	1.00	H, M, B	Wilson 1971
Belfast	41 351	4.20	4.50	1.07	R	Elwood J. H. and Nevin 1973
Northern Ireland	157 725	3.07	3.33	1.08	R	Elwood J. H. 1976
Cork	37 135	2.05	2.45	1.20	M, B	Spellman 1969, 1970
Rest of Europe						
Finland	621 026	0.32	0.38	1.19	R	Granroth *et al.* 1977
Sweden	159 500	0.37	0.72	1.95	R	Källén and Winberg 1968
Budapest	692 670	1.10	1.63	1.48	H, M, B	Czeizél and Révész 1970
North America						
British Columbia	135 730	0.58	0.87	1.50	R	
Alberta	123 377	0.58	1.01	1.74	R	
Manitoba	71 202	0.90	1.33	1.48	R	Elwood J. M. and Rogers 1975
New Brunswick	49 031	1.51	2.46	1.63	R	
British Columbia	243 149	0.64	0.84	1.31	R	Trimble and Baird 1978

Quebec	656 000	1.45	1.87	1.29	H, M	Horowitz and McDonald 1969
French	564 000	1.43	1.97	1.38	H, M	
British	57 000	1.77	1.42	0.80	H, M	
Jewish	6000	0.33	0.33	1.00	H, M	
Other	29 000	1.38	1.21	0.88	H, M	
Manitoba	94 167	1.20	0.99	0.83	R	Choi *et al*. 1972
Boston	311 437	0.98	1.26	1.29	H	Naggan and MacMahon 1967
New York State	1 580 499	0.61	0.67	1.10	M, B	Janerich 1973
Rochester, N.Y.	129 600	1.39	1.64†	–	M	Biggar *et al*. 1976
Rochester, Minn.	26 500	0.90	1.43	1.59	H	Kurtzke, Goldberg and Kutland 1973
Rhode Island	168 654	1.93	1.35	0.70	H	MacMahon, Pugh and Ingalls 1953
Iowa	58 686	0.58	0.95	1.64	H, M, B	Hay 1971
Rochester, Minn.	30 314	0.90	1.30	1.44	M, H	Haynes *et al*. 1974
Hawaii						
White	40 221	0.62	1.02	1.65	H, M, B	Morton, Chung and Mi 1967
Japanese	45 103	0.56	0.80	1.43	H, B, B	
US (12 hospitals)						
White	16 385	1.40	0.55	0.39	H	Chung and Myrianthopoulos 1968
Black	16 959	0.41	0.53	1.29	H	
Mexico City	38 783	1.78	0.94	0.53	H	Stevenson *et al*. 1966
Asia and Australia						
Japan	6 229 762	0.43	0.08†	–	M	Imaizumi 1974
Taiwan	25 814	1.17	0.16	0.14	H	Emanuel *et al*. 1972
Bombay	76 763	1.89	1.08	0.57	H	Stevenson *et al*. 1966
Singapore	8267	0.72	0.12	0.17	H	Stevenson *et al*. 1966
Melbourne	225 250	0.72	0.59	0.82	H	Stoller and Collman 1965
Africa						
Alexandria	9598	3.79	1.65	0.44	H	Stevenson *et al*. 1966

H Hospital records; M Mortality data; B Birth certificates; R Registry data.
Most rates are calculated per 1000 (live and still) births but some are per 1000 live births, † indicates prevalence is based on spina bifida deaths only and spina bifida/anencephalus ratio is omitted.

even within ethnic groups the rates vary between regions and this points to the action of environmental factors. Such factors may include differences in diet, including differences in mineral intake reflected by drinking-water composition, as in general the high prevalence areas have soft water (Penrose 1957). Socio-economic factors may also be partially responsible for the geographical variations observed.

Information on the prevalence of anencephalus in the rest of Europe comes mainly from hospital-based studies and any interpretation is in the light of this incompleteness of ascertainment. Surveys using multiple records are available only for a few cities. Penrose (1957) assembled a number of

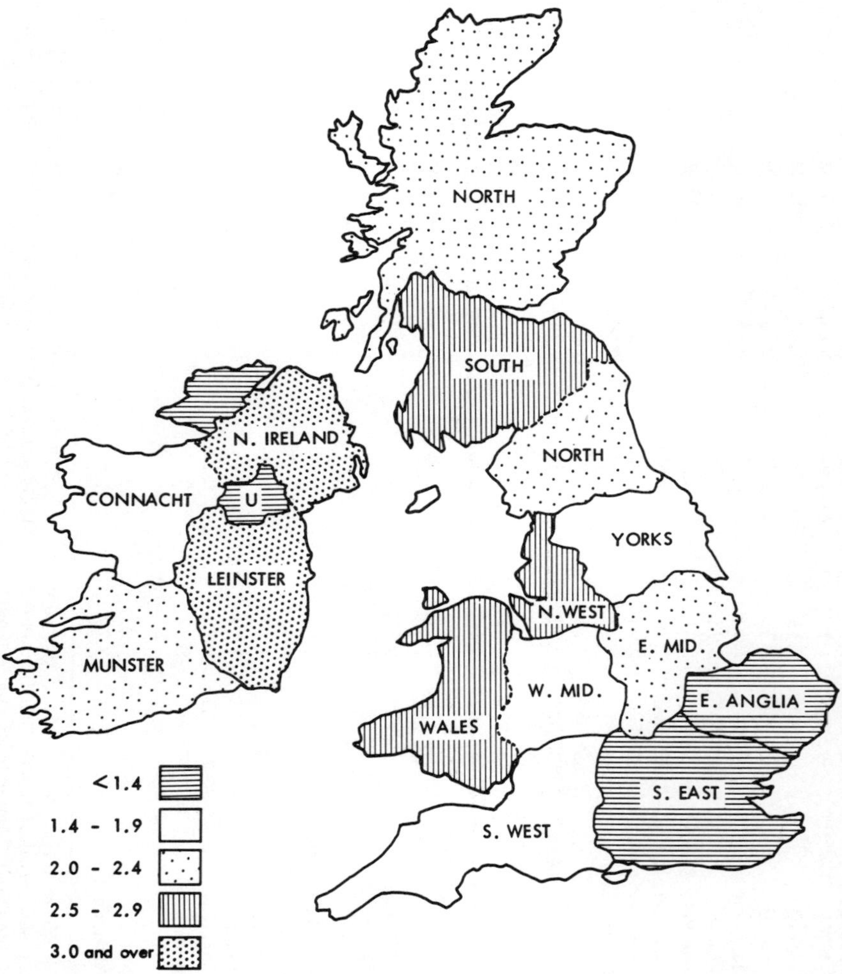

FIG. 10.1. Prevalence of anencephalus (stillbirths and infant deaths) per 1000 total births in the British Isles 1965–7. (Courtesy of *Developmental Medicine and Child Neurology*.)

small hospital studies and published an analysis of the pattern of anencephalus prevalence in Europe which is little changed by the addition of more recent information. Penrose showed that in most of western Europe from the Pyrénées to the Russian border the prevalence of anencephalus was less than 1 per 1000 births. An area of higher prevalence included Brittany and the Normandy coast of France, Holland, and Denmark. Small hospital studies have shown very high prevalence rates of anencephalus in Viipuri, Finland (3.0 per 1000) and in Naples, Italy (4.0 per 1000), but these reports require confirmation. High prevalence rates were recorded in Berlin and in Göttingen by Lenz (1965) in certain time periods. The findings of the World Health Organization survey of hospital births (Stevenson *et al.* 1966) and of the study in Budapest by Czeizel and Révész (1970) confirm the general pattern outlined by Penrose. Frézal, Kelly, Guillemot, and Lamy (1964) conducted a study of the prevalence of anencephalus in France in which they showed considerable regional variations within this country. This study was based on replies to questionnaires sent to hospitals and interpretations of the findings is difficult due to the different response rates for each hospital. However, the results confirm the earlier impression that the prevalence is high in the northern coastal areas of France and is lowest around Lyon. Recent community based studies in Sweden and Finland have shown very low rates for anencephalus of 0.4 and 0.3 per 1000 births respectively, and a prevalence rate of 0.72 per 1000 for spina bifida in Sweden.

North America

Detailed studies of hospital births in Boston and Providence and of all births in New York State excluding New York city have been made. These show prevalence rates of around 1 per 1000 births for anencephalus in recent years but much higher rates previously, as we will further discuss (Section 12). Within the United States, the available hospital data and the few community surveys show the rates are highest in the North-east and lowest in the West with anencephalus rates of around 0.5 per 1000 in Iowa and Los Angeles. Hewitt (1963) demonstrated an east-to-west gradient in infant death-rates from spina bifida and this is supported by the available series which show that spina bifida rates are higher than those of anencephalus, ranging from 1.6 per 1000 in Rochester, New York, to 1.0 in the State of Iowa. In Hawaii, the prevalence of anencephalus is 0.6 per 1000 in both the white and the Japanese population whereas spina bifida mortality rates are 1.0 and 0.8 respectively. Kurtzke, Goldberg, and Kurland (1973) noted an east-to-west decline in infant mortality rates attributed to anencephalus and spina bifida. The infant death-rate from spina bifida in recent years has been higher in the south-eastern than in the north-eastern states but prior to 1955 the mortality in south-eastern states was lower (Spiers 1973). Interpretation of anencephalic infant death statistics has little validity as the great majority of such infants are stillborn; similarly, interpretation of spina bifida mortality data is difficult as they reflect not only the true frequency of spina bifida but also the proportion of affected infants liveborn and the proportion dying within the first year. Thus, although the reported studies are consistent with the pattern of a decrease in prevalence of both defects from east to west, better quality data are required. Adams and Niswander (1968) reported a prevalence rate of 0.5 per 1000 for anencephalus in North American Indians, showing this ethnic group to have a lower prevalence rate than most of the white population. This may reflect the racial similarity of North American Indians to orientals who also have a low prevalence (Miller 1963). The Canadian Eskimos would be expected to fit this pattern but no data are available. Blacks have lower rates than whites in the United States; in a multicentre study, Chung and Myrianthopoulos (1968) reported rates of 0.4 per 1000 for anencephalus and 0.5 for spina bifida.

Other countries

Imaizumi (1974) analysed vital statistics, including stillbirths, for the whole of Japan and reported a mortality rate attributed to anencephalus of 0.4 per 1000 births. Other reports from Japan and from Hong Kong and the Philippines show similarly low rates, but the prevalence rate of anencephalus in Taiwan is 1.2 per 1000. Thus, although the prevalence of anencephalus in Asia is lower than in the British Isles, it is comparable to the prevalence in central Europe and in parts of North America. Rates for spina bifida in oriental peoples are much lower, being 0.1 per 1000 in Japan and 0.2 in Taiwan. Ethnic differences seem to be more important than geographical differences within Asia. In a hospital study from Singapore, Searle (1959) reported anencephalus rates of 6.5 per 1000 in births to Sikh parents, 2.2 in Europeans, and 1.2 in Malays. The rates in Chinese and Indians who were not Sikhs were much lower. In this study each ethnic group demonstrates prevalence rates similar to those seen in their areas of origin. Surveys from Australia estimate frequencies of anencephalus ranging from 0.5 to 0.8 per 1000 births which are similar to those in Asian countries and much lower than rates in the British Isles, but are comparable to rates in white South Africans and in western North America.

Naggan (1971) published a detailed study of anencephalus in Israel based on multiple sources of ascertainment. The overall prevalence is low, 0.9 per 1000, but is higher in mothers who came from parts of the Middle East outside Israel. Small hospital studies suggest that the prevalence in Iran and Beirut may be higher and very high rates of 3.8 per 1000 for anencephalus and 1.7 for spina bifida were recorded in Alexandria by the World Health Organization's hospital based study. Penrose (1957) reported the prevalence of anencephalus in coloured births in Johannesburg and Pretoria (0.2 per 1000) to be considerably lower than in white births (0.8), but Horner and Lanzkowsky (1966) report similar rates for the two groups in Cape Town. Henry and Mickel (1974) estimated the spina bifida prevalence in deliveries in a Durban hospital to be 0.46 per 1000 in African and 0.37 in Indian births.

Hospital studies from Central and South America show prevalence rates between 0.1 and 0.8 per 1000. Cruz-Coke (1972) calculated the prevalence of anencephalus in Chile from vital statistics as 0.13 per 1000 in 1959, but it rose steadily to reach 0.31 per 1000 in 1971. The lowest recorded prevalence rates of anencephalus in the world so far reported are in Chile, in blacks in Africa and in the United States, and in Finland and Sweden.

The ratio of the prevalence at birth of spina bifida to that of anencephalus in Europe and North America is usually around one (Table 10.1). However, in Singapore, Taiwan, and Japan this ratio is around 0.2 because the prevalence of anencephalus is similar to that in North America but the prevalence of spina bifida is much lower. A falsely high anencephalus-to-spina-bifida ratio could occur in hospital-based studies as mothers of anencephalics are more likely to be delivered in hospital, and in mortality statistics spina bifida will be underascertained; however the studies of Emanuel, Huang, Gutman, Yu, and Lin (1972) in Taiwan, although hospital based, have probably fairly complete ascertainment and show a spina-bifida-to-anencephalus ratio of 0.14. The spina-bifida-to-anencephalus ratios in Mexico City, Bombay, and Alexandria are around 0.5; these three series are based on relatively small numbers of hospital births and show fairly high rates of anencephalus which may be due to selective admission policies.

Canada

Prior to our own work, studies reported similar rates of anencephalus in eastern Canada as in the north-eastern United States, with rates of 1.5 per 1000 in Halifax (Alter 1963), and 1.5 in the province of Quebec where the prevalence of spina bifida was 1.9 per 1000 (Horowitz and McDonald 1969). In Manitoba, rates of 1.2 for anencephalus and 1.0 for spina bifida were reported by Choi, Klaponski, Ateah, and Nelson (1972) and Miller (1963) recorded rates for anencephalus in British Columbia of 0.7 per 1000 for the white population and 0.1 for native Indians.

We examined mortality data from anencephalus for the whole of Canada, excluding Newfoundland, the North-west Territories, and the Yukon, for the years 1943 to 1974. Over the whole period 1943 to 1974 the highest rate was in Prince Edward Island (2.04 per 1000) and the lowest in British Columbia and Saskatchewan (0.67 per 1000). However, this is not a simple east-to-west gradient as Ontario had the second highest rate of 1.42 per 1000. The geographical pattern has changed over time, as we will later discuss (Section 12). For the periods 1965–9 and 1970–4 the pattern is as shown in Fig. 10.2. Prince Edward Island has the highest rate, and there is a fairly steady decline across the country until a minimum is reached in Saskatchewan and Alberta, compared to which British Columbia has a higher rate. Nova Scotia has somewhat lower rates than the neighbouring provinces. Mortality data for Newfoundland from 1971 to 1974 show an anencephalus death rate of 1.28 per 1000 births which is similar to those of the other maritime provinces. This present pattern has existed since about 1955 (Fig. 10.3). If we consider the period from 1943 to 1954, the highest rates were in Prince Edward Island, but Ontario had the second highest rate

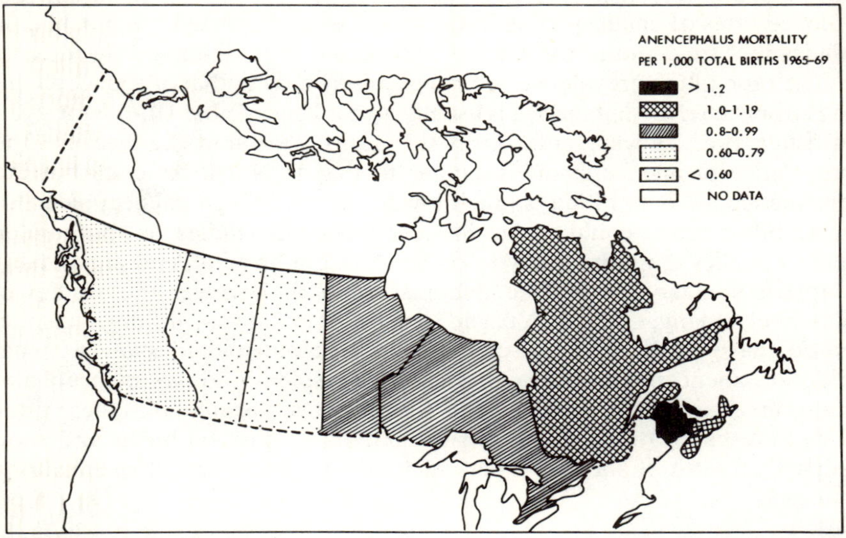

FIG. 10.2 Prevalence of anencephalus (stillbirths and infant deaths) per 1000 total births in Canada 1965–9.

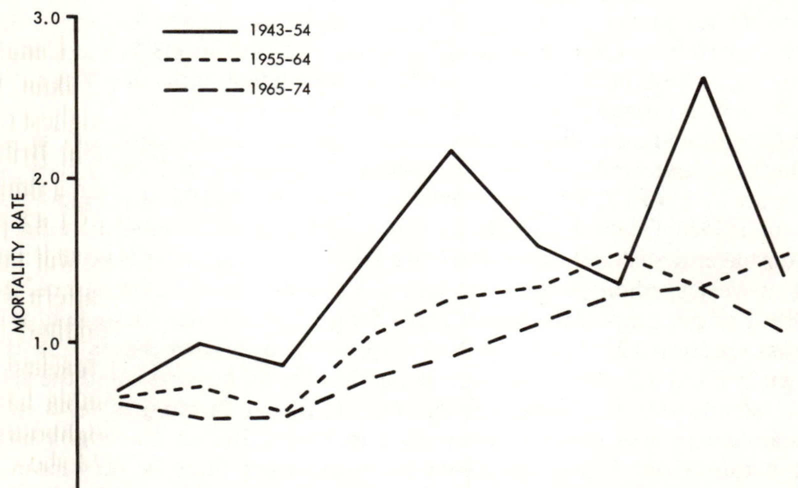

FIG. 10.3. Mortality rates (stillbirths and infant deaths) per 1000 total births attributed to anencephalus during three different time periods by province in Canada 1943–74.

followed by its neighbours, Manitoba to the west and Quebec to the east. The remaining eastern provinces of Nova Scotia and New Brunswick had somewhat lower rates, and the western provinces of Alberta, Saskatchewan and British Columbia had much lower rates, being less than half of that in Ontario.

We also examined the mortality rate from spina bifida from 1950 to 1970, although of course any interpretation of these data must be cautious as there may be large variations in diagnostic and certification practices and in treatment. However, the geographical distribution of spina bifida deaths is similar to that for anencephalus (Fig. 10.4). Quebec and Prince Edward

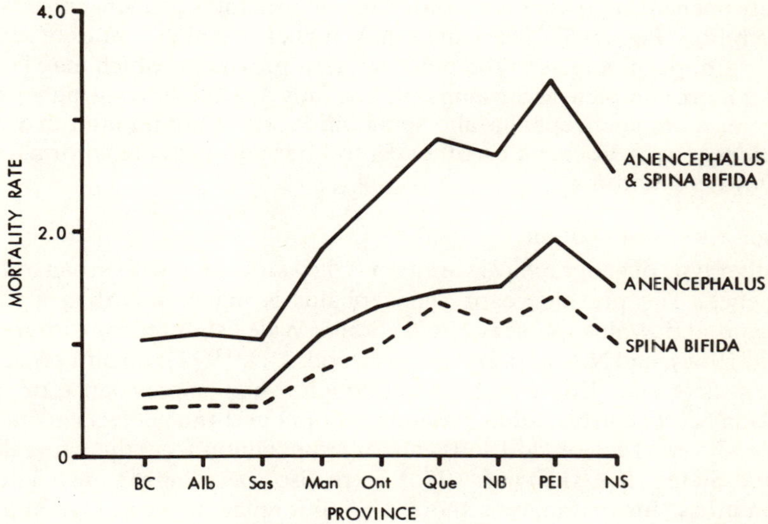

FIG. 10.4. Mortality rates (stillbirths and infant deaths) per 1000 total births attributed to anencephalus, spina bifida and both anomalies by province in Canada 1950–70.

Island show the highest mortality rates from spina bifida while New Brunswick and Nova Scotia have somewhat lower rates. The rates in Ontario and in Manitoba show a westward decline from the Quebec maximum and the lowest rates occur in Saskatchewan, Alberta, and British Columbia. This geographical pattern has not changed greatly in the time studied, although the rates in Ontario and Manitoba were almost as high as those in Quebec in 1950–4 and have declined relatively since then. The excess mortality in Quebec for spina bifida is more marked than that for anencephalus; mortality rates for anencephalus in Ontario exceeded those in Quebec in 1950–4.

The Congenital Anomalies Surveillance System has collated data from four provinces, New Brunswick, Manitoba, Alberta, and British Columbia since 1966. As described (section 9), from 1966 to 1969 this registry received stillbirth and death registrations and the Physician's Notice of Birth

Certificates. During this period, the prevalence rates of all recorded abnormalities were 21.8 per 1000 total births in British Columbia, 20.8 in Alberta, 19.7 in Manitoba, and 18.7 in New Brunswick (Elwood, J. M. and Rogers 1975). This maximum rate in the west was shown by several major groups of defects namely, those of circulatory, digestive, musculoskeletal, and genito-urinary systems, and by cleft palate, whereas Down's syndrome and clubfoot showed no interprovincial differences. The only defects showing an east-to-west decrease in prevalence were anencephalus, spina bifida, and, to a lesser degree, hydrocephalus. Since 1970, the registry also has received the hospital discharge record of each infant and this has led to much higher reported rates for many defects; however the geographical patterns are largely unchanged as are the recorded prevalence rates of anencephalus and spina bifida (Fig. 10.5). These data show higher prevalence rates of several major groups of defects in the more western provinces, which may largely reflect more complete ascertainment. The only defects showing higher rates in the east are anencephalus and spina bifida; there are no interprovincial differences in hydrocephalus, other central-nervous-system malformations, or Down's syndrome.

Urban–rural distribution

Another type of geographical variation is the association with urban or rural residence. The prevalence of anencephalus is higher in urban areas in England and Wales (Rogers 1969), South Wales (Laurence, Carter, and David 1968), and Northern Ireland (Elwood, J. H. 1972); no difference was seen in Scotland (Edwards 1958) although a higher prevalence of spina bifida in Scottish urban areas was noted. For neural-tube defects in Quebec (Horowitz and McDonald 1969) and for infant deaths from this cause in the United States (Kurtzke *et al.* 1973) there also was a higher prevalence in urban areas; further analysis showed no difference between high and low density urban areas. In Japan, mortality statistics show no rural-urban difference (Imaizumi 1974).

Interpretation of the geographical variations within Canada

The prevalence of birth of anencephalus shows a threefold variation between the Canadian provinces. This is essentially an east-to-west decline at present but in earlier years the highest rates were recorded in Ontario, Quebec, and Manitoba. The geographical distribution is shown by mortality data and is supported by information on prevalence and by comparisons of other Canadian studies such as those of Horowitz and McDonald (1969), Choi *et al.* (1972), and Trimble and Baird (1978). The mortality and prevalence rates from spina bifida are also higher in the east confirming the earlier report of Hewitt (1963). Although the available data are limited, the literature shows a similar east-to-west gradient in both anencephalus and spina bifida in the United States. The study of congenital abnormalities registered in four Canadian provinces indicates that this east-to-west decline in the prevalence at birth is not shared by any other major abnormalities.

Although this finding cannot be accepted without question, owing to possible differences in diagnosis and certification between the four provinces studied, it suggests that some geographically related factor is specifically associated with neural-tube defects. A similar situation may exist in England and Wales where the regional differences in the mortality rates from all congenital abnormalities are due almost entirely to differences in the mortality from neural-tube defects (Stocks 1970).

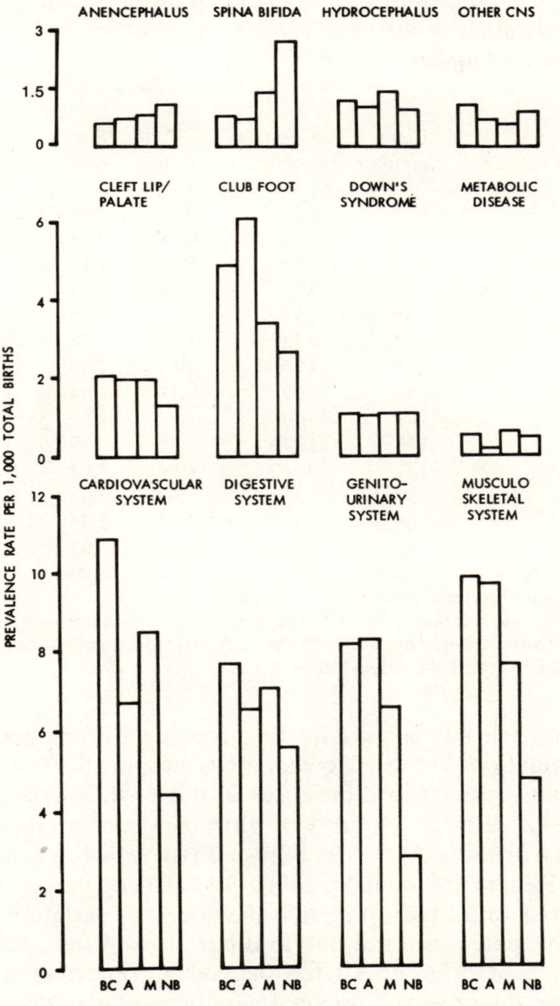

FIG. 10.5. Prevalence rates at birth per 1000 total births for twelve selected groups of congenital malformations reported by The Congenital Anomalies Surveillance System in four provinces of Canada 1970–1. BC. British Columbia; A, Alberta; M, Manitoba; NB, New Brunswick. The genito-urinary system group excludes hernia and phimosis.

In the Canadian 14-city study, we selected the cities to give a wide geographical range, from Vancouver in the west to Halifax in the east (Fig. 9.1). The prevalence rates of anencephalus per 1000 total births from 1950 to 1969 ranged from 0.62 in Regina, Saskatchewan, to 2.05 in St. John, New Brunswick; comparing each city's rate to that of Vancouver yields crude risk ratios of 1 for Vancouver (selected as the referent city), 0.78 for Regina, and 2.55 for St. John (Table 10.2). We used a multivariate method to compare

TABLE 10.2 *Crude and adjusted risks of anencephalus by maternal city of residence, relative to the risk in births to mothers in Vancouver, in 14 Canadian cities 1950–69*

Maternal city of residence	Cases number	Controls number	Rate	Crude risk ratio	Adjusted risk ratio and 95% two-sided confidence limits†
Vancouver	119	621	0.80	1.00	1.00
Calgary	103	547	0.79	0.98	0.97 (0.72–1.29)
Edmonton	148	653	0.95	1.18	1.17 (0.90–1.53)
Saskatoon	37	198	0.78	0.98	1.02 (0.68–1.53)
Regina	35	235	0.62	0.78	0.77 (0.51–1.16)
Winnipeg	149	442	1.49	1.76	1.74 (1.32–2.30)
Windsor	67	235	1.19	1.49	1.54 (1.08–2.19)
London	80	290	1.16	1.44	1.57 (1.13–2.20)
Kitchener	41	140	1.23	1.53	1.73 (1.14–2.64)
Hamilton	173	522	1.39	1.73	1.86 (1.41–2.45)
Ottawa	177	447	1.66	2.07	2.24 (1.69–2.97)
Quebec	138	356	1.62	2.02	1.67 (1.25–2.23)
St John	66	135	2.05	2.55	2.46 (1.71–3.53)
Halifax	57	170	1.40	1.75	1.59 (1.10–2.29)

Cities are in order from west (Vancouver) to east (Halifax).
† Maximum likelihood risk ratio (Gart 1970), after controlling for the joint confounding effects of all ten other factors included in the 14-city study, by stratification on a multivariate risk score (Appendix A.3; Elwood, J. M. and Mousseau 1978).

the rates for each city after adjusting for any differences between the maternal populations in regard to age, previous reproductive history, ethnic origin, and with respect to differences in the birth distributions by year, season, place of delivery, plurality of birth (single or multiple), and legitimacy status (Appendix A.2). The adjusted risk ratios so calculated ranged from 0.77 in Regina to 2.46 in St. John. For each city they were very similar to the crude risk ratios indicating that the inter-city variations in the prevalence of anencephalus are not due to differences in these factors.

It is unlikely that differences in the diagnosis or reporting of anencephalus would produce the observed regional variations. As we discussed (Section 8), anencephalus mortality data provide a reasonably good approximation to prevalence rates derived by more detailed studies, and there is no indication that the small error seen is greater in one part of the country than another. Hewitt (1963) suggested the east-to-west trend might be due to a greater frequency of consanguineous marriages in eastern Canada, using as evidence for this the higher mortality from diabetes and greater incidence of cystic fibrosis in the east. He also used a measure of the variance of birth weight of all livebirths based on the work of Morton (1958), who showed that populations with a greater degree of inbreeding should have a lower mean birth weight and an increased variance of the distribution of all births by birth weight. Hewitt found a positive correlation between an index of this variance and the provincial spina bifida mortality rates in 1955–9. However, calculation of this index for 1965–9 using Hewitt's method, demonstrates that there is a negative non-significant correlation with the corresponding provincial anencephalus rates ($r = -0.44$; d.f.$=7$; $P > 0.2$). In family studies (Record and McKeown 1949; Carter and Evans 1973), consanguinity has been demonstrated in less than 1 per cent of cases of anencephalus, and this seems an insufficient factor to contribute significantly to the geographical variation. We later show that two factors, the magnesium concentration in drinking water and mean income, account for 44 per cent of the total variation in mortality rates from anencephalus between 36 large Canadian cities (Section 19). The addition of longitude increased this proportion of the total variation explained to 69 per cent, but this is unhelpful because longitude has no direct meaning in biological terms. The correlation with income is consistent with the frequently reported association of high anencephalus rates and low socio-economic status. This association is quite strong in several areas: the ratios of anencephalus rates in the lowest to the highest socio-economic groups were 3:1 in Scotland, and 2:1 in Boston, based on occupational classes (Edwards 1958; Naggan and MacMahon 1967) and 2:1 in Montreal, based on mean rental value of housing (Horowitz and McDonald 1969). This socio-economic gradient is not restricted to high prevalence areas as it is present in Taiwan (Emanuel and Sever 1973). However, socio-economic status itself, like longitude, must be an indicator of some factor more closely related to the occurrence of anencephalus in biological terms. One group of factors which could relate both to the 'income' and 'longitude' factors are those related to nutrition. The studies of the quality of nutrition in mothers of anencephalics (reviewed in Section 18) have been inconclusive but they are very limited in scope and in size due partly to the practical problems of this type of research approach. One nutritional hypothesis, that of potato-blight infestation, has been fairly rigorously examined and found to be inadequate; there remains, however, a geographical association between high anencephalus mortality rates and high potato consumption. Several nutritional hypotheses related to factors which seem common enough to be worthy of further study such as folate deficiency, are suggested by the work of Hibbard and Smithells (1965) and by Smithells, Sheppard, and Schorah (1975). To see if any gross geographical differences in nutrition could be detected, data from a recent nutritional study of an approximately random sample of the Canadian population were examined (Nutrition Canada 1975). These data relate to samples of healthy pregnant women in each province and clearly would only indicate very major regional differences in nutrition; the samples were quite small (about 750 women in total). Estimates were available of total calorie intake, protein intake, urinary thiamine and riboflavine concentrations, serum vitamin-C and vitamin-A levels, calcium, vitamin-D and iron intakes, haemoglobin, transferrin and serum folate concentrations, mean corpuscular haemoglobin concentrations, and of the prevalence of clinical signs such as goitre. The only non-random regional difference was in the prevalence of goitre which was most common in the prairie provinces. There was no nutritional factor which showed an east-to-west trend suggestive of an association with neural-tube defects.

The striking geographical variations in the prevalence at birth of anencephalus have still to be adequately explained. The composition of drinking water may contribute to this variation but many other factors are likely to be involved (Section 19). The range in the prevalence rates in Canada is quite large with rates in eastern Canada being similar to those in New England and in much of Great Britain, while the low rate in British Columbia of about 0.7 per 1000 is of the same order as the rates in Australia and in the white population of South Africa. Interestingly, the rate in British Columbia has been stable over time, like that in Australia (Jones 1967), in contrast to the higher rates in eastern Canada which show large secular variations akin to the trends in the British Isles. This suggests the action of fairly stable, perhaps largely genetic factors, with the higher but less stable rates in the east possibly being caused by varying environmental factors.

11

Ethnic origin and migration

THE striking variations in the prevalence at birth of anencephalus and spina bifida in different places throughout the world have been discussed in Section 10. We now attempt to separate the contribution of the local environment from that of person-related characteristics. To some extent the former represent environmental and the latter genetic influences, but this is an oversimplification. An ethnic subgroup may have a characteristic disease pattern either because of genetic homogeneity or because of specific environmental influences such as dietary habits. Differences in disease patterns between geographically separate communities of the same ethnic group may be due not only to environmental influences but also to genetic differences as may arise through selective migration. On a large time scale selective outbreeding and intermarriage between different ethnic groups will change the gene pool but this process takes several generations.

In the British Isles, the prevalence rate at birth of anencephalus decreases from the north and west to become lowest in the south-east area of the country. This pattern might be related either to an environmental factor, and Penrose (1957) has suggested that the mineral content of drinking water might be such an agent, or it might be due to genetic differences between the populations of the different areas. The gross pattern suggests a higher risk in persons of Celtic (Welsh, Irish, Scots) origin than in those of Anglo-Saxon or Norman origin. This hypothesis is supported by the finding within Wales of prevalence rates for anencephalus in infants with two, one, or no parents of Welsh origin being 3.4, 3.1, and 2.6 per 1000 births respectively (Richards, McIntosh, and Sweenie 1972). In London, Carter and Evans (1973) found an excess of Irish parents of infants with anencephalus or spina bifida compared to control infants in London. This example of the geographical variation in the prevalence of anencephalus in the British Isles shows that it is very difficult to separate environmental and genetic effects. The scope for such studies is greater in Canada, because it is a much larger country and most of the population are descended from immigrants who came from Europe over the last 250 years. We now describe some findings from our study of 14 Canadian cities, chosen to cover a wide geographical range of about 5000 miles. Stillbirths and infant deaths from anencephalus, and a control series of livebirths, were selected on the basis of the mother's city of residence, as expressed on the birth certificate or stillbirth certificate. The question used on birth certificates—'to which racial group do you belong'—is the same as that used in Census, and its interpretation is discussed by Kalbach (1970). A footnote specifies the question as referring to ethnic origin through paternal descent and the replies 'Canadian' or 'American' are not acceptable and are coded as 'unknowns' except in the case of North American Indians or Eskimos who are coded specifically. Thus it is assumed that all persons can identify their ethnic origin; no consideration is given to time of immigration. The birth certificates of most provinces carry questions relating to both ethnic origin and the place of birth of the parents; unfortunately the place-of-birth information is not included in the computer-readable record. It is to be expected that there will be many inaccuracies in the ethnic origin recorded owing to complex family patterns and incorrect interpretation of the question. A more minor error may result from political national-boundary changes, as in Germany and Poland. The countries coded are assumed to have their present boundaries but the entry made may represent the country of allegiance at the time of the parents' birth. These errors are most likely to be random and so the observed differences between ethnic groups will under-represent the true differences. A systematic bias may result if parents of anencephalics are more or less likely to regard themselves as 'Canadian' than mothers of controls in the same ethnic group; this would occur if there were differences by social class or time of immigration. For the 1950–9 data such a bias is small as there are few unknown entries. A greater problem in the present data is the lack of information on parental origin of births in Ontario after 1960. The best estimates therefore, of the assocations of anencephalus risk with ethnic group are those based on 1950–9 information.

Analysis shows the crude mortality rate attributed to anencephalus varies from 0.67 per 1000 in births to mothers of Russian origin to 1.78 in those to mothers of French origin (Table 11.1). An important finding is that the crude risk ratios, namely the crude mortality rates relative to the rate in births to mothers from England and Wales, are very similar to the unconfounded risk ratios. The latter express the mortality rate relative to that for births to mothers from England and Wales after adjusting for all other study factors, amongst which are city of residence, maternal age and reproductive history. The crude and standardized risk ratios by city of residence are also similar (Table 10.2) so these two factors, place of residence and ethnic origin, have independent effects on the mortality rate from anencephalus. The geographical variation is not due to ethnic differences nor vice versa. The small differences between the crude and standardized risk ratios by ethnic group are consistent with these independent geographical effects (Table 11.1). Thus the risk ratio for offspring of French mothers, who live mainly in eastern Canada, is reduced after confounder control, while the risk ratio for offspring of Scandinavian and Oriental mothers, resident mainly in western Canada, is increased.

The differences in rates between different ethnic groups are small and only for the central European and Russian groups are the unconfounded relative risks significantly different from the risk in births occurring to the mothers from England and Wales. In general the ranking of mortality rates by ethnic group is similar to that expected from the prevalence rates of anencephalus in the country of origin. The highest risks, after confounder control, are seen in births to mothers from Ireland and Scotland; these are slightly but not significantly increased compared with the risk of anencephalus in births to mothers from England and Wales. Available census data suggest that these ethnic groups from the British Isles are similar with respect to socio-economic factors and time of immigration (Kalbach 1970). The crude mortality rates during 1950–9 for births to mothers from Ireland, Scotland, and England and Wales were 1.75, 1.47, and 1.56 per 1000. These rates are similar to mortality rates in England during the same time period but they are lower than those recorded in Scotland, Ireland, or Wales during 1950–9. The mortality rate in births to mothers of French origin is similar to the rate in births to mothers from England and Wales. The few available studies from France report much lower rates of 0.12 to 0.54 per 1000 in that country (Appendix A.1). Lower rates than in the French and British groups

TABLE 11.1 *Crude and adjusted risks of anencephalus by maternal ethnic origin, relative to the risk in births to mothers from England and Wales in 14 Canadian cities 1950—9*

Maternal ethnic group	Cases number	Controls number	Mortality rate per 1000 livebirths	Crude risk ratio	Adjusted risk ratio and 95% two-sided confidence limits†
England and Wales	219	589	1.56	1.00	1.00
Ireland	112	268	1.75	1.12	1.08 (0.82–1.43)
Scotland	99	283	1.47	0.94	1.04 (0.78–1.39)
France[1]	176	415	1.78	1.14	1.01 (0.79–1.30)
Germany[2]	76	295	1.08	0.69	0.80 (0.59–1.09)
Central Europe[3]	33	142	0.97	0.63	0.63 (0.41–0.97)
Scandinavia[4]	22	84	1.10	0.70	0.90 (0.54–1.51)
Mediterranean[5]	19	73	1.09	0.70	0.81 (0.47–1.40)
Russia	21	132	0.67	0.43	0.45 (0.28–0.74)
Oriental[6]	6	23	1.09	0.70	0.78 (0.31–1.97)
Other[7]	10	46	0.91	0.58	0.65 (0.32–1.33)
Canada and Unknown[8]	3	2	–	–	– –

Total cases = 796, total controls = 2352
[1] France and Belgium
[2] Germany, Holland, and Switzerland
[3] Austria, Bulgaria, Czechoslovakia, Estonia, Finland, Hungary, Latvia, Lithuania, Poland, Rumania, and Yugoslavia
[4] Denmark, Iceland, Norway, and Sweden
[5] Greece, Italy, Portugal, and Spain
[6] China, Japan, and 'other Asiatic'
[7] Includes North American Indians and Eskimos, Jewish and Negro groups
[8] Entries of Canada and the United States are coded as blanks
† Maximum likelihood risk ratio (Gart 1970), after controlling for the joint confounding effects of all ten other factors included in the 14-city study, by stratification on a multivariate risk score (Appendix A.3; Elwood, J. M. and Mousseau 1978)

are seen in births to mothers from central European countries which is in accordance with the low rates of anencephalus in the countries of origin.

Thus in general the anencephalus mortality rates seen in the European ethnic groups in Canada are similar at least in relative magnitude to those in the countries of origin with two notable exceptions. The rates in births to Irish and Scottish mothers are not much higher than in births to mothers from England and Wales and the rates for the French Canadian group are higher than those reported from France.

There are several possible reasons for the similarity of the anencephalic rates in French and British migrants. The socio-economic distribution of the French population in Canada is somewhat less favourable and this would increase the crude rate. However, Horowitz and McDonald (1969) found that the prevalence rate at birth of anencephalus was higher in births to mothers of British origin than in those of French origin within census tracts grouped by mean rental value in Montreal; the prevalence of spina bifida was lower in British mothers, and so there was no difference in rates for the two defects combined. Secondly, if the prevalence of anencephalus in France is in fact higher than that reported, the Canadian data do not necessarily point to environmental causes. The information concerning anencephalus in France is based, apart from a few small hospital studies, on the survey of Frézal *et al*. (1964). These authors sent requests to obstetricians in public hospitals in 99 French towns asking for the number of total births and the number of anencephalics born in their hospital from 1945 to 1955. Usable replies were received from 78 giving a non-response rate of 21 per cent. An obstetrician could easily obtain a reasonable estimate of total births, as these would be regularly counted and reported, but in many hospitals the numbers of anencephalics would be more difficult to count and a superficial attempt to provide such figures might underestimate the true prevalence rate. On the other hand, restriction of the study to hospitals only, and to public rather than private hospitals, might increase the reported rate due to women from the lower socio-economic classes being over-represented in public institutions. Similar low rates have been shown in other, albeit small, studies in France. At the 1961 Census, 99 per cent of women of French origin in the reproductive age groups were born in Canada (Table 11.2), most are at least second-generation Canadians as the expansion of the French Canadian population has been much more by natural growth from the seventeenth- and eighteenth-century arrivals than by recent immigration (Kalbach 1970). In fact, the French population may be regarded as the largest 'native' group and their mortality rate from anencephalus, therefore, should reflect any effect of the Canadian environment. Most mothers of British origin also were Canadian born (89 per cent), but the other European groups who have lower anencephalus rates, are predominantly post-Second World War migrants.

Despite the large differences seen between mortality rates from anencephalus in Ireland, Scotland, and Wales and England in recent years (Section 10), the rates in infants born in Canada to mothers originally from those four countries are very similar. The rates in infants born in Canada are lower than those observed during the same period in births in the British Isles. These findings suggest that over a few generations the originally high and diverse rates applicable to non-migrants resident in the British Isles are modified to a common lower rate. The level of the new rate is dependent on local environmental factors, as it varies between regions: thus in 1950–69 the anencephalus mortality rates in births to mothers from England and Wales were 1.7 per 1000 in the Maritimes and Quebec, 2.2 in Ontario, and 1.1. in the more western provinces. In births to French origin mothers the rates were slightly higher: 1.8 in Quebec and the Maritimes, 2.3 in Ontario, and 1.2 in the west, while for births to mothers from other European countries the rate in Ontario was 1.3 per 1000 and in the western provinces was 0.90, there being very few such mothers in Quebec and the Maritimes. At the present time, mothers originally from the British Isles living in eastern Canada show mortality rates from anencephalus in their offspring which are similar to those in the north-eastern United States and in parts of Great Britain, while mothers from the British Isles who live in western Canada show lower rates similar to those seen in Australia and in white South Africans.

The Canadian data clearly demonstrate that place of residence and maternal ethnic origin have independent effects on the anencephalus mortality rate, strongly suggesting the rates in ethnic subgroups are modified by migration. This conclusion is supported by other studies of Caucasian populations. For example, infants born in London to Irish parents have a higher prevalence rate of neural-tube defects than other infants born in London (Carter and Evans 1973), and a similar trend is seen in Birmingham (Leck 1969). Naggan and MacMahon (1967) found the highest neural-tube defect

TABLE 11.2 *Distribution of the female population of Canada aged 20—34 years at the 1961 Census by ethnic group and time of immigration*

Ethnic group	Total Number	Canadian born (per cent)	Immigration pre-Second World War (per cent)	Immigration post-Second World War (per cent)
Great Britain and Ireland	728 924	88.6	1.4	10.0
France	580 354	98.6	0.4	1.0
Germany	169 447	60.6	1.4	37.9
Scandinavia	37 602	65.1	1.4	33.4
Central Europe	60 551	61.7	5.3	33.0
Russia	63 941	85.6	2.6	11.8
Other European	103 404	30.0	1.6	68.4
Oriental	14 257	48.5	1.0	50.5
Other	24 987	86.7	1.4	12.0
All	1 783 467	84.4	1.3	14.3

After Kalbach (1970) and courtesy of The Queen's Printer, Ottawa rates in Boston occurred in births to mothers who were born in Ireland. Births to first generation Irish migrants, namely mothers of Irish descent but born in Boston, had lower rates but these were higher than the rates in births to non-Irish mothers. The lability of the prevalence rate of neural-tube defects in populations of British origin is shown by the contrasts between the high rates in Britain and the very low rates among the white population of South Africa, the population of Australia, and that of British Columbia (see Appendix A.1). Naggan's (1971) survey in Israel also demonstrates a rapid change in prevalence rates. Births to Jewish mothers now resident in Israel but who were born in Iraq, the Yemen, and Iran have higher neural-tube defect rates than births to mothers born either in Israel or Europe. However, by the next generation these differences had disappeared.

In contrast, prevalence rates for anencephalus in black and oriental populations appear to be quite stable even after major migrations. The black populations of South Africa (Penrose 1957) and the United States (Chung and Myrianthopoulos 1968) have similar low rates of anencephalus even though the environment and life-style of blacks in the United States is little different from that of the white population except for a lower socio-economic level which would be expected to increase the rate. Also, oriental groups in Singapore (Searle 1959) and Hawaii (Morton, Chung, and Mi 1967) have similar rates to the populations of their countries of origin, and Sikhs in India have a characteristically high prevalence rate even after migration from India to Singapore or to Britain (Searle 1959; Leck 1969).

12

Secular trends

Changes in the prevalence rate at birth of neural-tube defects with time have been reported in almost all well-studied areas. These may be divided into three types: long-term changes over ten or more years, short-term changes over a few years, and seasonal variations, which we shall consider separately (Section 13).

British Isles and Europe

Rogers and Morris (1971) described a period of high infant mortality attributed to spina bifida which occurred from around 1930 to 1943 in England and Wales. There was a similar trend in deaths from monstrosity although the latter rates are low, and the lack of data on stillbirths make these findings less certain than the reports from New England (MacMahon and Yen 1971). The male proportion of spina bifida deaths remained fairly constant at around 40 per cent suggesting no large change in diagnosis or classification, and no alteration in the case fatality rate owing to modifications in treatment would be expected at that time. No surveys of local areas of England and Wales cover this period, but high rates of anencephalus were observed in the early 1940s in Birmingham (Leck 1966) and Scotland (Edwards 1958). Mortality rates attributed to anencephalus and spina bifida in Northern Ireland, Scotland, and England and Wales show almost stationary rates for spina bifida and a small decline in anencephalus since 1960 (Fig. 12.1). The longest hospital series published is from Dublin, where data from the three main maternity hospitals were analysed from 1936 to 1965 (Leck and Rogers 1967) and from 1900 to 1965 (Elwood, J. H. 1973*a*, *b*). Over this period the prevalence of anencephalus rose from 1 per 1000 in 1900 to reach peak rates of 8 per 1000 in recent times (Fig. 12.2). Two periods of high rates, in 1938–41 and in 1960–1, are superimposed on this long-term trend and also the 1910–19 period showed a higher rate than did the adjacent decades. Spina bifida prevalence also rose, but to a lesser degree and peaks were seen in 1916–19, 1952–5, and 1960–1.

Data from Birmingham are available since 1936, and are drawn from a registry based on questionnaires completed by the attendant at all births in that city (Record and McKeown 1949; MacMahon, Record, and McKeown 1951; Leck and Rogers 1967; Leck 1966, 1972; Leck, Record, McKeown, and Edwards 1968). These statistics show the prevalence of anencephalus rose from 2.0 per 1000 in 1936–7, then to 2.81 in 1940–1, fell until 1948–9 (1.54), peaked again in 1956–7 (2.80), then progressively gradually

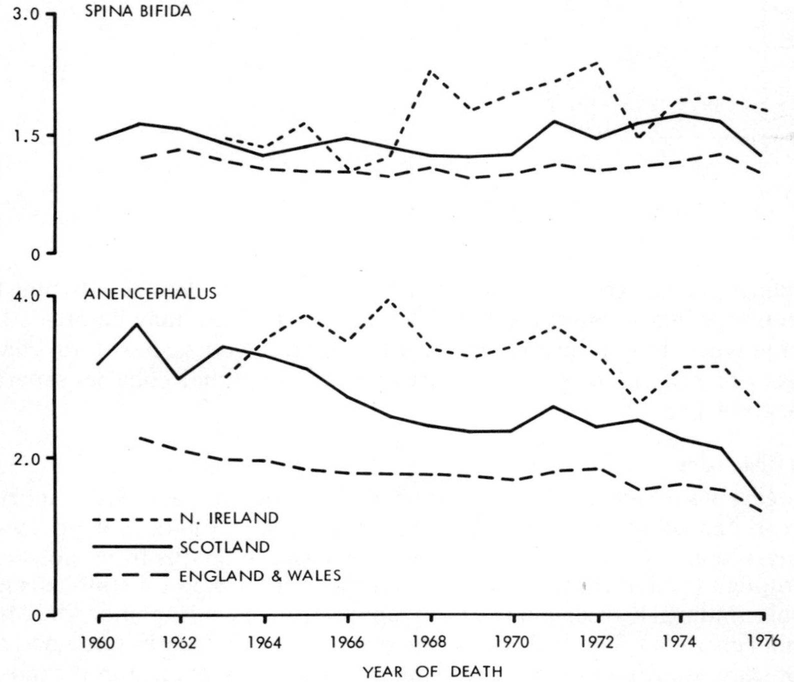

FIG. 12.1 Mortality rates (stillbirths and infant deaths) per 1000 total births attributed to anencephalus and spina bifida in Northern Ireland, Scotland, and England and Wales based on annual reports of the Registrars General 1960–76

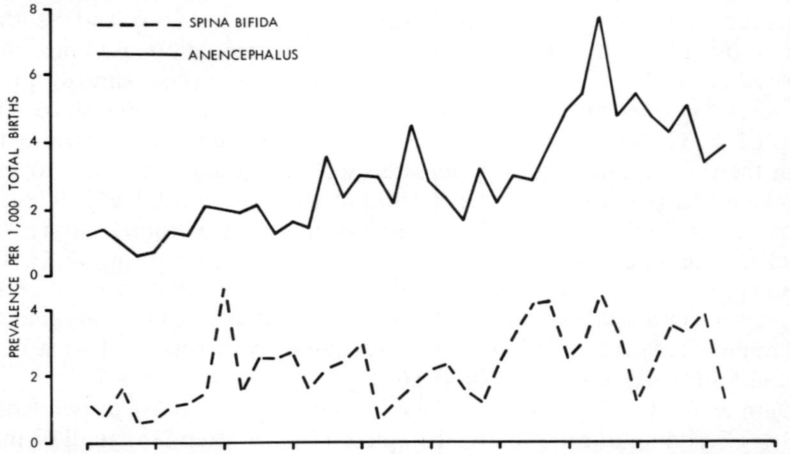

FIG. 12.2. Biannual prevalence rates (stillbirths and infant deaths) per 1000 total births attributed to anencephalus and spina bifida reported from the Rotunda Hospital, Dublin, 1900–75

declined until 1962–3 (1.56); the prevalence now appears to be increasing (Fig. 12.3). The 1956–7 peak was confined to females (Leck 1972). Spina bifida rates have shown broadly similar changes. Information on stillbirths attributed to anencephalus in Scotland since 1939 have been examined (Edwards 1958; Record 1961; Leck and Rogers 1967). More than 90 per cent of anencephalics in Scotland in 1958 were stillborn, hence exclusion of livebirths is probably of little consequence; however, in England and Wales in recent years the proportion liveborn has increased (Rogers and Morris 1973) so an apparent fall in prevalence might be expected if stillbirth data only are used. The Scottish data show a peak rate of 2.9 per 1000 in 1942, a fall to 2.3 in 1946–7 and then rise to a plateau of around 2.9 in 1958–61. Examination of the prevalence rates of anencephalus in first births only showed greater variation, with peaks in 1945 and 1952, and also winter rates

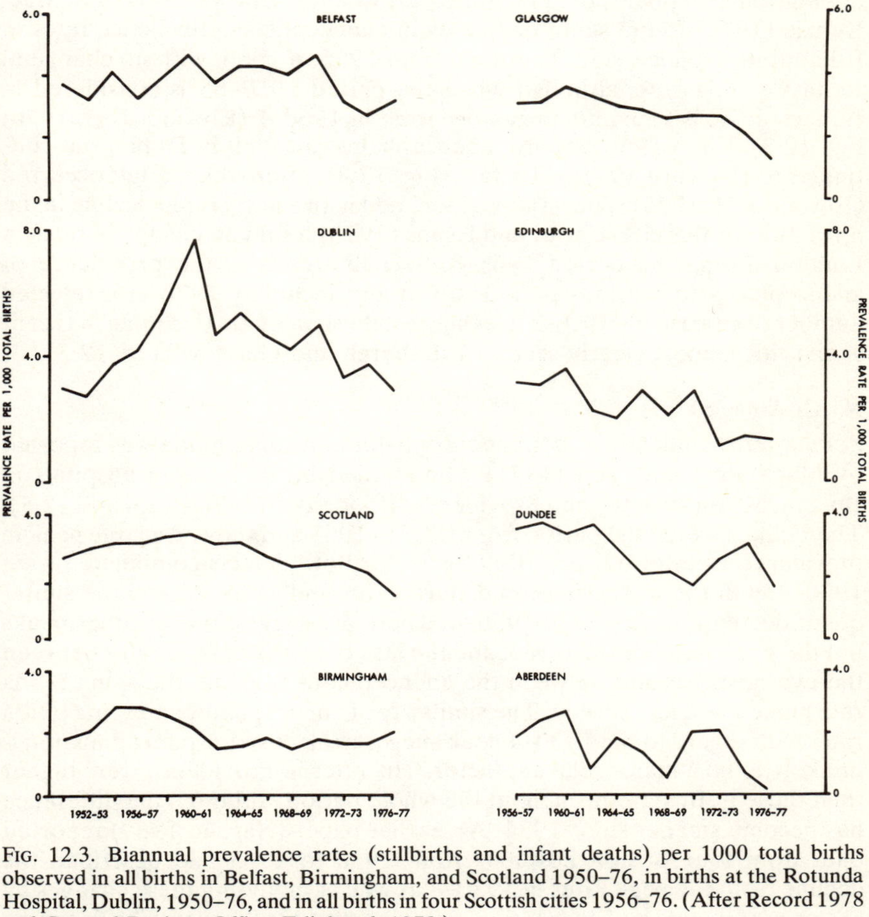

FIG. 12.3. Biannual prevalence rates (stillbirths and infant deaths) per 1000 total births observed in all births in Belfast, Birmingham, and Scotland 1950–76, in births at the Rotunda Hospital, Dublin, 1950–76, and in all births in four Scottish cities 1956–76. (After Record 1978 and General Register Office, Edinburgh 1978.)

varied more than summer rates (Edwards 1958). There was a lower male proportion in first births and in winter births indicating secular and seasonal changes may have affected mainly the prevalence of anencephalus in females. Record (1961) found the secular changes smallest in the maternal age group with the lowest rates (25–39 years) and largest in the parity group with the lowest rate (*para* 1); these changes occurred in all social classes. Secular trends in stillbirths and infant deaths attributed to spina bifida were similar to those described for anencephalus. Thus, there is a similarity between the secular trends in Dublin, Birmingham, and Scotland with maximal rates around 1940–2 and 1960–1 (1956–7 in Birmingham, 1960–1 in Dublin and Scotland) in all areas.

The other British studies may be examined against this background. Laurence *et al.* (1967) examined all births in most of South Wales using a special notification system; from 1956 to 1962 there was no apparent trend in either anencephalus or spina bifida prevalence. Elwood, J. H. and MacKenzie (1971) found slight decreases in anencephalus prevalence rates in Edinburgh, Dundee, and Aberdeen from 1956 to 1966, with no change in Belfast or Glasgow, although when the period 1950–65 is considered in Belfast, a rise is seen and a peak occurred in 1960–1 (Elwood, J. H. 1970; Fig. 12.3). From 1966 onward, anencephalus rates fell in Dublin but continued to rise until 1971 in Belfast (Fig. 12.3), after which a fall occurred (Elwood J. H. 1975). The latter is associated with a fairly rapid decline in the birth rate for this city. Carter and Evans (1973) found no change in rates in London during the period 1965–8. Secular trends in the prevalence of anencephalus for various periods up to and including 1976 in a selected number of cities in the British Isles suggest these rates are declining in recent years; this is most clearly seen in Edinburgh and Glasgow (Fig. 12.3).

North America

A long-term epidemic of both anencephalus and spina bifida was reported by MacMahon and Yen (1971) who studied births in large hospitals in Boston, Massachusetts, and Providence, Rhode Island (Figs 12.4 and 12.5). Their data covered the period from 1885 to 1965 and showed a large peak in prevalence rates of 6.0 per 1000 births for both defects combined during 1930–4 with the increasing trend starting around 1915–20 and the subsequent decrease lasting until 1950–4. There are suggestions of other peaks but the small numbers involved, and the lack of consistency in rates between the two hospitals and between the anencephalus rate and the spina bifida rate make these less certain. The similarity of anencephalus and spina bifida rates with regard to the 1930–4 peak suggests selective hospital admission is unlikely to be a major relevant factor. The rates in Providence were higher than those in Boston throughout the whole period, although the difference has become smaller since 1934. An earlier paper (Naggan 1969) reported data from four Boston hospitals from 1930 to 1965 and described the decline from the peak rates in 1930–4 as well as analysing these changes by ethnic group, paternal occupation, and maternal birth-order. The declining

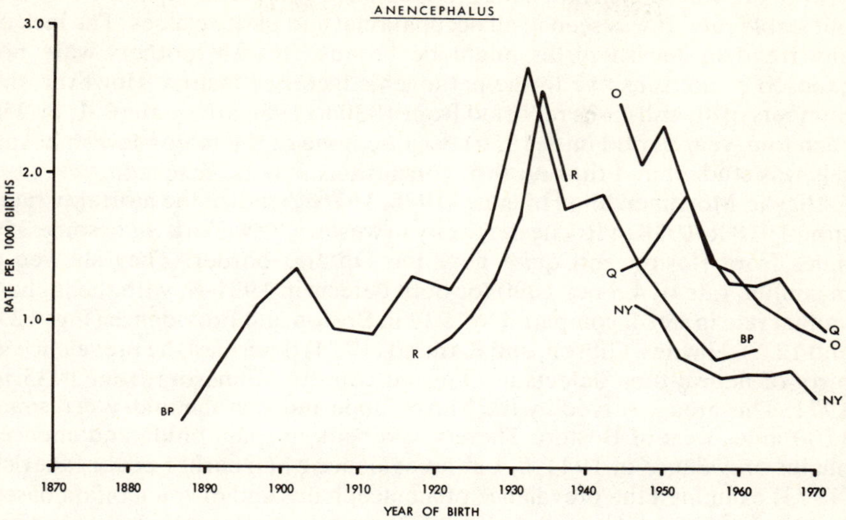

FIG. 12.4. Secular trends in the prevalence rate or mortality rate (stillbirths and infant deaths) per 1000 total births attributed to anencephalus in several areas of North America. BP, Boston and Providence hospitals (MacMahon and Yen 1971); R, Rochester, New York State (Biggar *et al*. 1976); NY, New York State excluding New York city (Janerich 1973); and O, Ontario and Q, Quebec (Elwood, J. M. 1976*b*).

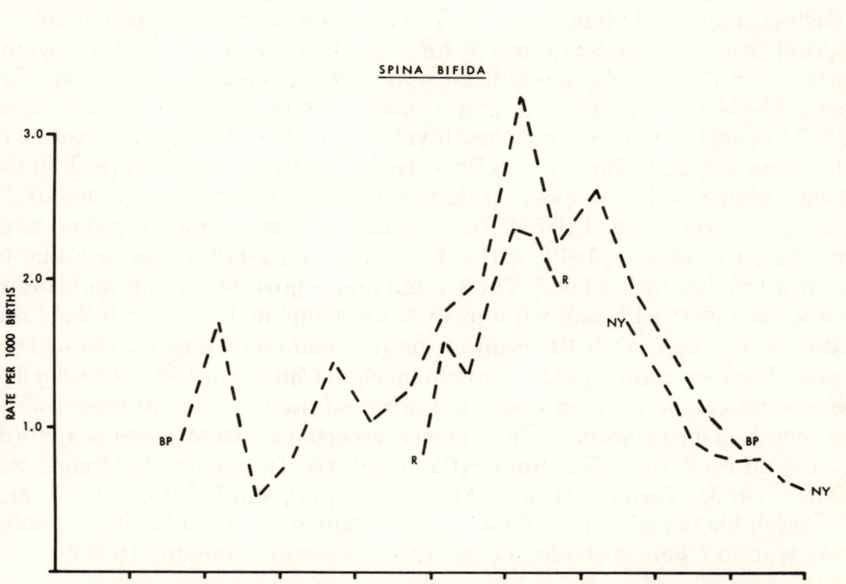

FIG. 12.5. Secular trends in the prevalence at birth per 1000 total births of spina bifida in several areas of North America. Key and sources as in Fig. 12.4.

prevalence was seen in all ethnic groups except Jews, who experienced a low but stable rate. It was seen in all occupational and parity classes. The lack of any trend in Jewish births might be because Jewish mothers were not exposed or not sensitive to the pathogenic factor or factors. However, the numbers of Jewish cases reported from 1930 to 1950 are small (0, 1, or 2 in each four-year period until 1950) because none of the major Jewish hospitals was studied and thus no firm conclusions may be reached.

Biggar, Mortimer, and Haughie (1976, 1976*a*) studied the mortality rates from 1918 to 1938 in Rochester, a city in western New York State some 350 miles from Boston and quite near the Ontario border. They showed a maximum rate of 4.5 per 1000 for both defects in 1931–4, with the highest annual rate in 1934, compared to 1932 in Boston and Providence (Figs 12.4 and 12.5). Haynes, Gibson, and Kurland (1974) described the prevalence at birth of neural-tube defects in Olmsted county, Minnesota from 1935 to 1971. This area is served by the Mayo Clinic and is in the mid-West, some 1100 miles west of Boston. There was a peak in spina bifida and anencephalus prevalence in 1944–5, but no evidence of an earlier peak. Janerich (1973) examined the prevalence of anencephalus and of spina bifida based on a registry which has collated stillbirth and livebirth notifications in New York State, excluding New York City, since 1945. The annual rates for both conditions declined from 1945 in a similar fashion to the Boston–Providence rates. The anencephalus rate declined from 1.1 per 1000 in 1945–7 to 0.62 per 1000 in 1957–9, stabilized around 0.65 during the period 1960–8 and declined again to 0.50 in 1969–71. The spina bifida rate fell throughout the period from 1945 onward except for a small rise in 1963–5. Age-specific rates for both abnormalities indicate a rise in prevalence in births to mothers aged 15–24 years in 1963–5, and a small increase in births to those aged 25–34 years in 1966–8. Thus the prevalence in New York State declined in the same way as in Boston and Providence but there is a small peak in the 1960s seen mostly for spina bifida in offspring of mothers aged under 25 years. Kurtzke *et al.* (1973) found small rises in infant mortality rates attributed to anencephalus and spina bifida and a fall in the rate due to hydrocephalus during 1962. The United States introduced different coding for spina bifida with and without hydrocephalus in 1962 which later was adopted by the Eighth Revision of the *International Classification of Diseases*. The new coding practice commenced in Canada in 1969. This change seems unlikely to have produced the reported rise in spina bifida mortality, as increases in spina bifida prevalence ascertained from hospital records were reported for 1972 from Atlanta (Boris, Blumberg, Feldman, and Sellers 1963), Vermont (Lucey, Mann, Simmons, and Friedman 1964) and Philadelphia (Ingalls and Klinberg 1965), and an increase in anencephalus was seen in Charlottesville, Virginia (Solowy and Shephard 1971).

Other countries

Information concerning the long-term secular variations in neural-tube defect prevalence in other countries is sparse. No trend was apparent in the frequency of anencephalus in France from 1945 to 1955 (Frézal *et al.* 1964) or Budapest from 1963 to 1967 (Czeizel and Révész 1970). Rogers and Morris (1971) examined national infant mortality rates from spina bifida in several European countries and described no definite change in France from 1950 to 1968, a 1954–5 peak in West Germany over the study period 1952 to 1968 and a 1952–3 peak in the Netherlands, studied over the period 1948 to 1968. Lenz (1965) described several small hospital studies which found peaks in anencephalus mortality in 1930 to 1934 in Hamburg (studied from 1930 to 1963), in 1945 to 1949 in Berlin (studied from 1934 to 1954) and in 1941 to 1945 in Göttingen (studied from 1931 to 1954). Apart from the higher rates in the mid-1950s in West Germany and the Netherlands, which occurred just before rises in neural-tube defect prevalence in Birmingham, Dublin, and Scotland, there is little concordance between the secular trends in different European countries.

Stoller and Collmann (1965) report a low but stable prevalence of anencephalus in Melbourne from 1943 to 1962, and Wei and Chen (1965) a constant rate in Taiwan from 1955 to 1962. In Israel, there was a large decline from 1958 to 1968 in the prevalence of spina bifida and of anencephalus which was independent of changes in maternal parity (Naggan 1971). The trend was more marked for spina bifida than for anencephalus. Cruz-Coke (1972) described a rapidly increasing rate of anencephalus in Chile from 1960 to 1971 based on national vital statistics but the rate there is still very low. A hospital study in Santiago from 1961 to 1964 also found a low rate of 0.30 per 1000 (Stevenson *et al.* 1966). Thus, in most regions for which data are available the prevalence of anencephalus is declining at present, with the exception of Chile. Whether these trends represent permanent reductions in prevalence or only troughs of underlying long-term cycles is not yet known. Monitoring of changes over the next few years may answer this question.

Canada

The annual mortality rate from anencephalus per 1000 total births in Canada has fallen from 1.56 in 1943 to 0.89 in 1974 (Fig. 12.6). This trend has been fairly regular since 1954; before that time the rate could be interpreted as being steady from 1943 to 1949 and rising from 1950 to 1953, or else as rising irregularly from 1943 to a peak in 1951 and then falling. In view of the large geographical variations in anencephalus mortality rates in Canada, we examined the secular trends in the provinces of Quebec, Ontario, and British Columbia, in the Maritime provinces combined (Nova Scotia, New Brunswick, and Prince Edward Island) and in the Prairies combined (Manitoba, Saskatchewan, and Alberta). The secular trends show considerable differences between regions (Fig. 12.7). The anencephalus rate in Ontario has had the greatest fall, from 2.48 per 1000 in 1943–4, to 0.65 per 1000 in 1973–4. The rate in the Prairie provinces has fallen less markedly and that in British Columbia showed no change over the 28-year period. In the Maritimes, the rate rose from 1943–4 to 1949–52 and then fell slowly. Examination of the rates for the smaller provinces separately shows the Manitoba rate had a sharp peak in 1951–2 and the rate in Prince Edward Island declined throughout the whole period. Thus in all provinces except British Columbia there has been a downward trend in anencephalus mortality rates since the early 1950s. From 1943 to this time rates were falling in Ontario and in Prince Edward Island but rising in the other provinces, which thus showed their highest frequencies around 1950. All the maximum rates did not occur in the same year nor do they show a geographical pattern; however, it is interesting that the rate in British Columbia also peaked in 1951 and 1952, despite the absence of any long-term trend.

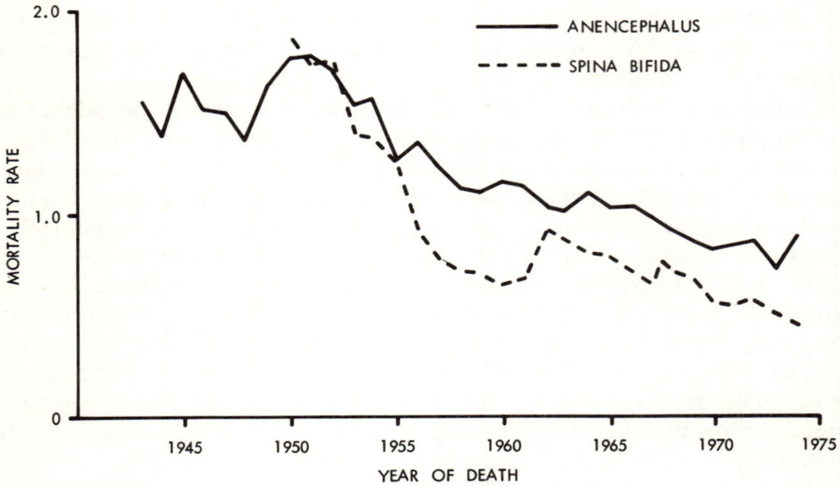

FIG. 12.6. Annual mortality rates (stillbirths and infant deaths) per 1000 total births attributed to anencephalus 1943–74 and spina bifida 1950–74 in Canada (excluding Newfoundland, the North-west Territories, and the Yukon).

Comparison of the trends in anencephalus mortality rates in Ontario and Quebec with those of adjacent areas in the United States (Fig. 12.4) shows that in Ontario the decline since 1943 parallels those seen in Boston and Providence and in New York State. The rates are considerably higher and it seems possible that a peak may have occurred prior to the earlier years studied. The trend in Quebec is clearly different with a maximum in 1951–4.

The annual mortality rate from spina bifida has fallen from 1.87 per 1000 total births in 1950 to 0.46 in 1974 (Fig. 12.6). From 1950 to 1955 the mortality rates attributed to anencephalus and to spina bifida are similar, but the spina bifida rate subsequently fell more rapidly and has remained below that of anencephalus. The fall in spina bifida mortality was interrupted by a sharp rise during 1961–2 which was then followed by a gradual decline. The standard error of each of the annual rates is approximately 0.04 per 1000, and the increase from 0.68 per 1000 in 1961 to 0.93 in 1962 is significant. The period of most rapid decrease in spina bifida mortality was from 1950 to

1960 which seems too early to be due to the changes in surgical treatment introduced in the late 1950s. The annual spina bifida mortality rate has shown similar changes since 1950 in all regions of Canada (Fig. 12.8). In all regions there was a rapid fall from 1950 which ended around 1957 in British Columbia, the Prairies and the Maritimes, in 1958 in Ontario and in 1960 in Quebec. This was followed by a rise in the early 1960s which peaked in the Maritimes, Quebec, and Ontario in 1962 and in 1963 in British Columbia and Manitoba. Only in Alberta and Saskatchewan was there no such rise.

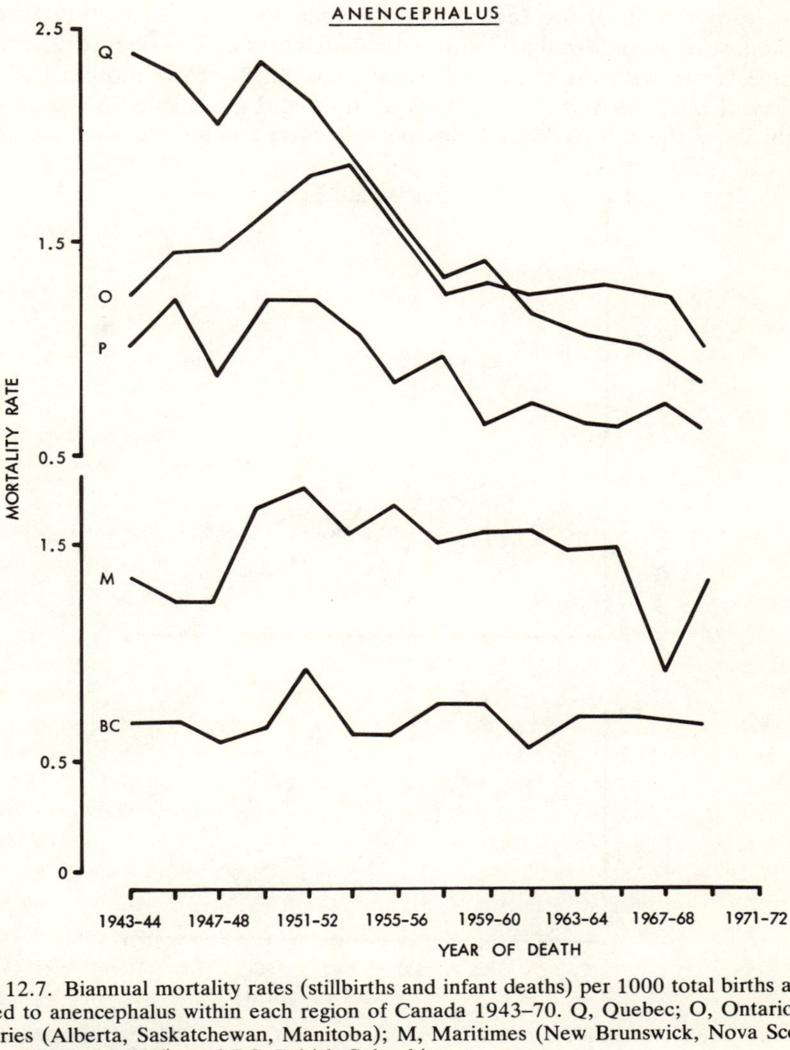

FIG. 12.7. Biannual mortality rates (stillbirths and infant deaths) per 1000 total births attributed to anencephalus within each region of Canada 1943–70. Q, Quebec; O, Ontario; P, Prairies (Alberta, Saskatchewan, Manitoba); M, Maritimes (New Brunswick, Nova Scotia, Prince Edward Island); and BC, British Columbia.

The Canadian 14-city study allowed us to examine other factors related to the secular trend in anencephalus mortality. The control series of livebirths for this investigation were taken from births in the years 1952, 1957, 1962, and 1967 and so quinquennial periods are compared. The mortality rate was 1.76 per 1000 births in 1950–4, and 1.06, 1.01, and 0.91 per 1000 in subsequent quinquennia. The relative risk for 1965–9 is thus 0.52, compared to a reference risk of one in 1950–4. The adjusted risk ratios, controlled for all other variables included in the study, are 1.0, 0.64, and 0.80, and 0.67 for sequential quinquennia (Table 12.1). The adjustment alters the overall decrease from a crude figure of 48 per cent to 33 per cent, showing that a proportion of the secular trend is due to changes in other factors studied, such as maternal age and parity distributions. The degree of secular change varies with the sex of the infant, the parity of the mother and the season of birth. Both the vital statistics data and the results of the 14-city study show the fall over time has been greater for female anencephalics

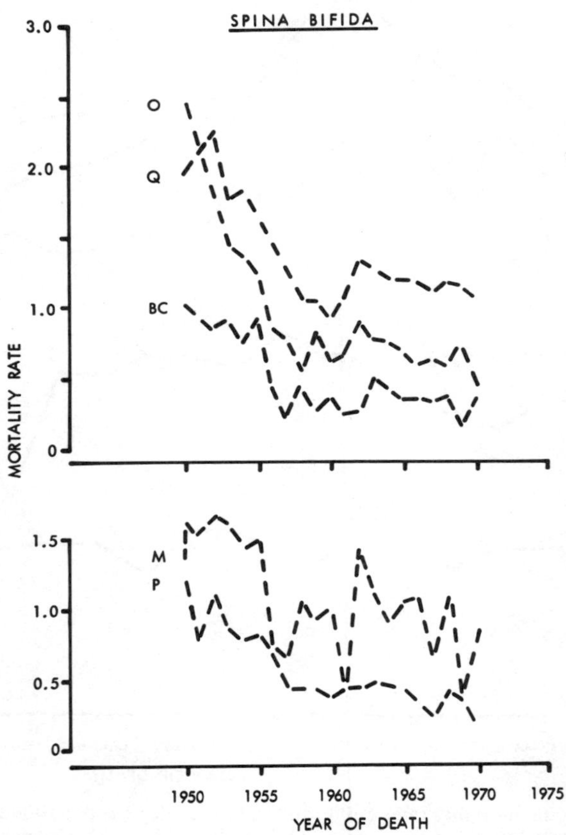

FIG. 12.8. Annual mortality rates (stillbirths and infant deaths) per 1000 total births attributed to spina bifida within each region of Canada 1950–70. Key as in Fig. 12.7.

resulting in an increase in the male proportion (Section 14). The 14-city study also shows this decline has been restricted to first births; thus the greatest fall in rate (68 per cent) has occurred in the rates for female first births, with lesser decreases for later female births (42 per cent), later male births (38 per cent) and male first births (28 per cent) as illustrated in Fig. 12.9. The secular trend has been more marked for winter than for summer births (Section 13).

TABLE 12.1 *Crude and adjusted risks of anencephalus by year of birth, relative to the risk in births during 1950—4, in 14 Canadian cities*

Year of birth	Number of cases	Number of controls	Mortality rate per 1000 livebirths	Crude risk ratio	Adjusted risk ratio†
1950–4	469	1117	1.76	1.00	1.00
1955–9	317	1255	1.06	0.60	0.64
1960–4	341	1420	1.01	0.57	0.80
1965–9	262	1206	0.91	0.52	0.67

Test of linear trend in adjusted risk ratios (Mantel 1963) yields $Z = -3.51$, $P = 0.008$
† Maximum likelihood risk ratio (Gart 1970), after controlling for the joint confounding effects of all ten other factors included in the 14-city study, by stratification on a multivariate risk score (Appendix A.3, Elwood, J. M. *et al*. 1978)

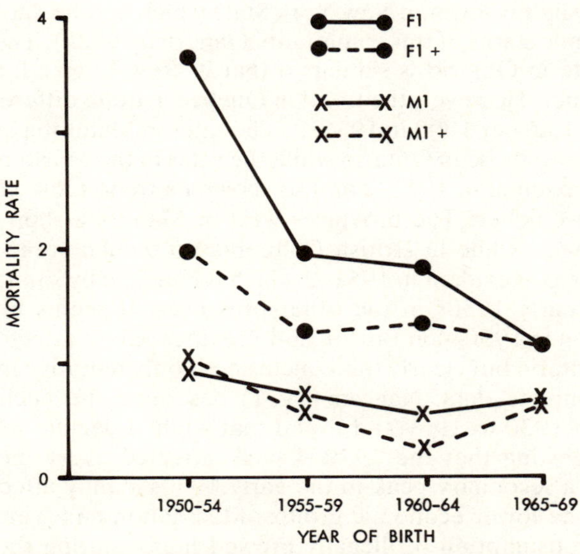

FIG. 12.9. Estimated mortality rates from anencephalus per 1000 total births by time period, sex, and birth order—Canadian 14-city study. Trends for each subgroup except male first births are statistically significant. F1, female first births; F1+, female later births; M1, male first births; M1+, male later births.

A secular trend in the frequency of a congenital malformation may be due to changes in the maternal at risk population over the same time period, to influences which affect all mothers in the population simultaneously such as exposure to an epidemic of infectious disease, or to influences which affect the mothers before the pregnancy in question. If these latter factors operate at a certain age, for example in the early childhood of the mother or at puberty, the occurrence rates will be related more clearly to the mother's year of birth than to the year in which the affected offspring are born. This will produce a birth cohort effect. Such influences may alter the age and parity distributions of mothers of affected infants (Section 21). The secular trends in anencephalus and spina bifida prevalence have been interpreted as suggesting that mothers who had inadequate nutrition in early childhood have a significantly greater lifetime risk of bearing affected infants (Emanuel and Sever 1973; Baird 1974; Janerich 1974). The Canadian data are broadly consistent with this postulate although they do not specifically support the hypothesis.

Interpretation of secular trends

The dramatic secular changes in the frequency of anencephalus in certain areas of North America, summarized in Fig. 12.4, show the peak prevalence rate of 2.7 per 1000 births in 1932 in Boston and Providence. The data from Rochester, New York from 1918 to 1938 show a similar peak, in 1934, and after 1945 the decreasing trend seen in New York State (which includes Rochester) is similar in slope to that in Boston and Providence. The rates are consistently slightly lower in New York State which may be due to the higher socio-economic status of this community (Janerich 1972*a*). The trend in the mortality rate in Ontario is similar to that in New England, although the rates are higher. However, the trend in Quebec in quite different showing a peak rate of 1.85 per 1000 in 1951–3. The rates in Manitoba have followed similar trends to those in Ontario while the rates in the Maritimes rose from 1943 to a maximum in 1951–2 and so showed a trend more closely resembling that in Quebec. The provinces west of Manitoba show less marked secular changes, while in British Columbia no secular trend is apparent, although a peak is evident in 1951–2 which is matched by similar short-term rises in the early 1950s in the other provinces. It seems likely that the epidemic seen in 1930–4 in Boston and Providence also affected New York State and Ontario but clearly this conclusion is only tentative in the absence of more complete data. Naggan (1971) described the declining rate in Boston from 1930 to 1969 and found that while a decline was seen in all groups, suggesting that the 1930–4 peak affected every mother in that community, a secondary peak in the early 1940s mainly affected births to mothers in the lower economic groups. MacMahon and Yen (1971) suggested the consumption of illegally brewed liquor during the prohibition period (1920–33), or else the economic depression of 1929 to 1936, could have contributed to the epidemic; however, they note the epidemic began before the depression and that a quick decline after the end of prohibition would have been expected and was not in fact observed. The economic depression also affected Canada, but this does not easily account for the maximum rates in Ontario and Manitoba being in the 1940s; furthermore, Quebec and the other provinces were similarly affected.

There is some evidence for a high rate of anencephalus and spina bifida in Great Britain in the 1930s or early 1940s (Rogers and Morris 1973; Leck and Rogers 1967; Elwood, J. H. 1973*a, b*) which raises the question of a possible world-wide pandemic, or at least an epidemic affecting the British Isles and North America and perhaps Europe as well. It is impossible to make a firm conclusion, but this is an intriguing idea and relationships to pandemics of infectious diseases such as influenza or to certain effects of wars and economic depressions are worthy of further research. On the other hand, it is striking that as well as showing long-term trends, prevalence rates vary over quite short periods of time of a few years or so and these trends vary greatly between countries and between areas within one country. The observations of these short epidemic periods which may be localized to one area suggests that in the search for causative factors attention should be paid to environmental or biological agents which demonstrate large qualitative or quantitative variability in time and space. In contrast, the 60 year period of the Boston–Providence epidemic and the possibilities of this being accompanied by periods of high prevalence in other countries, suggests a role for a widely distributed aetiological factor. The failure to show consistent relationships with identifiable factors such as notifiable infectious diseases leaves the field open to further study. From a health-planning perspective, the current decline in the prevalence of these defects is convenient but should not lead to complacency. As the causes of the decline are unknown and as the rates have been very labile, they could well increase again in the near future.

13

Seasonal variation

SEASONAL variations in the frequencies of congenital malformations are of interest as if present they may indicate the action of environmental agents such as climate, dietary agents, or infections. Historically, the evident seasonality of congenital cataract (Gregg 1941) led to the demonstration of an infectious aetiology associating this defect with maternal rubella infection in early pregnancy.

The first well-documented study of seasonality in the prevalence of anencephalus is that of McKeown and Record (1951) who showed a winter excess of affected births in Birmingham from 1930 to 1947 and in Scotland from 1939 to 1946. Information on the date of last menstrual period was available for the Birmingham series and the months of conception associated with the greatest risk were from April to June. Winter excesses of affected births have also been observed in Belfast (Elwood, J. H. 1970) and London (Carter and Evans 1973). Seasonal trends in Birmingham have changed over time with a summer excess in 1955–60 and the winter excess reappearing in 1965–9 (Leck and Record 1966; Leck 1972). A similar diminution of the trend in Scotland is evident between 1938–66 and 1967–72 (Edwards 1958; Record 1961; Fedrick 1976*a*). Rogers and Weatherall (1976) showed a maximum anencephalus prevalence rate in pregnancies with the last menstrual period in February to April in England and Wales in 1964 to 1965, and from 1968 to 1972, with less variation in 1966 and 1967. Summer excesses of anencephalic births were observed in South Wales (Laurence *et al*. 1968) and in Aberdeen (Elwood, J. H. and MacKenzie 1971). Smaller studies show no seasonal trend in Liverpool (Smithells *et al*. 1964), Southampton (Williamson 1965), Edinburgh or Dundee (Elwood, J. H. and MacKenzie 1971). However negative results from small studies are not informative; for example a study of 100 affected births analysed using harmonic methods has only about a 22 per cent chance of detecting a seasonal trend whose range is 20 per cent above and below the mean rate (Walter 1977).

In contrast to the winter excess of affected births seen in the British Isles, albeit with some inconsistencies by region and in time period, is the failure of most North American surveys preceding our Canadian study to find any seasonal variation (Table 13.1). Demonstration of no trend or a summer excess in several quite large studies strongly suggests the situation in North America differs from that in the British Isles. It is more difficult to reach conclusions with respect to other countries but winter excesses have been

TABLE 13.1 *North American studies of seasonal trends in anencephalus and spina bifida (after Elwood, J. M. 1975)*

Study	Place	Sources	Time period	Number of cases		Period of maximum occurrence	Reported significance of trend	Winter: summer ratio
MacMahon, Pugh and Ingalls 1953	Rhode Island	H	1936–52	Anencephalus	326	July-Dec.	N.S.	1.00†
				Spina bifida	426	Oct.-Mar.	N.S.	1.06†
Alter 1963	Halifax Nova Scotia	H, C	1946–55	Anencephalus	74	Sept.-Feb.	N.S.	1.24‡
	Charleston South Carolina	H, C	1946–55	Anencephalus	34	Sept.-Feb.	$P<0.01$¶	2.67‡
Naggan 1969	Boston Massachusetts	H	1930–65	Anencephalus	305	Apr.-June	N.S.	0.85†
				Spina bifida	393	July-Sept.	N.S.	0.93†
Silberg, Watson and Martin 1968	Missouri	B	1953–64	Anencephalus	252	Apr.-Sept.	N.S.	0.84†
				Spina bifida	715	Oct.-Mar.	N.S.	0.15†
Horowitz and McDonald 1969	Quebec	H, C, B	1956–65	Anencephalus	1497	Dec.-June	N.S.	>1.00§
				Spina bifida	2077	Dec.-June	(Edwards Test)	
Cassady 1969	Alabama	C, B	1961–6	Anencephalus	367	None	N.S.	1.02†
Choi *et al*. 1972	Manitoba	H, C, B	1964–8	Anencephalus	113	Mar.-Aug.	N.S.	>1.00§
				Spina bifida	93	Dec.-Feb.		

N.S. = non-significant ($P>0.05$)
H = hospitals
C = stillbirth and infant death notifications
B = birth certificates

† Ratio of incidence rates
‡ Ratio of number of cases
§ Insufficient data to calculate ratio
¶ Based on χ^2 statistic comparing two 6-month periods

recorded in Germany (Tünte 1965), and Italy (Beolchini and Bailo 1965), Norway (Verstege 1971), and Sweden (Sandahl 1977), but not in Hungary (Czeizel and Révész 1970). Studies from the Southern hemisphere are of particular interest. The largest is a study of 194 cases of anencephalus in the state of Victoria, Australia which showed no regular seasonal trend (Collmann and Stoller 1968).

Spina bifida has been less extensively studied with regard to seasonality, but in general the findings are similar to those for anencephalus. Winter increases in the prevalence of spina bifida have been observed in Birmingham since 1950 (Leck 1972), Manchester (Guthkelch 1962), and in a nationwide study in Great Britain (Slater, Watson and McDonald 1964). In England and Wales from 1964 to 1972, there was a winter excess of affected births with the maximum prevalence rates associated with the last menstrual period falling in April to June, that is two months later than the peak for anencephalus (Rogers and Weatherall 1976). As with anencephalus, the seasonal trends were most marked in 1964 to 1965 and 1968 to 1972. A summer excess was present in South Wales (Laurence *et al*. 1968). However, no seasonal variation was found in Birmingham from 1940 to 1947 (McKeown and Record 1951) and Edwards (1958) found no seasonal variation in spina bifida stillbirths in Scotland from 1939 to 1946. The winter excess of affected births in Belfast was more marked for fatal cases of spina bifida than for those who survived over one year (Elwood, J. H. and Nevin 1973). Studies from America have shown no seasonal trend in spina bifida births (Table 13.1). A winter excess was found in Hungary (Czeizel and Révész 1970).

Analysis of trends by season

Information should be obtained on all births in a defined population. The use of birth dates, and of dates of the last menstrual period, may give different results because a seasonal factor influencing survival *in utero* may affect birth dates but not conception dates of malformed infants. Any effect of a true aetiological seasonal factor may be masked if birth dates only are used. In general, published works do not show any consistent differences between results from these two data sets, and birth dates yield similar conclusions to conception dates if adjusted for mean gestation time. Use of date of birth produces the effect expected by introducing a source of random error, namely, to dilute any true seasonal variation in conception dates and make it more difficult to recognize a trend. For example, Rogers and Weatherall (1976) and Sandahl (1977) were able to demonstrate seasonality more clearly by using the date of the last menstrual period rather than the date of birth in their surveys.

Most published analyses apply chi-square tests to monthly, quarterly, or biannual totals of affected births. However, the 12-monthly chi-square value tests any departure from homogeneity of the monthly rates and does not distinguish between regular and irregular variations, while the value of other statistics will vary with the choice of three- or six-monthly periods. We have used statistical methods which assume a regular annual cycle of rates with one maximum and one minimum point. Edwards (1961) suggested the first such method based on fitting a harmonic curve to the data. However this method considers only the number of cases per month and is inaccurate if the monthly number of total births varies, which is usually the situation in practice. A simple adjustment overcomes this (Elwood, J. M. 1975), but we prefer a method which adjusts for a changing birth population and for varying month length and also incorporates a test for the adequacy of the fitted curve as a model for the data (Walter and Elwood, J. M. 1975). The analysis requires a knowledge of the monthly numbers of affected and total births. A harmonic curve is fitted and the maximum amplitude of the curve together with the date of this maximum are estimated. Two chi-square statistics are calculated, one with two degrees of freedom testing significant departure of the fitted curve from linearity and secondly, a goodness of fit statistic with nine degrees of freedom testing for departure of the observed monthly totals of affected cases from the numbers predicted by the fitted curve. An important practical problem is the likelihood of detecting a seasonal trend in a relatively small study. Walter (1977*a*) has derived power expressions for the Edward's model which also are approximately true for the Walter–Elwood method. If there is a true seasonal amplitude of 10 per cent, which seems a typical value, a study of 1000 cases will have only a 50 per cent chance of demonstrating this trend at the conventional 5 per cent level of significance (Table 13.2). As most published studies report smaller numbers and use less powerful statistical methods such as simple chi-square tests, the inconsistencies in published results are not surprising. Further discussion of methodological issues in seasonal analysis is presented in Appendix A.2.

TABLE 13.2 *Probability of detecting a simple harmonic seasonal variation, at the 0.05 significance level, by Edward's test, for a given amplitude* A *and number of affected births studied* N.

	Amplitude A (per cent)				
Number of cases studied N	1	2	5	10	20
50	5	5	5	7	13
100	5	5	6	9	22
250	5	5	7	15	50
500	5	6	10	27	82
1000	5	6	15	50	99
5000	7	13	60	100	100
10 000	9	22	90	100	100
100 000	50	99	100	100	100

From Walter (1977*a*).

Seasonal variation of anencephalus in Canada

We examined the seasonal variation of anencephalus deaths by month in Canada for the period from 1954 to 1972, based on 8871 cases. For the period from 1954 to 1962, a significant trend with a maximum mortality rate in January to March was present but for the later period from 1963 to 1972 no significant trend was seen (Elwood, J. M. 1975). Examination of the data by individual year within these periods did not change this conclusion. Comparison of the mortality rates from anencephalus in winter (October to March) and in summer months (April to September) in each year from 1954 to 1972 shows a higher rate in winter in each year up to 1962 (Fig. 13.1).

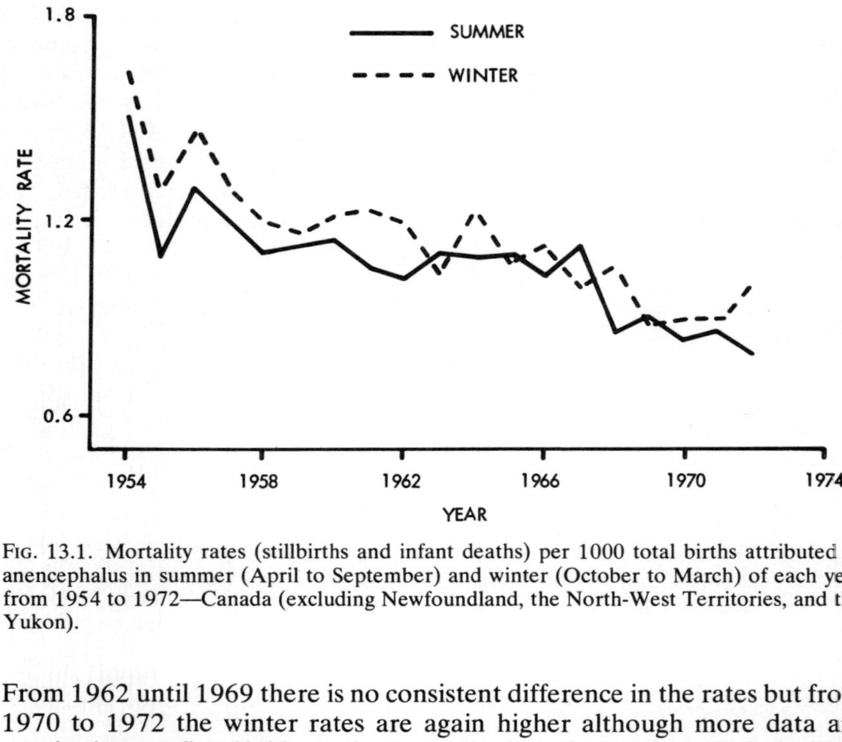

FIG. 13.1. Mortality rates (stillbirths and infant deaths) per 1000 total births attributed to anencephalus in summer (April to September) and winter (October to March) of each year from 1954 to 1972—Canada (excluding Newfoundland, the North-West Territories, and the Yukon).

From 1962 until 1969 there is no consistent difference in the rates but from 1970 to 1972 the winter rates are again higher although more data are required to confirm if this marks the beginning of another period of winter excess. During the 1954 to 1962 period, the mean annual mortality rate was 1.21 per 1000 total births and the range in monthly rates was 1.37 in January to 1.01 in May (Fig. 13.2). The maximum amplitude of the fitted curve is 11.3 per cent in December (that is, the maximum rate is 11.3 per cent higher than the mean), the fitted trend is significant ($\chi = 12.5$ d.f. $= 2p<0.01$), but the goodness of fit test also is significant ($\chi^2 = 28.2$ d.f. $= 9p<0.01$). Thus we conclude that there is a seasonal trend which is not adequately described by simple harmonic model, and on inspection of the data there is evidence of bimodality. For the period from 1963 to 1972, the mean rate was 0.99 per 1000 and the range from 1.06 in February and March to 0.88 in July and December. The fitted curve has a maximum amplitude of 5.8 per cent in January, which is not statistically significant (χ^2 trend = 1.7, d.f.=2, $p>0.25$, χ^2 goodness of fit=16.6, d.f.=9, $p>0.05$). Our results are consistent with a trend for maximum birth-rates of anencephalus to be in winter, but this became less marked after 1962 than in earlier years. However, seasonal variation may now be becoming more pronounced.

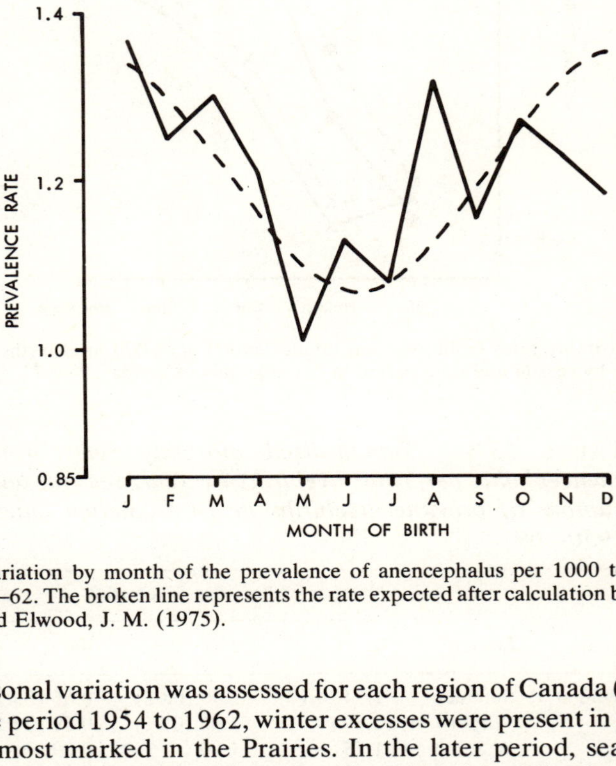

FIG. 13.2 Variation by month of the prevalence of anencephalus per 1000 total births in Canada 1954–62. The broken line represents the rate expected after calculation by the method of Walter and Elwood, J. M. (1975).

The seasonal variation was assessed for each region of Canada (Fig. 13.3). During the period 1954 to 1962, winter excesses were present in all regions, and were most marked in the Prairies. In the later period, seasonality is reduced in all regions but is still maximal in the Prairies. The peak month of occurrence is earlier in the Prairies than elsewhere; November rather than December to March. If we assume a mean gestational period of 36 weeks, as found in the Canadian 14-city study, and assume that initiation of anencephalus occurs at four weeks of gestation, then maximum rates of incidence are in May to June in Quebec and in February to April in the Prairies. Thus seasonal variation of anencephalic births clearly is present in Canada although it is not identical for every year and in all regions. We looked for possible modifying factors in the 14-city study. These data also show a winter excess which persists after control for the confounding effects of seven other variables studied (city of residence, maternal age, ethnic group, numbers of

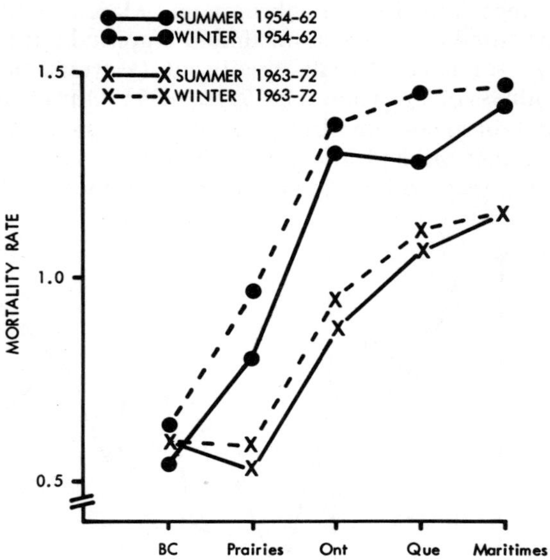

FIG. 13.3. Mortality rates (stillbirths and infant deaths) per 1000 total births attributed to anencephalus by season and time period in five regions of Canada 1954–72

TABLE 13.3 *Standardized mortality rates from anencephalus per 1000 livebirths by year, season, and number of previous livebirths in 14 Canadian cities, 1950—69*

		Number of Previous Livebirths		
Years	Season	0	1–3	4+
1950–9	Summer	1.54 (0.12)	1.06 (0.05)	0.66 (0.07)
	Winter	2.70 (0.61)	1.06 (0.06)	0.59 (0.05)
	W:S ratio	1.75	1.00	0.89
1960–9	Summer	1.24 (0.12)	1.10 (0.08)	0.85 (0.07)
	Winter	1.96 (0.31)	1.15 (0.08)	0.90 (0.08)
	W:S ratio	1.58	1.05	1.06

Standard errors of rates in parentheses.
Summer = April to September   Winter = October to March
Rates are derived by direct standardization over 5 strata of a risk score based on city of residence, maternal age, ethnic group, previous stillbirths and infant deaths, legitimacy status, multiplicity of birth, and place of confinement (home or hospital), using the total number of controls in each stratum as the standard population.

previous stillbirths and infant deaths, legitimacy, and plurality). The winter and summer mortality rates by year of birth and by the number of previous livebirths show the winter excess to be restricted to first births (Table 13.3). The variation by season in first births is very marked, the winter rates being 75 per cent higher than the summer rates in 1950–9 and 58 per cent higher in 1960–9. As birth order and the sex distribution of anencephalics are correlated, we also examined seasonality by sex of infant. However, the seasonal variation is similar in both sexes, and the winter excess is present in only first births of either sex.

Interpretation

In Canada, the winter-to-summer ratio of anencephalus mortality rates was 1.10:1 in 1954–62, and 1.06:1 in 1963–72, the trend being statistically significant only in the earlier period. Secular changes in seasonal variation have also been noted in the British Isles. The overall mortality rate in Canada was higher in the earlier time period but in neither Canada nor the British Isles is there a consistent association between the presence of significant seasonal variation and a high prevalence or mortality rate of anencephalus. The Canadian data were studied in the two time periods 1954–62 and 1963–72 and the change in seasonal pattern with the year of division of the data suggests that there may be differences in ascertainment. Between 1960 and 1962, the various provinces altered their registration policies to include stillbirths from 20 weeks rather than from 28 weeks of gestation, but analysis of the later data with restriction to gestation periods over 28 weeks does not alter our findings. There are no other known differences in ascertainment or recording procedures between these two time periods. We have demonstrated that seasonal variation persists after simultaneous control for several other factors including maternal reproductive history and ethnic group. One possible confounding factor which was not included in our analysis is social class. However, the seasonal variation seen in the United Kingdom is independent of this factor also (Record 1961; James 1972). Seasonal variation is modified by birth order as well as by year of birth. In the results presented, birth order was based on the number of previous livebirths as the effect of the numbers of previous livebirths and of previous stillbirths on a mother's risk of bearing an anencephalic infant are different. In Canada, the winter excess is virtually restricted to first births which show a marked seasonal trend with winter to summer mortality ratios after confounder control of 1.72 in 1950–9 and 1.58 in 1960–9. An increased seasonal trend for first births was reported by McKeown and Record (1951) and MacMahon, Pugh, and Ingalls (1953) but is not seen in more extensive data from either Birmingham (Edwards 1958) or Scotland (Record 1961). British studies suggest that spina bifida occurrence also varies seasonally with the peak conception times perhaps being a few weeks later than those of anencephalus (Rogers and Weatherall 1976).

No acceptable hypothesis explaining seasonal variation has yet been put forward. Both the British and Canadian studies suggest that the period of highest risk for conception is from February to June. Obvious candidates for causative factors, or at least indicators of such agents, are climate, infections, and dietary habits. In the British Isles, estimated conception dates of anencephalics were shown to have a negative association with maximal air temperature in Belfast and in four Scottish cities (Elwood, J. H. and MacKenzie 1971), and a positive association with hours of sunshine and daylight in Scotland (Record 1961). In all regions of Canada, maximum daily temperatures and sunshine hours are in July and are minimal in January to February. Maximum rainfall is in October to December in the maritime areas and in British Columbia, and in June to August elsewhere. Thus there is no apparent association of the period of highest anencephalus risk with these meterorological variables in Canada. Most studies comparing the trends in anencephalus prevalence rates with the prevalence of infectious diseases have shown no association, although there are some reports of an increased risk after influenza during pregnancy. In Canada, most common infectious diseases have their peak incidence rates rather earlier than the calculated peak in conception dates, but their effects could well be delayed and very little information is available on infectious agents other than those of the major notifiable diseases. Renwick (1972, 1973) suggested seasonal variation may be due to maximum consumption of blight-damaged potatoes at the end of the winter, when stored potatoes are eaten, and that the lack of seasonal variation in previous North American studies might reflect less storage of potatoes than in the British Isles. Besides other evidence against this hypothesis, trends by season are not more marked in the areas of high potato-blight prevalence in Canada (Elwood, J. M. 1976*a*).

A seasonal variation may be consistent with the water-composition hypothesis as in hard-water areas there is an appreciable drop in the mineral concentrations of water in the spring owing to the fast flow of snow melt-water and relatively small holding reservoirs; in soft-water areas there is less seasonal change in water composition. A seasonal trend would thus be expected in the Prairies but not in Quebec or the Maritime provinces. There seems to be no other evidence of an association in time between anencephalus rates and changes in water hardness; the anencephalus mortality rates in Canadian cities have changed over time despite the constancy of water composition, and no change in anencephalus rates followed softening of the water supplies in St Helens, England (Fielding and Smithells 1971). Thus if a water factor causes some of the geographical variations in anencephalus prevalence, any effect may be on a long-term basis. A dietary factor might explain the seasonal variation, for example if the intake of an important nutrient were reduced in the winter months. A relative lack of fresh vegetable products would produce maximum deficiency in the spring. Alternatively, intake of some toxic agent might be maximal at that time. Such ill-defined hypotheses are difficult to test. Knox's (1972) study of the temporal associations between dietary constituents and anencephalus occurrence found significant positive associations with the consumption of canned peas and cured meat products, and negative associations with consumption of cheese, fresh meat, and apples. The concept of a dietary agent is attractive as the secular and geographical variations may be explicable by differences in climate, food storage, and cooking habits. The limitation of the seasonal trend to first births indicates the need to consider more complex hypotheses than these.

14

Distribution by sex

In most communities, anencephalus and spina bifida are seen more frequently in females than in males. Sex distribution may be presented as the sex ratio, namely the ratio of the numbers of male to female cases, or as the proportion of all cases which are male or female. A proportion is simpler to handle statistically than a ratio and so we have expressed sex distribution as the 'male proportion'. Within Caucasian groups, the male proportion ranges from 0.23 in Belfast, Northern Ireland, to 0.46 in Sydney, New South Wales (Table 14.1). In Canada, the male proportion of 0.32 seen in data for 1943 to 1969 is similar to that reported in other North American studies but higher than in most British surveys. Higher proportions (0.44) are seen both in Israel and in Jewish births in Boston (Naggan and MacMahon 1967), and in Oriental populations where the range is from 0.48 to 0.53. Spina bifida exhibits higher male proportions and a narrower range of variation from 0.34 in Manitoba and Iowa to 0.47 in South Wales, and in British Columbia (Table 14.2). Most large studies have results in the 0.38 to 0.48 range. Israeli and Japanese reports show similar values.

An inverse relationship between the male proportion of anencephalus and the prevalence rate at birth was suggested by Searle (1959) and Naggan (1971), who showed that in Singapore, Israel, and Boston the ethnic groups with lower prevalence rates of anencephalus had higher male proportions. Male proportions of 0.25 or less are found in the high prevalence areas of Belfast, Dublin, and South Wales while several groups with high male proportions have low prevalence for example, blacks in the United States, Orientals, and Australians. The Canadian data and world literature lend some support for this hypothesis but there are inconsistencies. The mortality rates in the nine provinces of Canada (excluding Newfoundland) from 1943 to 1969 ranged from 0.68 to 2.17 per 1000 but there was no trend in the male proportion (Table 14.1). More detailed analysis to take account of simultaneous secular trends still reveals no variation (Elwood, J. M. 1976). The association between the prevalence rate and the male proportion for anencephalus in several series is summarized in Fig. 14.1. A weighted regression analysis of male proportion against prevalence rate based on all 40 studies does reveal a negative association with a correlation coefficient r of -0.61 ($p<0.001$). However, as is indicated by inspection of the scatter diagram, while the negative association is evident in British and European studies, no association is seen within the North American group ($r=-0.14$, $p>0.5$). It is clear also that the male proportions seen in Japan, Taiwan,

TABLE 14.1 *Sex distribution of anencephalus in selected series*

Area	Anencephalus Total number†	Rate‡ per 1000	Per cent male	Reference
British Isles				
Birmingham	366	2.31	32	Record and McKeown 1949
Liverpool	177	3.27	29	Smithells, Chinn *et al.* 1964
London	578	1.41	29	Carter and Evans 1973
Oxford	177	1.49	34	Fedrick 1976
Southampton	27	1.95	26	Williamson 1965
South Wales	362	3.55	25	Laurence *et al.* 1968
Belfast	175	4.20	23	Elwood, J. H. and Nevin 1973
Cork	76	2.05	30	Spellman 1969
Dublin	977	4.20	25	Coffey 1974
England and Wales	16 045	1.90	29	Registrars General (various years) and Rogers and Morris 1973
Scotland	5825	2.95	26	
Northern Ireland	923	3.41	28	
Europe				
Hungary	277	1.10	33	Czeizel and Révész 1970
Finland	196	0.32	38	Granroth *et al.* 1977
France	369	0.54	40	Frézal *et al.* 1964
Sweden (Lund and Malmo)	66	0.64	36	Böök and Rayner 1950
United States				
Boston	305	0.98	29	Naggan and MacMahon 1967
Birmingham, Alabama	367	0.83	36	Cassady 1969
Iowa	34	0.58	29	Hay 1971
Los Angeles	48	0.49	35	Smilkstein 1962
New York State	2205	0.86	32	Gittelsohn and Milham 1962
Rhode Island	326	1.93	30	MacMahon *et al.* 1953
Rochester, Minn.	26	0.90	12	Haynes *et al.* 1974
Virginia	23	1.00	39	Solowy and Shepard 1971
Rochester, New York	180	1.39	28	Biggar, Mortimer & Haughie 1976
Canada 1943–69 all	13 825	1.26	32	Elwood, J. M. 1976
British Columbia	586	0.68	33	
Alberta	664	0.79	29	
Saskatchewan	415	0.69	32	
Manitoba	659	1.19	32	
Ontario	5357	1.54	30	
Quebec	4726	1.41	34	
New Brunswick	598	1.41	32	
Nova Scotia	665	1.38	31	
Prince Edward Island	155	2.17	33	
Other areas				
Mexico City	29	1.78	38	Stevenson *et al.* 1966
Alexandria	36	3.79	33	
Bombay	66	1.89	29	

TABLE 14.1 *continued*

	Anencephalus			
Area (continued)	Total number†	Rate‡ per 1000	Per cent male	Reference
Singapore	64	0.77	48	Searle 1959
Japan	2661	0.43	52	Imaizumi 1974
Taiwan	30	1.17	53	Emanuel *et al.* 1972
Sydney	67	0.74	46	Jones 1967
State of Victoria	196	0.74	35	Collman and Stoller 1968
Israel	462	0.86	44	Naggan 1971

† Excluding any of unknown sex.
‡ Prevalence at birth or mortality rate per 1000 total births.

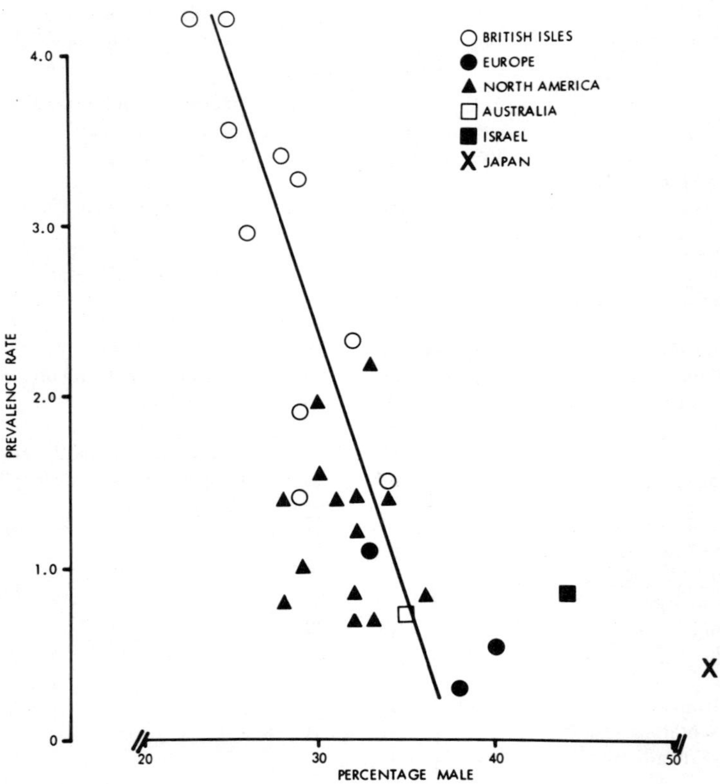

FIG. 14.1. Anencephalic male proportion and corresponding population prevalence rate or mortality rate per 1000 total births from anencephalus in selected series (studies of less than 100 cases excluded).

Singapore, and perhaps Israel are higher than those in North American and European populations with similar prevalence rates. This suggests a difference between Caucasian and other racial groups. No association is seen between the prevalence rates of spina bifida and its male proportion; a weighted correlation analysis of the 21 reports available (Table 14.2) yields a coefficient r of 0.26 ($p>0.2$), and there is no significant difference between the male proportions in Oriental and Caucasian populations even though there is a greater difference in prevalence rates for spina bifida than for anencephalus. Oriental and Caucasian populations show two major differences with regard to neural-tube defects: Oriental populations have a higher male proportion of anencephalus (Table 14.1) and a lower ratio of spina bifida cases to anencephalus (Table 10.1). Accordingly, we examined the data for all Caucasian populations for an association between the male

TABLE 14.2 *Sex distribution of spina bifida in selected series*

Area	Total number†	Spina bifida: Prevalence rate per 1000	Spina bifida: Per cent Male	Reference
British Isles				
Birmingham	389	2.46	43	Record and McKeown 1949
Liverpool	256	3.54	46	Smithells and Chinn 1965
London	631	1.54	44	Carter and Evans 1973
Southampton	59	3.22	39	Williamson 1965
South Wales	425	4.13	47	Laurence *et al*. 1968
Belfast	185	4.50	38	Elwood, J. H. and Nevin 1973
Northern Ireland	525	3.33	48	Elwood, J. H. 1976
Cork	91	2.45	44	Spellman 1969
North America				
Boston	393	1.26	40	Naggan and MacMahon 1967
Iowa	56	0.95	34	Hay 1971
New York State	3021	1.18	43	Gittelsohn and Milham 1962
Rochester, Minn.	39	1.30	33	Haynes *et al*. 1974
Rhode Island	388	2.30	45	MacMahon *et al*. 1953
Quebec	1228	1.87	43	Horowitz and McDonald 1969
Manitoba	93	0.99	34	Choi *et al*. 1972
British Columbia	597	0.87	47	McBride 1977
Other areas				
Hungary	572	1.63	42	Czeizel and Révész 1970
Mexico City	24	0.94	50	Stevenson *et al*. 1966
Bombay	44	1.08	41	Stevenson *et al*. 1966
Japan	503	0.08	44	Imaizumi 1974
Israel	314	0.60	42	Naggan 1971

† Excluding any of unknown sex.

proportion of anencephalus and the spina-bifida-to-anencephalus ratio, but found no consistent relationship.

In the Canadian 14-city study, the mortality rates from anencephalus showed independent associations with city of maternal residence and with maternal ethnic origin (Sections 10 and 11). There was no association between male proportion and city of residence. With regard to ethnic origin, the results are equivocal (Table 14.3). Mothers of oriental origin have a low mortality rate from anencephalus and a high male proportion (0.54) similar to those reported from Japan and Taiwan, while mothers of British or Irish origin show higher mortality rates and male proportions of 0.28 to 0.24, similar to those seen in the British Isles (Table 14.1). Mothers of French origin show both a higher mortality rate and a lower male proportion than is reported in France. However, other groups show more irregular variations and there is no statistically significant association between the mortality rate and the male proportion over all 11 ethnic groups defined. Restriction of the analysis to the 1950–9 period, and control for parity, made no difference to this result.

TABLE 14.3 *Numbers of stillbirths and deaths from anencephalus, mortality rate per 1000 births and male proportion by maternal ethnic origin, 14 Canadian cities 1950–9*

Ethnic Origin	Number	Anencephalus rate	Male Proportion
France	255	1.56	0.29
Ireland	153	1.50	0.28
England and Wales	319	1.44	0.28
Scotland	132	1.22	0.24
Mediterranean	34	1.14	0.44
Germany	128	0.97	0.25
Scandinavia	31	0.90	0.16
Central Europe	47	0.90	0.40
Oriental	13	0.88	0.54
Other	18	0.67	0.50
Russia	36	0.64	0.25

Weighted correlation coefficient = -0.39 $p>0.2$.
Ethnic origin defined as in Table 11.1.

Effects of length of gestation

The male proportion increases with gestational age and birth weight. In the Canadian 14-city study, the male proportion increased steadily from 0.26 in anencephalics delivered at under 33 weeks of gestation to 0.37 at 42 or more weeks of gestation. Consequentially, the male proportion is usually higher in infant deaths than in stillbirths (Böök and Rayner 1950; MacMahon and McKeown 1952; Coffey and Jessop 1957; MacMahon *et al.* 1953; Laurence *et al.* 1968). Most surveys of liveborn anencephalics show male proportions between 0.4 and 0.5. Naggan (1971) found no difference in the male proportion (0.44) between liveborn and stillborn anencephalics in Israel, while Czeizel and Révész (1970) found a male proportion of 0.32 in both live and stillborn anencephalics in Hungary. Such results could be due to under-reporting of early stillbirths, but in Naggan's study the total stillbirth rate was not lower than expected. MacMahon and McKeown (1952) suggested that the change in sex ratio with gestational age is due to the earlier onset of hydramnios in the mothers of female anencephalics, and MacMahon *et al.* (1953) recorded hydramnios in 45 per cent of mothers of female anencephalics and in 35 per cent of mothers of males. In pregnancies without hydramnios there was a decrease in the male proportion with increasing gestational age. Under-reporting of early stillbirths may be a factor leading to high male proportions in some surveys, such as the early study of Böök and Rayner (1950), the questionnaire-based study of Frézal *et al.* (1964), and the small hospital study of Jones (1967).

Secular variation

Rogers and Morris (1973) reported a secular increase since 1968 in the male proportion of anencephalus in England and Wales, Scotland, and Northern Ireland. This was due to the female mortality rate falling with little concomitant change in the male anencephalic mortality rate. Leck (1972) demonstrated that the short-term rise in the prevalence of anencephalus in Birmingham during 1955–9 occurred only in females. Similarly, in New York State the variations in the prevalence rates for anencephalus from 1945 to 1971 were much more marked for females although the secular trends in spina bifida rates were similar in the two sexes (Janerich 1975).

In Canada, in our studies of both the whole country and the selected 14 cities we found a slight increase in the male proportion of anencephalics over time. Annual sex specific mortality rates from anencephalus in Canada from 1943 to 1970 are shown (Fig. 14.2) on a semi-logarithmic scale so that the same proportionate decrease in rate is shown by the same slope. It is evident that the secular trends are very similar for each sex and in particular the period of high mortality from 1950 to 1954 is seen in both sexes. The slope of the fitted linear regression line is greater for females than for males, but the difference is not statistically significant ($0.1 > p > 0.05$). Thus although there is a small increase in the male proportion over time no striking differences in the female and male trends are evident.

Birth order and season of birth

In the case-control study of 1391 anencephalics and 5000 control livebirths in 14 Canadian cities, the mortality rate from anencephalus varied by year and season of birth, maternal city of residence, maternal ethnic origin, and with the maternal history of livebirths, stillbirths, and infant deaths. These factors, and others having no association with anencephalus risk such as maternal age, legitimacy and plurality of birth, were examined with reference to the sex distribution of the anencephalus cases. There was no variation in sex distribution with maternal city of residence. The male proportion showed a small non-significant increase over time, conforming with the trend shown in the national data. In first births the mortality rate from anencephalus was higher and the male proportion (0.27) was significantly lower than at higher birth orders (0.44). This difference has been shown elsewhere (McKeown and Lowe 1951; MacMahon and McKeown 1952; MacMahon *et al.* 1953; Edwards 1958), although it is not seen in Belfast (Elwood, J. H. 1970). In the Canadian data the difference was seen with reference to the number of previous livebirths; despite the greatly increased risk of anencephalus to infants of women who had had a previous stillbirth or infant death, the sex distribution did not vary with these factors.

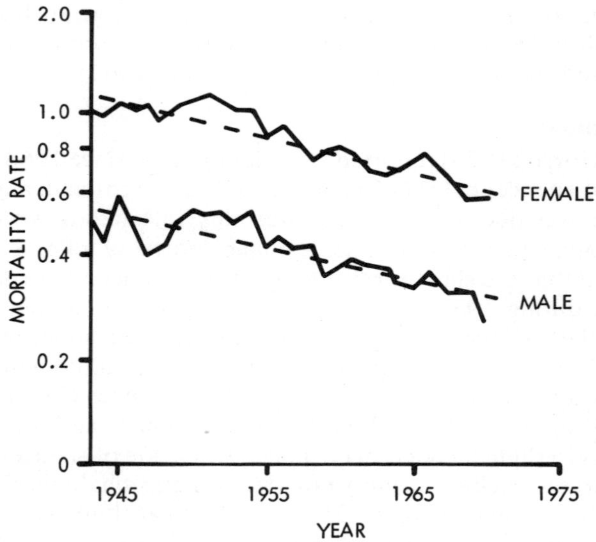

FIG. 14.2. Annual mortality rates (stillbirths and infant deaths) per 1000 total births attributed to anencephalus by sex—Canada 1943–70. (Courtesy of Academic Press.)

The prevalence of anencephalus was higher in winter births and this relationship was modified by birth order, being restricted to first births. However in both first and later births the male proportion is similar in anencephalics born in winter and in summer; hence any seasonal factor is modified by birth order but not by sex. Of the ten factors studied the sex distribution of anencephalus varies with only three, namely year of birth, birth order, and ethnic origin.

Interpretation

In British and European populations the male proportion of anencephalus appears to be higher in communities having a low prevalence rate at birth.

However, this trend is not seen in comparisons of different provinces of Canada nor is it discernible by comparison of reports from different areas of the United States. Nonetheless, there are variations in the sex distribution of anencephalus between different ethnic groups in Canada, although a consistent association with the mortality rate has not been shown. The suggestion of an inverse association between anencephalus prevalence and male proportion was made originally on the basis of comparisons between different ethnic groups residing in the same area—Singapore, Boston, or Israel (Searle 1959; Naggan and MacMahon 1967; Naggan 1971). If such an inverse association did hold specifically between ethnic groups it might explain the observations that a negative association between prevalence and male proportion is seen when countries of Europe or regions of the British Isles are compared, as their place of residence is strongly related to ethnic origin, and yet is not seen if different areas of Canada and the United States are compared, as in these countries geographical region is a poor indicator of ethnic distribution. Clearly more data are required to explore this possibility. If this were the case, it would suggest that the factors influencing sex distribution were closely related to those responsible for ethnic differences, while the factors governing geographical differences in prevalence independently of ethnic origin have no effect on the sex distribution.

An inverse association between the male proportion and prevalence rate with respect to secular trends was suggested by Janerich (1975) and is supported by the data from New York State, Birmingham (Leck 1972), England and Wales (Rogers and Morris 1973), and the whole of Canada. However, while in Canada there was a slight increase in the male proportion over time, this was of a similar size in British Columbia where there was no decrease in the mortality rate, as in Quebec where there was a large decrease in prevalence. Over the time period of the epidemic in Boston and Providence (MacMahon and Yen 1971) there was no change in the sex distribution of anencephalus (Yen 1975). It appears that secular variations in prevalence rates and in sex distribution may not be consistently linked but may occur coincidentally.

It is conceivable that the female excess seen in anencephalus and in spina bifida could represent only a phenotype but chromosomal studies confirm that female anencephalics are genotypically female (Nakano 1973, Polani and Claireaux 1959, Polani 1959). Anencephalics as presently recorded represent those which have survived to 20 or 28 weeks of gestation. Thus a female excess at this time may represent either more females being affected, or more males being lost before this gestational age. Polani (1959) studied six early abortuses with anencephalus and all had a male chromosome configuration, and Bell and Gosden (1978) reported on 15 spontaneous abortuses with neural-tube defects of which nine were male and six female, including a probable case of Turner's syndrome. Creasy and Alberman (1976) report 11 abortuses of over 30 mm crown–rump length with neural-tube defects, five being male, four female, and two of unknown sex, and in preliminary data from a large study of all spontaneous abortuses seen at

Vancouver General Hospital, British Columbia, Poland and Harris (1978) describe 35 with neural-tube defects of whom seven were male, 11 female, and three had triploid configuration; a further 14 could not be classified. In total these studies describe 48 affected spontaneous abortuses of known sex of which 27 (56 per cent) were male, suggesting that the female excess seen in registered stillbirths and livebirths with neural-tube defects may be due to the abortion rate before 20 weeks of gestation being greater for affected males than for females.

Female foetal rats are more sensitive to the teratogenic effects of acetazolamide than are males (Scott, Butcher, Kindt, and Wilson 1972), illustrating that sex modification of the effects of a teratogen does occur. Janerich (1975) hypothesizes that if anencephalus is caused by a deficiency of gonadotrophins, a female foetus may be more sensitive to such deficiency because in normal pregnancies the levels of chorionic gonadotrophins are higher in both maternal serum (Brody and Carlström 1965) and in amniotic fluid (Younglai and Lin 1973) if a female foetus is being carried. Other possible reasons for the female predominance involve genetic mechanisms. The hypothesis of multifactorial inheritance, in its simple form, does not explain the observed sex distribution. It predicts that siblings of male cases should be more often affected than those of female cases, and also that the male proportion should be greater in areas of high prevalence. The first of these predictions is not supported by observation (Section 26) while the evidence about the second is equivocal. Knox (1970) proposed a sex-linked genetic model which is compatible with a large female excess but again this hypothesis in its original form is not supported by the Canadian observations (Section 27). A modification of this hypothesis involving interaction of the foetus with tissue derived from a previous pregnancy (Knox 1974) predicts that the sex distribution of the births immediately preceding an anencephalic birth should vary with the sex of the anencephalic. This was suggested by the data of Record and McKeown (1950) but is not seen in the study by Carter *et al.* (1968) as discussed by Clarke, Hobson, McKendrick, Rogers, and Sheppard (1975*a*). Clarke *et al.* also propose a hypothesis based on interactions with a cell rest from the previous pregnancy, and this interaction between the cell rest and the subsequent conceptus may be more severe if the two elements are of unlike sex; if cell rests, like hydatidiform moles, are mostly female, then male foetuses will be more severely affected and thus more often aborted than are female foetuses.

Thus one of the most consistent observations on the epidemiology of anencephalus and spina bifida, namely the marked female predominance in most Caucasian populations, remains unexplained. If as we have suggested the sex distribution is more closely linked to ethnic rather than geographical factors, the explanation may lie in a complex genetic model rather than in a sex-specific environmental teratogen. The sex distribution is one of the few factors by which anencephalus and spina bifida differ. Further study of the several hypotheses already proposed may provide some clarification.

VIII

Environmental factors

ALTHOUGH the cause of the great majority of birth defects is largely unknown, the importance of environmental factors has been highlighted by the relationship between intrauterine viral infection with rubella and infant cataracts first recognized by Gregg (1941), and the epidemic of limb-reduction deformities in newborns whose mothers had taken thalidomide, a presumed harmless sedative drug, during pregnancy (Lenz 1961; McBride 1961). Animal research has demonstrated convincingly that mammalian embryos are susceptible to environmental agents (Shepard, Miller, and Marois 1975; Wilson 1977). As the human foetus cannot be studied under controlled conditions akin to those of the teratology laboratory, epidemiological observations relating birth-defect occurrences to postulated causative agents in the environment are particularly important from the viewpoint of elucidating aetiology and to protect the community from future harmful effects. Investigation of suspected environmental factors is fraught with problems of which one of the most difficult is assessing the timing of human embryogenesis. The so-called critical periods have a considerable range of variation and estimates of the time of conception often are inaccurate owing to unreliable histories given by a significant proportion of women. Storage of drugs, chemicals, or infectious agents in tissues may mean that the time of initiation of embryological defect and exposure are not coincident and this may mask a real causal association. We now consider some of the pertinent epidemiological evidence concerning associations of anencephalus and spina bifida with the taking of drugs during pregnancy, socio-economic status and occupation, maternal infections, and the composition of food and water. Lastly we look briefly at the concept of time–space clustering of these defects which relates to the classic epidemiology of infections and crowd diseases as described by Greenwood (1935) and others.

15

Drug use and maternal illness in pregnancy

AVAILABLE reports associating the taking of drugs specifically during pregnancy and subsequent occurrence of anencephalus and spina bifida are mostly non-specific. Obtaining satisfactory relevant data in human populations is extremely difficult even for drugs obtained by medical prescription and is virtually non-existent in relation to the large number of drugs self-prescribed and purchased directly from pharmacies or shops. Further complicating factors are the numerous brand names and combinations of different drugs contained in one tablet favoured by the pharmaceutical industry. Wilson (1977*a*) estimates that around 5 per cent of developmental defects in man today may be attributable to drugs and environmental chemicals. In some surveys, mothers of anencephalics reported having taken drugs of all types, including non-prescription drugs, more frequently than controls but no one specific type was identified (Laurence *et al.* 1968; Clarke, McKendrick, and Sheppard 1973; Clarke *et al.* 1975). Richards (1969) found mothers of anencephalics in South Wales stated they took salicylates in early pregnancy more often than did controls. The reports by Thiersch (1952, 1956) and others (Melzer 1956; Warkany, Beaudry, and Hornstein 1959; Emerson 1962) implicating amniopterin, a powerful folic antagonist sometimes taken by women to induce abortion, confirms drug teratogenicity and this also applies to antimitotic cancer chemotherapeutic agents such as methotrexate (Milunsky and Gaynor 1968) and busulfan (Abramovici, Shaklai, and Pinkhas 1978) which cause acute biochemical disturbance. Woman taking oral contraceptives have elevated vitamin-A levels and Gall (1972) has suggested on the basis of animal data, that excessive doses of the fat-soluble vitamins A, D, and K may be dangerous to the foetus. Much greater doses of the water soluble vitamin-B compounds and vitamin C appear non-toxic. Anencephalus and spina bifida do not form a predominant part of the spectrum of abnormalities described in the foetal alcohol syndrome (Jones, Smith, Ulleland, and Streissguth 1973), in the offspring of epileptic women taking lysergic acid diethylamide (Smithells 1976), or of women taking warfarin (Pettifor and Benson 1975; Warkany 1975). One case of anencephalus in association with cleft lip and palate out of a series of nine malformed infants born to mothers taking a number of anticonvulsive drugs was reported by Biale, Lewenthal, and Aderet (1975).

There do, however, seem to be stronger grounds for implicating the use of sex hormones with occurrences of birth defects (Nora and Nora 1973, 1975) due to inadvertently taking oral contraceptives during early pregnancy.

Although these drugs are the most widely used hormone preparations they are not associated with an increased frequence of anencephalus and spina bifida. Nora and Nora's first report (1973) described ten children having multiple congenital defects involving the vertebrae, anus, cardiac system, trachea and oesophagus, renal system, and limbs (the VACTERL syndrome) and two children with the Di George syndrome whose mothers had taken either oestrogen–progestogen or progestogen-only compounds in early pregnancy. A study of 7723 infants in the Greater Boston area whose mothers had reported using oral contraceptives concluded that these drugs present no major teratologic hazard (Rothman and Louik 1978). Gal, Kirman, and Stern (1967) obtained histories of drug ingestion retrospectively from 100 mothers of spina bifida infants and 100 matched controls. Some 19 women in the study group compared with 4 controls reported having taken a hormonal pregnancy test during the second to eleventh week of foetal life. The usual test was one tablet orally for two or three successive days, these tablets containing relatively large doses of synthetic hormones. For example, Primodos has 10 mg of norethisterone acetate and 0.02 mg of ethinyloestradiol while one tablet of Amenorone Forte contains 50 mg of ethisterone and 0.05 mg of ethinyloestradiol. This significant finding was later confirmed with respect to neural-tube defects (Gal, Sharman, and Pryse-Davies 1972) and it now appears also to relate to congenital heart disease (Levy, Cohen, and Fraser 1973). A few authors have published negative findings (Laurence, Miller, Vowles, Evans, and Carter 1971), but the United Kingdom Committee on Safety of Medicines (1975) issued a circular recommending that these hormone preparations be no longer used (Greenberg, Inman, Weaterall, Adelstein, and Haskey 1977). Synthetic progesterone preparations are sometimes prescribed during pregnancy for threatened or habitual abortion (Roberts and West 1977) but there is no evidence of their effectiveness and foetal virilization and teratogenesis may occur in any subsequent offspring (Shearman and Garrett 1963).

Clomiphene, a drug used to increase the release of pituitary gonadotrophins and hence to stimulate ovulation may produce multiple ovulation and sometimes multiple pregnancy. A number of cases of neural-tube defects in offspring of mothers who had received clomiphene have been observed (Dyson and Kohler 1973; Barrett and Hakim 1973; Sandler 1973; Field and Kerr 1974*a*; Nevin and Harley 1976; Ahlgren, Källén, and Rannevik 1976). Any real association between usage of this drug and an increased malformation risk has not yet been conclusively demonstrated as the reported cases may be due to chance association only (Elwood, J. M. 1974*a*). The prospective studies of pregnancies preceded by clomiphene therapy find low malformation rates (Goldfarb, Morales, Rakoff, and Protos 1968; Hack, Brish, Serr, Insler, Salmony, and Lunenfeld 1972) but as James (1977) points out, these women are self-selected usually on the basis of subfertility. If anencephalus and spina bifida are more common in subfertile women a spurious association with this drug would be expected. Furthermore, there is some evidence that the subfertile patients described may have a high spontaneous abortion rate and not necessarily a true below-average conception rate. Of the seven prior pregnancies not preceded by clomiphene therapy and considered by James (1977), two resulted in spontaneous abortion, two were anencephalic and there were three normal livebirths. As just described, hormone imbalance produced by ingesting high doses of synthetic preparations in early pregnancy for the purpose of a diagnostic test seems to be teratogenic hence hormone imbalance associated with subfertility or conditions such as the Stein–Leventhal syndrome (Barrett and Hakim 1973) may predispose to foetal malformation in any future pregnancy. A study of 414 sibships in which at least one infant (stillbirths plus deaths) had anencephalus or spina bifida and a random sample of 1362 unaffected sibships in British Columbia showed that the affected sibships were larger (Elwood, J. M. and McBride 1979). Furthermore, there were more births than expected after the affected birth and shorter intervals between births prior to the affected births. Thus mothers of anencephalic and spina bifida infants appear to have higher fertility than comparison mothers in this province of Canada.

It has been suggested that anaesthetic agents may be associated with an increased risk of neural-tube defects and also of spontaneous abortion and involuntary infertility based on surveys of operating room personnel. An increased incidence of cleft palate in C-57 black mice exposed to halothane has been reported (Smith, Usubiaga, and Lehrer 1971), but most teratological work so far has not demonstrated large increases in embryotoxicity in relation to anaesthetic agents such as nitrous oxide or methoxyflurane (Corbett, Beaudoin, Cornell, Endres, and Page 1974). A national study of occupational disease among operating-room personnel was made by mail questionnaire in the United States based on 49 585 exposed and 23 911 unexposed individuals (American Society of Anesthesiologists 1974). Women exposed to operating room conditions exhibited higher rates of congenital defects, cancer, hepatic disease, renal disease, and spontaneous abortion. An above-average malformation rate also was found in unexposed wives of male anaesthetists. Among the offspring of exposed nurse-anaesthetists and female physician-anaesthetists there was a 60 per cent ($p=0.01$) and 100 per cent ($p=0.13$) increase of congenital abnormalities respectively; for children born to the wives of exposed male physician-anaesthetists the increase was 25 per cent ($p=0.04$). Cohen, Bellville, and Brown (1971) reported increased spontaneous abortion rates in operating-room staff but the numbers of malformed infants are too small to permit any valid conclusions. Corbett, Cornell, Endres, and Lieding (1974) surveyed 621 nurse-anaesthetists and found of those continuing to work during pregnancy 16.4 per cent had malformed children compared with 5.7 per cent in those who did not work during their pregnancies; this difference is significant ($p<0.005$). From the findings of these and other investigations (Askrog and Harvald 1970, Knill-Jones, Rodrigues, Moir, and Spence 1972) it seems teratogenic effects may result from anaesthetic gases or from other factors common to operating-room staff. A second national study in the United

States is planned for 1978. Some supporting data have been reported from India (Mikakhur 1978) and England (Pharoah, Alberman, and Chamberlain 1977). Also, Tomlin (1978, 1978*a*) described five children having serious congenital abnormalities of the central nervous system or musculoskeletal system whose fathers were anaesthetists in the Birmingham area and suggested they may be linked to occupational exposure to waste pollutant gases. These conclusions have been questioned and in another study Knill-Jones, Newman, and Spence (1975) found no excess of major congenital malformations among 5175 offspring of British male anaesthetists. The malformations described are not homogeneous and cover a wide spectrum of unrelated defects, some probably acquired such as hydrocephalus secondary to meningitis and others are known metabolic conditions (McPherson, Smith, and Vessey 1978; Rushton 1978). The case, therefore, implicating waste anaesthetic gases as teratogenic is unproven but requires further study.

Smoking

While an association between maternal smoking and low birth-weight probably is causal and now well authenticated, there are only a few studies which have examined the possibility of a relationship with birth defects. Three report associations between maternal smoking and neural-tube defects. Andrews and McGarry (1972) found increased frequencies not only of neural-tube defects but also of gastrointestinal defects and cleft lip and palate in smokers compared to non-smokers. A Canadian survey noted more neural-tube defects occurred in births to women who were heavy smokers (Choi and Klaponski 1970). A case–control study based on several hospitals in Connecticut estimated that women who smoked more than 20 cigarettes per day during pregnancy had a relative risk of 1.6 for congenital defects in their offspring compared with women who did not smoke at all during pregnancy (Kelsey, Dwyer, Holford, and Bracken 1978). For anencephalus, spina bifida, and hydrocephalus the relative risks were 1.3 and 1.8 for women smoking 1 to 20 cigarettes a day and 21 or more cigarettes a day during pregnancy respectively. These risks remained after controlling for maternal age, parity, and social class in the analysis. Kelsey and colleagues calculated from their data that if cigarette smoking was causally related to congenital malformations of all types the population attributable risk would be 3 per cent assuming a relative risk among all smokers of 1.1 or alternatively a relative risk of 1.6 among smokers of more than 20 cigarettes daily and no increased risk compared with non-smokers for women who smoke less than 20 cigarettes daily. This effect, even if accepted, is small.

Maternal illness

Regarding maternal illnesses or other exposures, there is little firm evidence definitely relating such events during pregnancy with anencephalus or spina bifida. Richards (1969) noted a higher frequency of accidents during pregnancy. Several studies have found no increased incidence after exposure to X-rays (Record and McKeown 1949; Laurence *et al.* 1968; Smithells *et al.* 1964; Böök and Rayner 1950; Richards 1969). Infants born to women having diabetes mellitus are reported to have an excess of congenital malformations including neural-tube defects. Soler, Walsh, and Malins (1976) studied 701 such infants born in Birmingham between 1950 and 1974; 8.1 per cent had some type of anomaly, a rate three to four times higher than in the normal population. This agrees with findings from Copenhagen (Molsted-Pedersen, Tygstrup, and Pedersen 1964) but other investigators have not observed this relationship (Farquhar 1965; Richards 1969). Wilson and Vallance-Owen (1966) found 13 of 14 mothers of infants with spina bifida had increased antagonism to insulin associated with plasma albumin compared to 14 of 50 control mothers of similar age and parity. Kučera (1971) collected information on 7101 foetuses and infants delivered to women having diabetes mellitus from 47 reports in the literature; some 340 (4.8 per cent) had some type of congenital defect compared with 7124 (1.7 per cent) abnormal infants out of 431 764 control births (live and still) from the World Health Organization survey (Stevenson *et al.* 1966) which he selected as a comparison group. Although anencephalus occurred in births to diabetics the question of whether diabetic mothers have an increased risk of a specific type of congenital defect in their offspring is unclear. The caudal regression syndrome, also called the diabetic embryopathy syndrome (Williamson 1970), is a possibility (Assemany, Muzzo, and Gardner 1972); this comprises aplasia of the femora, agenesis of the lumbar and sacral vertebrae, joint abnormalities, and other defects of the ear, mouth, and palate and sometimes the humerus. Owing to this rather involved picture it follows that reports implicating oral hypoglycaemic agents as teratogenic are difficult to interpret even though these drugs are embryotoxic in mice, rats, and rabbits (Wilson 1973). Insulin also is teratogenic in some animals but not in man unless the individual has experienced insulin coma psychiatric therapy (Wilson 1973).

Blood groups

The small amount of work examining maternal blood groups has not produced any striking findings although only ABO and Rh groups have been considered to date. Coffey and Jessop (1957) reported an excess of group-O and a deficiency of group-B mothers having anencephalic infants compared to a control group, but other studies have not confirmed these differences (Smithells *et al.* 1964; Smithells and Chin 1965; Wilson 1971). Investigations of Rh groups suggest that there may be an excess of negative individuals among women having children with spina bifida but the data are inconclusive.

Hyperthermia

Two studies from Seattle describe a possible association between pyrexia in early pregnancy and neural-tube defects (Smith, Clarren, and Harvey 1978;

Miller, Smith, and Shepard 1978). Smith and colleagues examined retrospectively a sample of mothers ascertained by reporting a positive history of pyrexia of 38.9 °C or over during early pregnancy; their offspring had a high prevalence of neural-tube defects, but a small number of mothers ascertained prospectively and having hyperthermia from pyelitis had no neural-tube defects in subsequent births. Miller and colleagues compared retrospectively 63 mothers of anencephalic infants with a control group comprising 64 relatives or female friends. Some 7 per cent out of the 63-case group reported a positive history of fever in pregnancy due to febrile illness (five cases) or sauna bathing (two cases) and none of the control group reported any such events. Heat stress induces neurological defects in animals (Section 2). However, the prevalence rates of anencephalus in Finland and Sweden, where sauna bathing is popular, are among the lowest in the world for Caucasian populations. This hypothesis, although interesting, requires other supporting evidence of a causal relationship before any counselling is given to patients and the general public (Lancet 1978*a*). A small retrospective Canadian study compared the incidence of febrile episodes in early and in late pregnancy in women having infants with a variety of malformations and found an excess of early fever only in mothers of infants with microphthalmia (Fraser and Skelton 1978). Infections such as influenza would produce hyperthermia (Chance and Smith 1978) as would certain occupations such as laundry work (James 1978*a*); McDonald (1958) comments on the latter in her survey (27 laundry workers having four affected births each with different defects—one anencephalus, one hypospadias, one congenital heart disease, and one hydrocephalus) and there is no specificity for anencephalus rather than any other defect.

16

Socio-economic status and occupation

STEVENSON, statistician at the General Register Office, London, devised a social class classification in 1911 which has been used extensively to examine disease trends in the United Kingdom. This system divides the population into five social classes depending on two criteria relating to the head of the household namely, occupation and general standing in the community. Non-working wives take the social class of their husband, single working women of their father, children of their father, and certain groups such as members of the Armed Forces are separately classified; illegitimate births and the unemployed are not included. The classification has been used by the Registrar General since the census of England and Wales in 1921. These five social classes are:

Class I	Higher professional and administrative occupations
Class II	Other professions
Class III	Skilled workers (manual and non-manual)
Class IV	Semi-skilled workers
Class V	Unskilled workers

This arbitrary division takes no account of personal circumstances or life-style. Various modifications of this system have been made and other countries have similar classifications usually related to income or educational attainment. Social class and socio-economic status are, however, theoretical concepts still awaiting clear definition (MacMahon and Pugh 1970). Investigations, therefore, should use any social class gradients found with respect to a particular condition or disease as a starting point for formulating more specific hypotheses and not as an end result *per se.* An association with social class may arise by a direct relationship to one of many factors: occupation is one important component and others include the frequency of infections, chronic illnesses, parasitic infestation, spontaneous abortion, age at marriage, use of contraception, spacing of births, alcohol consumption, smoking, and exposure to atmospheric pollution and many other toxins. The early recognition of marked social class effects for infections like tuberculosis where the mortality rates are higher in classes IV and V compared with classes I and II demonstrate strong environmental effects. Thus if a condition of unknown aetiology exhibits a similar trend by social class, a search for environmental causes may be fruitful.

Most studies in the British Isles show anencephalus and spina bifida to be more common in the lower socio-economic groups (Williamson 1965; Richards, Roberts, and Lloyd 1972; Elwood, J. H., and Nevin 1973; Carter and Evans 1973). The range of risk is from two- to fourfold in social classes IV and V births compared with births to women of classes I and II who have the lowest risk. Similar trends are seen in Boston (Naggan and MacMahon 1967) based on a classification according to father's occupation (Warner, Meeker, and Eelis 1957) and in Montreal (Horowitz and McDonald 1969) based on a classification according to mean rental of census tracts (Fig. 16.1). Blishen's (1967) socio-economic index is commonly adopted to examine social class effects in Canada. Several authors have demonstrated that this social class effect persists after controlling for maternal age and parity, geographical region, and ethnic group (Richards *et al.* 1972; Fedrick 1970; Naggan and MacMahon 1967), but no investigator has found a particular aetiological agent to account for this social class association. Several suggest poor nutrition is a likely factor. Baird (1974) and Emanuel and Sever (1973) implicate poor nutrition in the mother's childhood as a cause of increased risk of bearing an anencephalic infant throughout life and stress the observation that mothers of anencephalics are of shorter stature than others, even within the same social group. It might be expected that in a population where nutrition did not vary with social class there would be no social class effect, and the lack of an association between anencephalus prevalence and father's occupation in Israel (Naggan 1971) and in Jews in Boston (Naggan and MacMahon 1967) in interesting. However, in Israel this lack of association may reflect absence of concordance between current social class and that in childhood typical of a new innovative society, while in the Boston data the number of Jewish cases is too small to estimate reliably class-specific rates. Anencephalus is more common in the lower socio-economic groups in Taiwan (Emanuel and Sever 1973) and probably also in Japan. This is interesting as a socio-economic gradient might be expected to be absent in a low prevalence area. Imaizumi (1974) divided his data into six classes based on the occupation of the head of the household. These were: Class I, agriculture only; Class II, agriculture with other work; Class III, self-employed; Class IV, white collar; class V, blue collar; and Class VI, other. The lowest mortality rate from anencephlus was in class II and the highest in class IV while for spina bifida the highest rate was in class I and the lowest in class III. An exception to most British studies is that of Record and McKeown (1949) who found no social class effect in Birmingham. This survey did not adopt the Registrar General's social class classification but used a classification of city wards into three social groups depending on a sanitary index, average rateable value, housing densities, and population densities for each ward. Leck (1972) also observed no significant social class gradient in the frequencies of neural-tube defects but cases were less common in the professional and managerial classes in Birmingham at the time of the study.

Fedrick (1976) examined the occupational component in her Oxford survey by comparing the occupations of the index fathers as described on the birth certificates of 151 anencephalics and the occupations of all fathers in the same area during the period 1965–71. Although numbers are small there was a significantly higher risk in offspring of fathers working in the paper and printing trades (relative risk of 6.72), painters and decorators, transport workers who were mainly truck drivers, and members of the Armed Forces. These occupations associated with an above-average risk possibly point to some chemical or toxic agent being involved. Aylett (1973, 1974) a family doctor in Corsham, Wiltshire, found that in a localized outbreak of 18

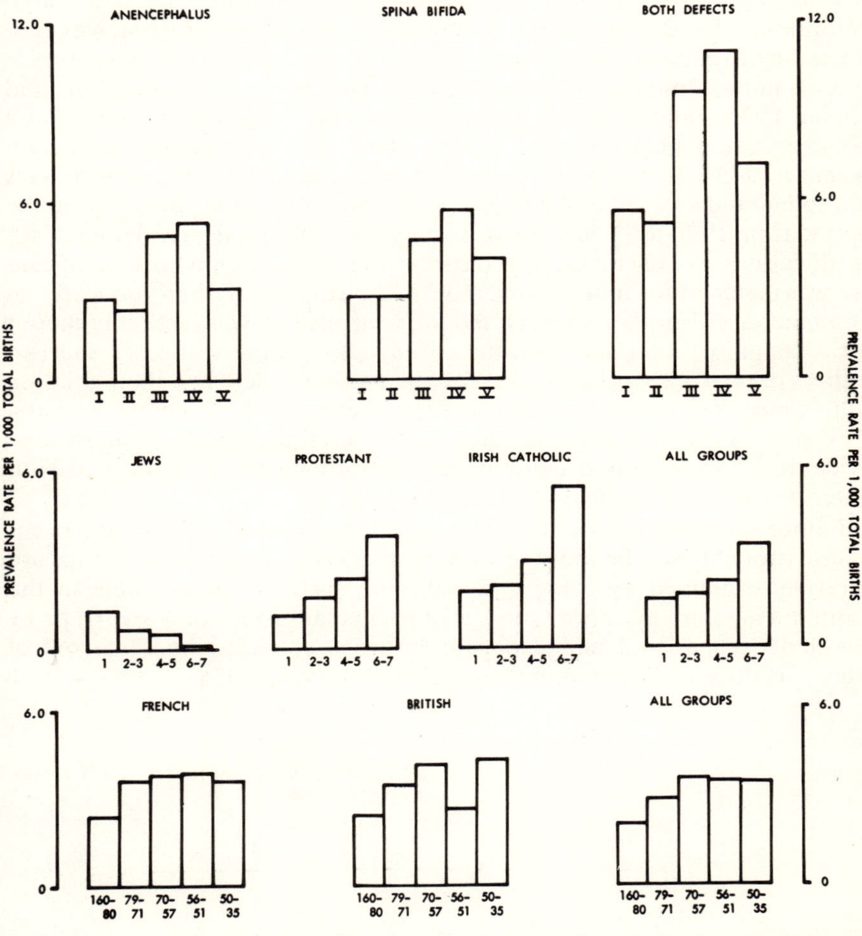

FIG. 16.1. *Top*: socio-economic gradients associated with anencephalus, spina bifida, and both defects combined in Belfast 1964–8 (Registrar General's social-class classification); *middle*; for both defects combined in different ethnic groups in Boston 1930–65 (Naggan and MacMahon 1967; classification by occupation from Warner *et al*. 1957); and *bottom*: for both defects combined in different ethnic groups in Montreal 1961–5 (classification by mean rental of census tract; Horowitz and McDonald 1969).

infants with anencephalus and spina bifida occurring in 979 births over five years, offspring of rubber workers had an increased risk. There were four cases of anencephalus alone, one case of anencephalus with spina bifida, five of spina bifida alone, seven of spina bifida with hydrocephalus, and one with hydrocephalus alone (Aylett, Robert, and Lloyd 1974). The conclusion is based on four out of these 18 infants (22 per cent) having fathers who worked with rubber, compared with an expected value of 6.3 per cent calculated from 150 male rubber workers living in Corsham out of a total male workforce of 2400. A matched case–control interview study examining the association of central nervous system malformations and vinyl-chloride-monomer exposure in Kanawha County, West Virginia, was conducted by Edmonds, Anderson, Flynt, and James (1978) following earlier reports in the United States of a possible relationship (Edmonds, Falk, and Nissim 1975; Infante 1976). There are some 40 polyvinylchloride (PVC) polymerization plants in the United States (Environmental Protection Agency 1975). Some 46 infants having neural-tube defects (anencephalus 23, spina bifida 15, other CNS defects 8) born in the study area during the period from 1970 to 1974 were ascertained from hospital records and death certifications. For each case two controls were selected from birth certificate records matched for four factors, month of birth, race, father's educational attainment, and mother's age. Of the two controls, one was randomly chosen for a telephone interview with the parents. Two fathers of cases and two fathers of controls worked at a PVC plant at the time when their children were conceived; none of the mothers in either group had ever worked at a PVC plant. Edmonds and colleagues concluded there was no demonstrable evidence of an increased neurological malformation rate associated with parental exposure to vinyl-chloride-monomer.

Future studies relating neural-tube defect prevalence and parental occupation probably will be more rewarding if specific occupational groups are carefully examined by using national data, such as are available in the United Kingdom, by cohort surveys of particular groups of workers, or by detailed occupational and exposure histories collected by case–control studies (Office of Population Censuses and Surveys 1978).

17

Infections

THE possible role of maternal infections in early pregnancy in causing neural-tube defects has been investigated epidemiologically by three methods: case–control studies of mothers of affected infants and comparison groups of mothers, cohort studies in which one group of mothers has a history of a specific infection or a symptomatic illness, and by examination of time association between epidemics of infectious diseases and neural tube defect prevalence. More indirect evidence of a possible infectious aetiology in man is given by studies of clustering in time and space and from laboratory experiments. One of the most closely examined defects is the rubella syndrome, which, however, does not include anencephalus and spina bifida (Gregg 1941; Dudgeon 1976). The influenza virus has been extensively studied both in laboratory animals and in man.

Failure of the neural tube to close occurs in chick embryos inoculated with influenza A virus when two days old (Hamburger and Habel 1947). Viral antigens have not been found in the affected neural tissues but they are identifiable in the chorion and amnion and at a later stage of embryogenesis in the extraneural ectoderm and gut; the infected tissues, however, are not malformed hence influenza virus infection may act by altering metabolic pathways essential for neural-tube closure (Johnston, Klasnja, and Johnston 1971. Sever, J. L. (1975) noted that although a number of infectious agents can reach the human foetus only five have been shown to produce congenital malformations in man. These are varicella, rubella, cytomegalovirus, herpes virus hominis, and Venezuela equine encephalitis virus and none of the associated increased birth defect frequencies includes anencephalus and spina bifida. The only other agent producing neural-tube defects in animals apart from influenza A is Newcastle disease virus. This again causes failure of neural-tube closure in chicks (Robertson, Williamson, and Blattner 1955) and antigen to this virus is found in cells of the caudal neural tube (Williamson, Blattner, and Robertson 1965).

How frequent are infections during pregnancy in women? The Collaborative Perinatal Research Study followed 60 000 pregnancies and found between 3 per cent and 22 per cent of mothers had infections ranging from cytomegalovirus (3–20 per cent), herpes virus hominis types I and II (0.15–1.5 per cent), epidemic rubella (2–4 per cent), non-epidemic rubella (0.1–0.2 per cent) toxoplasmosis, and syphilis (Kurent and Sever 1973). These in turn affected between 1.2 per cent and 3 per cent of foetuses and the most common were cytomegalovirus (1–2 per cent) and epidemic rubella (0.2–0.4 per cent). During non-epidemic rubella periods around one or two children for every 10 000 pregnancies were born with defects compatible with the rubella syndrome. There was no evidence from this work that prenatal infection played a prominent role in the causation of anencephalus and spina bifida. If we consider other epidemiolgical observations, Record and McKeown's (1949) survey of 755 infants with central nervous malformations in Birmingham found no reported cases of rubella, influenza, or other viral infection in pregnancies of either the case or the control mothers. This seems surprising, even if the mothers' exposure was similar to that of the whole population and suggests their method, namely retrospective inquiry from the mothers after delivery, may have been unsatisfactory.

Campbell (1953) in Belfast, used a prospective method by asking mothers attending antenatal clinics if they suffered from influenza between 15 December 1950 and 31 January 1951, during which time there was an influenza A epidemic. A symptom complex, including fever and muscle pains severe enough to require bed rest, was used to define the disease. The stillbirth and total abnormality rates of the 164 exposed mothers was greater than those of the non-exposed mothers. However, the malformation rate was not maximal when exposure was in the first or second month of pregnacy and was not specifically increased for any particular abnormality. Coffey and Jessop (1959) interviewed mothers after pregnancy and found more acute illnesses, of any type, during the first or second trimester in mothers of anencephalics than in controls. Laurence *et al.* (1968), conducting retrospective interviews in South Wales from 1960 to 1962, reported more episodes of 'influenza' in mothers of infants with neural-tube defects (30 of 551, compared with 4 of 277 controls). Richards (1969) using a similar method to study 279 cases born in South Wales in 1964 to 1966, found no association with illness in pregnancy, but identified positive associations with salicylate ingestion and poor diet. Choi *et al.* (1972) used retrospective interviews in a case–control study of 77 mothers of infants having neural-tube defects and 150 control mothers having unaffected offspring in Manitoba. There was a positive history of influenza during the first trimester for 13 out of the 77 (17 per cent) compared with four out of the 150 controls (3 per cent); this difference is statistically significant. Walker and McKee (1959), in Iowa, used post-delivery interviews and post-delivery estimations of haemagglutination-inhibition titre to measure exposure to Asian influenza amongst 398 mothers and found no difference in the prevalence of anomalies between mothers with and without histories of symptomatic infection. Wilson *et al.* (1959) adopted similar methods prospectively to study 126 mothers in Los Angeles with similar negative results. In this survey there was no significant correlation between antibody titre levels and clinical symptoms, while in Walker and McKee's survey 98 per cent of mothers with symptoms (158) had positive titres, but so did all of another group of 101 mothers irrespective of their history. Hardy, Azarowicz, Mannini, Medearis, and Cooke (1961) examined 671 mothers at pre-natal clinics in Baltimore during the period from 1957 to 1958, after the onset of the

Asian influenza epidemic. Each mother was questioned regarding influenza-like symptoms and blood tests for antigen to Asian influenza A were performed at each visit. Some 56 per cent of the mothers (375) reported having had clinical symptoms of whom 94 per cent were serologically positive; however 75 per cent of those who gave no history were also serologically positive. Using the serological criterion alone, the attack rate was so high that the unexposed group was quite small. Abortion and stillbirth rates, in those with serologically confirmed clinical influenza and in those with serological positive tests only, were higher than for the serologically negative group. Total malformation prevalence rates were 3.0, 5.9, and 1.3 per cent respectively. In relation to the stage of pregnancy at which infection occurred, the total malformation prevalence rates were 10.7, 4.3, and 2.5 per cent for the first, second, and third trimesters. Although these results are suggestive, none is statistically significant.

Three studies relying on a history of relevant symptoms obtained during the pre-natal period all refer to the Asian influenza epidemic of 1957 to 1958 in Great Britain. Pleydell (1960) found malformations in three (7 per cent) of 41 mothers who had had influenza compared to 14 (1 per cent) of 1030 mothers with no history of infection. Manson, Logan, and Loy (1960) reported malformation rates in 4.3 per cent of 163 mothers with influenza compared to 2.8 per cent of 5611 controls. Doll *et al.* (1960) studied 175 mothers who reported having had influenza and compared the stillbirth and malformation rates in those with influenza in the first trimester (3.2 per cent of 63 infants), those with influenza before the last menstrual period (3.0 per cent of 66), and in those who were classified as not having influenza on the basis of detailed inquiries (2.0 per cent of 48). Saxen, Hjelt, Sjostedt, Hadosalo, and Hadosalo (1960) surveyed a large number of mothers in Finland using antenatal inquiry. Amongst 446 exposed to influenza, as diagnosed clinically during the first trimester, the total anomaly prevalence was 2.9 per cent, compared to 1.6 per cent with second-trimester exposure, and 2.2 per cent of 2573 mothers with no exposure. These differences are not significant. McDonald (1958, 1961) investigated 3296 women interviewed at antenatal clinics in Watford and St Albans, England. The prevalence of major anomalies of all systems was 6.1 per cent in the 148 mothers who had a febrile illness in the first 12 weeks which was not significantly greater than the prevalence in mothers without illness.

The difficulties involved in such studies are serious. First, retrospective surveys requiring the mother to recall events some months previously are open to random error in recall, and also to bias, in that mothers of affected infants tend either to under or to over report symptoms. Prospective surveys have to be very large to include enough mothers in both the exposed and non-exposed groups. The definition of an infection and the criteria for exposure are difficult to judge. There is some evidence from these studies that spontaneous abortions are increased after a symptomatic infectious disease but the effect on the prevalence at birth of malformation is unclear.

Another approach is to examine changes in the malformation prevalence rates in the whole population after a major epidemic in which the attack rate is high. For example, in the study by Doll *et al.* (1960), the monthly anencephalic stillbirth rates in Scotland from 1950 to 1959 were higher in May to December 1958 and in April to July 1959; these authors concluded that the first peak was concordant with influenza epidemicity in August 1957 to April 1958. Record (1961) analysed the seasonal trends in the same data for the period from 1939 to 1958 in relation to the incidence of influenza and the notifiable infectious diseases reported eight months previously. The distributions of anencephalus conception dates and of measles and rubella incidence rates were similar, but this is regarded as coincidental in view of the many investigations of rubella teratogenesis, none of which has shown any association with neural-tube defects. Leck (1963) studied the prevalence of abnormalities in Birmingham 26 to 40 weeks after the major influenza epidemics in 1957, 1959, and 1961. This large study showed a significantly increased prevalence of cleft lip, oesophageal atresia, anal atresia, and exomphalos during the relevant time periods but no increase in the prevalence of neural-tube defects. The attack rate of influenza in Birmingham was estimated as 20 per cent. Leck also re-analysed the Scottish data for anencephalus used by Doll *et al.* (1960) taking more careful account of the seasonal trends in births, and concluded no increase occurred after these influenza epidemics. A further study by Leck (1971) analysed all types of congenital abnormalities occurring in all total births in relation to epidemics of influenza in Birmingham during the period from 1957 to 1962 and in England and Wales from 1965 to 1968. The data allowed separating infants born in high-risk periods into four groups by gestational age at the time of the influenza epidemic. Although increased frequencies of some defects were observed they were not restricted to infection at the critical gestational period for embryotoxicity with respect to the epidemic. The prevalence of anencephalus for example in the data for England and Wales was 1.3 per 1000 births during the high-risk period and 1.5 during the low-risk period. The Birmingham data exhibited a significant increase in the prevalence of cleft lip without cleft palate (0.7 per 1000 in the high-risk period and 0.4 in the low-risk period) but Leck concluded this association was unlikely to be causal.

In most of the case–control and cohort studies mentioned there was no control for socio-economic status. As this factor is likely to affect both the prevalence of abnormalities and of infectious disease, this means that even where a positive association is found it may reflect other variables related to socio-economic status, such as dietary differences. The studies of time trends in total populations avoid this problem, and thus the lack of association between influenza and neural-tube defect prevalence in the largest survey of this type (Leck 1963) provides good evidence that influenza does not contribute greatly to the total prevalence of these defects. However, several surveys do suggest a small increased risk of these defects after exposure to influenza, and the studies of population data cannot exclude this association.

The possible role of viral agents other than influenza has been little investigated. Those that have been studied do not manifest neural-tube defects as part of any syndrome complex. Microcephaly (South, Tompkins, Morris, and Rawls 1969) has been described in association with infection by herpes simplex. A large epidemic of echo 9 virus in Minnesota in 1957 did not result in an excess of malformed infants (Kleinman, Prince, Mathey, Rosenfield, Bearman, and Syverton 1962). Coxsackie B3 and B4 infections were thought to be associated with a small increase in cardiac defects by Brown and Evans (1967) based on 900 pregnancies observed over seven years. Suggestions that mumps virus is a cause of congenital defects have not been confirmed (Rhodes 1961). In 1974 a severe epizootic of bovine congenital arthrogryphosis and hydrancephaly in cattle occurred in New South Wales around the same time as a cluster of neural-tube defects in the human population (Field 1976). The animal infections were related to antibodies to akabane virus but viral studies of the mothers of malformed infants were negative. A prospective survey of 48 000 individuals has been reported from Finland (Koskimies, Lapinleimu, and Saxén 1978) in which 274 mothers of malformed children were found to have more seroconversions than 274 paired control mothers owing to an increase in infections by herpes complex viruses 1 and 2, cytomegalovirus, varicella-zoster virus, and toxoplasma. The case group also reported more diseases in total during pregnancy, a greater intake of drugs and a greater number of previous abortions.

Although work to date associating the occurrence of anencephalus and spina bifida with certain bacterial and viral infections has been essentially negative, it must be emphasized that studies designed to test this hypothesis are most difficult in practice. Apart from problems relating to the numbers of affected and non-affected pregnancies to be studied, the mother is often unaware of her pregnancy until after the first month of gestation by which time these defects have already occurred in the foetus. Until epidemiology and other disciplines can identify more closely possible teratogenic organisms, the microbiologist cannot be asked to screen the entire field of known bacteria and viruses.

Obviously, the causal relationship may be more complicated and perhaps involves infections during early childhood and not necessarily illness occurring during the affected pregnancy. Infection by a slow virus or an atypical reaction to a common agent such as measles and the later manifestation of subacute sclerosing panencephalitis and possibly multiple sclerosis are examples from other fields. It may be possible to obtain early abortuses from spontaneous or therapeutic abortions and to examine the products of conception at 4–8 weeks of gestational age. If an infectious aetiology is postulated then the causative organism should be present in an affected embryo of this age if anencephalus and spina bifida are initiated according to the generally accepted embryological timetable. A case–control study of such early affected and non-affected embryonic material taking great care to avoid secondary infection during the collection process might identify organisms present in the former but absent in the latter group. Such a study, although technically very difficult, would require only a small number of specimens to be examined. Replication also should not pose any great problem.

18

Diet

THERE is much evidence from laboratory experiments demonstrating the production of neurological malformations in animals by alteration of the diet (Warkany 1971; Lemire, Beckwith, and Warkany 1978). Factors implicated include both deficiencies and excesses of vitamins, trace elements, and other agents (Table 2.2). Epidemiological studies in man have considered aspects such as general calorie deficiency, food additives, ingestion of blighted potatoes, and tea drinking as well as attempting to confirm the findings of animal teratology in human populations.

Coffey and Jessop (1957) examined the mothers of 137 infants with anencephalus and 192 controls soon after delivery in Dublin. The mothers of anencephalics had lower haemoglobin and lower total plasma protein levels. These indices are very non-specific, and may only reflect a social class effect; more of the fathers of anencephalics than of control infants were unemployed. Richards (1969) in South Wales found mothers of infants with central nervous system defects more frequently reported a diet in the first trimester which was regarded as 'unbalanced' as compared to mothers of normal infants matched for age, parity, social class, area of residence, and date of delivery. These results were based on post-partum interviews and are thus open to considerable error in recall. The average weight of mothers of the anencephalics was greater than for the matched controls. An indirect approach to the dietary hypothesis was used by Knox (1972). He compared variations in the stillbirth rate attributed to anencephalus in England and Wales by year and season from 1961 to 1967 with data on the consumption of various foodstuffs, using intervals of five to nine months between consumption and month of birth. The problem of finding nominally statistically significant correlation coefficients by chance was dealt with by partitioning the association seen into three components namely, that part due to variation between years, between seasons (three month periods) and a residual covariance. Only if a correlation was found in each component as well as in the total was any causal association considered. Significant negative correlations were found with cheese, apples, and total meat consumption, suggesting a beneficial effect of higher protein intake or possibly a confounding effect of social class. Significant positive correlations were found between anencephalus prevalence and the consumption of large white bread loaves, total cereals, ice cream, canned peas, canned meat, cooked meats, and corned beef. Knox points out that preserved meat products contain nitrites and nitrates and suggests that the canning process may produce compounds similar to known carcinogens and teratogens. He shows the sharp drop in the consumption of cured meats after the Aberdeen typhoid outbreak in 1964 was associated with a drop in anencephalus prevalence, and also the regions of England and Wales with the highest rates of anencephalus also have high canned meat consumption.

Animal experiments readily demonstrate that restriction of total calorie intake, especially protein, leads to a reduced birth-weight, a reduced brain-weight and abnormal brain function (Dobbing 1974; Smart and Dobbing 1971). Human experiments along these lines, following strict scientific protocols, are not possible and the main body of data on man relates to examinations of prisoners of war and the experiences of communities during periods of wartime hardship. Thus, Antonov (1947) found that the mean birth-weight of infants born during the siege of Leningrad was 500 g below normal. If adequate food intake was consumed throughout the last trimester of pregnancy, even if restriction existed during the first and second trimesters, Smith (1947) observed that birth-weight was near normal. A survey of a large community who experienced the Dutch hunger winter of 1944–5 as a result of the Second World War has been reported (Stein, Susser, Saenger, and Marolla 1975, Stein and Susser 1976). The results are based on the study of a cohort of Dutch men born during the famine period and later called up at age 19 years for military service. Findings from psychological, medical, and physical examination carried out at the time of military induction were linked to nutritional deprivation in pregnancy and early life. A significant excess of central nervous system abnormalities was found in relation to severe famine exposure early in gestation. The relative risk was 2.0 based on eight cases of spina bifida and hydrocephalus ascertained compared to an expectation of four cases (Stein and Susser 1976). Although findings from this large study point towards some relationship between an increased neural-tube defect prevalence and maternal nutritional deprivation in early pregnancy, they must be heavily biased by survivorship into adult life as only a proportion of all male infants born during the Dutch hunger winter would have lived through this period. Also, no data on stillbirths in 1944–5 are available. We would expect the survival rate of male infants with malformations to be lower than those without malformations and if this were so, the relative risk reported would underestimate the true association. A test of the hypothesis that malnutrition early in the mother's life may lead to neural-tube defects in her offspring, as described in general terms by Baird (1973, 1974), Emanuel and Sever (1973), and Janerich (1972, 1972*a*), would be an analysis of pregnancy outcomes of women who had experienced the Dutch famine *in utero* or as young children. However, the study by Stein and colleagues considered only men and was not designed to test this hypothesis.

Hibbard and Smithells (1965) performed formiminoglutamic acid (FIGLU) excretion tests on the mothers of 73 infants with central nervous system abnormalities, delivered in Liverpool. Some 66 per cent of these mothers had test results showing folate deficiency. A subset of 35 mothers were matched with mothers of normal infants by age, parity and time of conception and gestation; in this group 69 per cent of the mothers of affected children compared with 17 per cent of mothers of normal children had folate deficiency. Leck, Iles, Sharman, Toe, and Wadsworth (1974) compared the blood levels of folate, vitamin A, and serum carotenoids in normal mothers in early pregnancy with the blood levels in the puerperium and with an estimate of intake taken from a dietary history in the puerperium. The correlation coefficients between the blood levels in early pregnancy and in the puerperium were fairly high (+0.50 or over) which suggests that measurements after birth may give some indication of the nutritional status of the mother in early pregnancy. One of the methods frequently adopted to produce anencephalus in animals is the use of excess vitamin A. Gal *et al.* (1972) compared post-partum vitamin A levels in two small studies. In the first they compared measurements on mothers of 56 liveborn infants with spina bifida referred for surgical treatment to those on 21 mothers of normal infants, matched by age, sex of the baby, and 'reproductive history'. They found six of the control cases showed extremely low vitamin A levels but this group was all analysed on the same day. After excluding these six, they showed that mothers of the index cases had significantly higher levels of vitamin A than did the control mothers. They also report a second study of 36 mothers of infants with various types of neural-tube malformations and 31 control cases; again the mothers of cases had higher vitamin A levels, although the difference was nonsignificant. The mean values for the index and control cases were 64 μg and 42 μg per 100 ml respectively in the first study and 47 μg and 39 μg per 100 ml in the second study. As all samples were taken at the same time after birth and analysed in the same laboratory, the differences in the levels in the mothers of the cases in the two studies is difficult to understand and is not commented on in the paper. These authors also describe results of a study of 200 foetal liver samples, including 14 from infants or abortuses with neural-tube malformations. The vitamin A concentration in healthy foetuses increases with gestation and the concentration in the livers of foetuses with neurological malformations was somewhat higher than that of healthy foetuses, although this difference was not significant. Other workers have not found any correlation between neural-tube defect prevalence and nutritional deficiencies including folic acid levels estimated in maternal blood (Scott, Whalley, and Prichard 1970; Hall 1972, 1977).

A prospective survey to examine the nutrition of women in their first trimester and their subsequent pregnancy outcome was initiated in Leeds in 1969–70. Estimates of serum folate, red-cell folate, white-blood-cell vitamin C, riboflavin saturation index, and serum vitamin A were made in over 900 women (Smithells, Sheppard, and Schorah 1976). All these indices exhibited a social class gradient being highest in classes I and II. In five mothers who had offspring with neural-tube defects (three anencephalics, one spina bifida, and one spina bifida and hydrocephalus) plus one microcephalic, significantly low levels of red-cell folate and white-blood-cell vitamin C were demonstrated. Further testing of this dietary hypothesis by preconceptual vitamin supplementation of mothers who have already had one or more infants with neural-tube defects is being undertaken.

Fedrick (1974) described a positive correlation between the prevalence of anencephalus in 18 countries and the annual consumption of tea per capita. In the British Isles a greater amount of tea per capita is consumed by lower socio-economic groups (classes IV and V) who have above-average neurological malformation rates. Fedrick then identified 558 married women resident in England and Wales who had delivered a stillborn anencephalic infant in 1969, and for each woman obtained four controls, two of whom had had a stillbirth attributed to some cause other than anencephalus and two a livebirth. The controls were matched for marital status, time of delivery, area of residence, age, and parity. A questionnaire, including questions on tea drinking, was mailed to each subject. Some 83 per cent of the index mothers and 80 per cent of the control mothers replied, and there was a statistically significant excess risk of anencephalus associated with drinking three or more cups per day; this increased risk was seen in all social classes. It occurred, however, only in regions of the country with high or medium prevalence rates, and Fedrick suggests there may be an interaction between tea drinking and the use of soft water.

Potato blight

Renwick (1972) put forward a hypothesis that the causal agent in anencephalus and spina bifida is an unidentified teratogen present in blight-infested potatoes. This disease of potato blight is due to a fungus, *Phytophthora infestans.* He based his hypothesis on several sets of observations including an apparent geographical association between world-wide prevalence rates of neural-tube defects and potato-blight frequency. The teratological evidence was the experimental production of anencephalus-like defects in the offspring of South American cotton-eared marmosets (*Callithrix jacchus*) fed a diet containing extracts of blighted potatoes (Poswillo, Sopher, and Mitchell 1972) and other evidence where malformations or death occurred in offspring of animals such as rats given solanine (Nishie, Gumbmann, and Keyl 1971), chicks given indoleacetic acid, a plant hormone present in blighted potatoes (Fehrmann and Dimond 1967), or cytochalasin B (Linville and Shepard 1972), a chemical associated with some potato mould infestations. A detailed enunciation of the hypothesis is set out in Renwick's (1972) original paper.

Epidemiologically, there is a general similarity between the geographical distribution of the prevalence of anencephalus and spina bifida and the frequency of potato blight. Both demonstrate high rates in Ireland, an east-to-west decline in Canada and the United States and a west-to-east decline in Europe. Renwick suggested the excess of defects in offspring of mothers in the lower social classes may be related to the greater consumption of poor quality potatoes and the greater degree of exposure due to preparing food for large families, working with no domestic help in overcrowded and poorly ventilated kitchens. The mode of spread of the toxin, probably a chemical, is postulated to be by skin absorption whilst peeling potatoes and by ingestion. The observed increased risk in siblings may be due to the mother's exposure to a common poor diet over a considerable period of time while genetic factors produce the female excess, twin discordance and ethnic differences.

As regards the teratological data, the anomalies illustrated in a report of the marmoset experiment (Poswillo, Sopher, Mitchell, Coxon, Curtis, and Price 1973) are cranial dysostosis and macrencephaly (Lemire *et al.* 1978). A second set of experiments were conducted (Poswillo *et al.* 1973) in which three groups of female marmosets each were fed different potato diets. The first group (six animals) received white potatoes, the second (seven animals) received a mixture of blemished and poor quality white potatoes, and the third group (five animals) received potatoes infected in the laboratory with bacteria (*Erwinia cartovora*) responsible for the plant disease of 'black leg'. No major defects occurred in any group. The results of the original experiment, therefore, could not be replicated. Ruddick, Harwig, and Scott (1974) also reported negative results after feeding rats with blighted potatoes. Swinyard and Chaube (1973) carried out extensive studies using a variety of animals, rats, rabbits, and rhesus monkeys, who were fed blighted potatoes, glycoalkaloids and solanidine; no neural-tube defects were observed in subsequent offspring.

This hypothesis received much attention subsequent to its publication in 1972. If correct and if perhaps 95 per cent of cases of anencephalus and spina bifida are preventable by potato avoidance as Renwick (1972*a*) later wrote, then three associations should be present in other independent sets of data. First, anencephalus and spina bifida prevalence should be highest in areas of high potato consumption and high blight prevalence. Secondly, as blight is an epidemic disease there will be a time series correlation between blight and malformation prevalence rates. And thirdly, anencephalus and spina bifida prevalence will vary by season owing to the consumption of stored blighted potatoes and this variation will be maximal in areas and in years of high blight prevalence.

Many inconsistencies in the geographical variations of neural-tube defects and potato blight were pointed out. Emanuel (1972) showed that the prevalence of neural-tube defects in Taiwan was quite high, despite the very low potato consumption, and the defects were most common in the lowest socio-economic classes, as in Britain, while potato consumption in Taiwan was probably the highest in the upper classes (Emanuel and Sever 1973). Studies of the postulated association in time between blight epidemics and neural-tube defect occurrence were reported from Scotland (Smith, Watt, Boyd, and Holmes 1973; Kilnen and Hewitt 1973), New South Wales (Field and Kerr 1973), Canada (Elwood, J. M. 1973*a*, 1976*a*), Ireland (Elwood, J. H. and MacKenzie 1973; Masterson, Frost, Bourke, Joyce, Herity, and Wilson-Davies 1974), and Boston and Maine (MacMahon, Yen, and Rothman 1973). These studies found the associations between neural-tube defect prevalence and blight prevalence, although significant in a few areas, were inconstant. Irish data from the largest Dublin maternity unit, the Rotunda Hospital, and estimates of the number of blight outbreaks recorded by the end of June during each year exhibit no significant variation attributable to blight with or without adjusting for the linear trend with time (Fig. 18.1 and Table 18.1). The amount of blight infestation was based on specimens collected by potato inspectors and blight was verified by microscopic examination (McKay 1957). In Canada, the eastern provinces of Nova Scotia, Prince Edward Island, New Brunswick, and Quebec have a higher mortality from anencephalus and spina bifida than the rest of the country and are also major potato-producing areas with a high prevalence of late potato blight (Cox and Large 1960). The consumption of potatoes per capita, 1.55 kg per week in 1966, is about 80 per cent of that in Britain (Dominion Bureau of Statistics 1969). However, there is no correlation between annual anencephalus mortality rates and potato blight severity, even if different lag periods between the occurrence of affected births and blight epidemics are examined or if interprovincial movements of potatoes are taken into account. Also, seasonal variations in anencephalus mortality are no more marked after years of severe blight (Elwood, J. M. 1973*a*, 1976*a*).

Despite the accumulation of observations which did not support his hypothesis, Renwick (1973) attempted to explain the lack of correlations between neural-tube defect prevalence and the frequency of potato blight observed in widely separated areas of the world, modified his original hypothesis to consider possible effects of teratogens found in foods other than potatoes, and strongly advocated in scientific journals as well as in the lay press that women should avoid eating potatoes prior to and during pregnancy. Apart from initiating several teratological and epidemiological studies, this publicity had other effects including a decline in the consumption of potatoes, the introduction of new measures for quality control by the Potato Marketing Board of the United Kingdom, and questions in the House of Commons as to whether people should discard diseased, damaged, or discoloured potatoes (Renwick 1972*a*, *b*). Renwick argued that even if his hypothesis were wrong, the risks of publicity were trivial compared with the potential benefit which would result from widespread acceptance of his advocated policy.

Epidemiological case–control studies were carried out in Liverpool (Clark *et al.* 1973), South Wales (Roberts, Revington, and Lloyd 1973) and New York State (Spiers, Pietrzyk, Piper, and Glebatis 1974). The Liverpool study based on 83 schoolchildren with spina bifida found no significant difference in the amount of potatoes consumed by their mothers compared with a matched control group of mothers having healthy children, although the likelihood for inaccuracy in interviews asking about events several years previously makes this negative finding of little value. The Welsh study of 240 infants born with neural-tube defects in Glamorganshire during the years 1964 to 1966 found no association between the consumption and storage of home-grown potatoes by their parents compared with the matched control

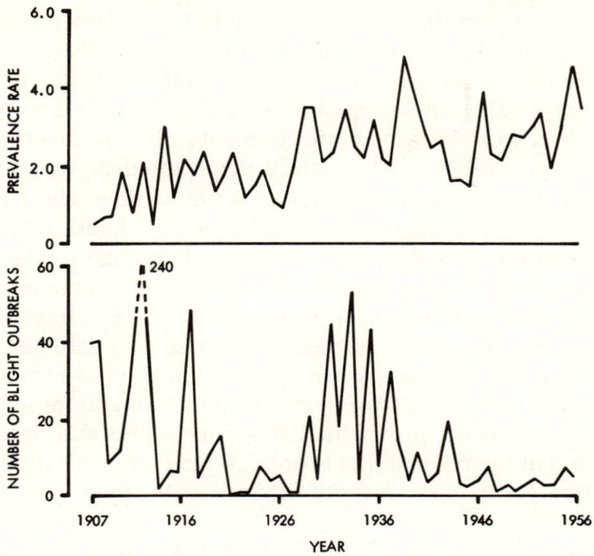

FIG. 18.1. Annual prevalence of anencephalus per 1000 total births reported from the Rotunda Hospital, Dublin (*top*) amd the total number of potato-blight outbreaks recorded by the end of June of each year in the Republic of Ireland (*bottom*) between 1907 and 1956. (Courtesy of *Nature*.)

TABLE 18.1 *Analysis of variance of the association between the annual prevalence of anencephalus in births reported from the Rotunda Hospital, Dublin, 1908–57 and the frequency of blight outbreaks in the Republic of Ireland during the previous year after allowing for secular trend*

Source of variation	Degrees of freedom	Sums of squares	Mean square	*F* ratio value
Linear trend	2	312.70	156.35	—
Linear trend and blight	3	313.05	104.35	—
Extra attributable to blight	1	0.35	0.35	Not significant
Residual	47	38.55	0.85	—
Total	50	351.60		

$y = a + b_1$ (year) $+ b_2$ (blight frequency)
where y = annual prevalence rate of anencephalus
$a = 1.075 \pm 0.347$
$b_1 = 0.044 \pm 0.009$
$b_2 = -0.003 \pm 0.004$

group. The American case–control telephone interview survey of 265 mothers of infants with neural-tube defects and 549 matched control mothers did not support the potato-blight hypothesis. Prospective intervention trials are the most valid method of testing a hypothesis in man, and the best test of Renwick's hypothesis would be a randomized study, with one group of mothers being encouraged to avoid potatoes and a control group not given such advice. However, the publicity already given to this issue would have compromised such a study if mounted at that time. Lorber (1974) described a series of nine pregnancies in women who already had at least one previous child with a neural-tube defect. These women avoided potatoes throughout their next pregnancies and two had further births with anencephalus or spina bifida. Nevin and Merrett (1975) advised all parents of infants with anencephalus and spina bifida born at a Belfast hospital from July 1972 onwards to avoid potatoes as soon as they decided on another pregnancy. Some 88 mothers were followed up, on whom 27 reported having avoided potatoes and 61 reported that they did not modify their diet. In the potato avoiders the prevalence of anencephalus and spina bifida was 8.7 per cent and in the normal diet group 3.6 per cent. This difference is not significant, but is in the opposite direction to that expected by the hypothesis.

Thus, most evidence to date, does not support the potato-blight hypothesis. Natural teratogens, however, probably exist and Renwick has developed his work to examine the Brassicae group of vegetables and their relationship to goitrogens and thyroid disease as well as to congenital defects (Renwick 1974; Renwick, Possami, and Munday 1974). Related chemicals such as ethylene thiourea can produce neural-tube defects in rats (Khera 1973). A dietary hypothesis as the explanation for the occurrence of neural-tube defects is attractive as it is compatible with several aspects of the epidemiology of these malformations. Better quality case–control studies are one approach to identifying possible embryotoxic substances. Confirmation of agents so identified in more than one geographical area of the world might warrant intervention trials.

19

Drinking-water composition

SEVERAL studies have investigated a possible relationship between the occurrence of neural-tube defects and the composition of drinking water. Initially, these investigations considered water 'hardness', a quantity traditionally used by water engineers which reflects the amount of insoluble carbonates present. Hardness is produced mainly by the concentrations of calcium and magnesium and in our studies we calculated a hardness index from the levels of these two elements (Elwood, J. M. 1977). However, hard and soft waters differ with respect to many minerals, owing to differences in source water and in the uptake or deposit of minerals in the distribution system which includes domestic water piping.

Penrose (1957) suggested that the geographical differences in the prevalence of neural-tube defects might reflect the presence or absence of trace elements in the water supply, noting that some areas of high prevalence, like Glasgow, had very soft water. Fedrick (1970) compared population rates for anencephalus in ten areas of Great Britain with analyses of water composition from various sources, and found significant negative correlations between anencephalus prevalence and total hardness, pH, and the calcium and sodium content of the water supplies. She also showed states of the USA having low and high infant mortality rates attributed to spina bifida had different mean water-hardness values with the high prevalence areas having softer water. Her study was based on routinely available data and the comparisons of different water components involved varying numbers of areas. No estimates of other relevant differences between the areas, for example with respect to maternal age, parity, or socio-economic status, were possible. Stocks (1970) examined data relating to stillbirths and deaths in the first year of life attributed to all congenital abnormalities in the fifteen hospital regions of England and Wales. The total malformation rates were higher in the north and west (Liverpool, Wales, and Manchester regions) and lowest in the south-east (Oxford, South-west, and North-west Metropolitan regions). Virtually all of this difference was due to a similar north–south decrease in the rates for anencephalus, spina bifida, and hydrocephalus, there being only random differences in the rates for other abnormalities. Comparisons of the regional prevalence for congenital abnormalities of the central nervous system with death rates of women aged from 25 years to 54 years showed large positive correlations (the correlation coefficients *r* being greater than 0.80) with death rates from chronic rheumatic heart disease, coronary disease, other heart disease and vascular lesions of the central nervous system and somewhat weaker associations (*r* values from 0.62 to 0.75) with death rates from nephritis and nephrosis, stomach cancer, and bronchitis. No significant associations were seen between central nervous system defect prevalence rates and other causes of death in adults or between non-central-nervous-system defect prevalence rates and any of the above causes. Stocks suggested that these distributions all might reflect associations with water hardness.

In a detailed study, Lowe, Roberts, and Lloyd (1971) found a negative correlation ($r = -0.40, p < 0.01$) between prevalence rates for central nervous system malformations in the 48 local authority areas of South Wales from 1964 to 1966 and total water hardness, which ranged from 20 to 270 parts per million. To examine individual defects, the areas were grouped into eight larger geographical units; the correlations with hardness were -0.81 ($p < 0.05$) for all central nervous system abnormalites, -0.92 ($p < 0.1$) for spina bifida, and -0.45 ($p < 0.05$) for anencephalus. Repeating the analysis by considering families of non-manual workers and manual workers separately showed the associations held in both occupational groups although the correlation coefficients were smaller. They also studied the perinatal mortality rates for anencephalus from 1963 to 1967 in the 58 county boroughs of England and Wales. These showed a negative association with water hardness ($r = -0.22, p < 0.05$) and a stronger association with calcium concentration ($r = -0.29, p < 0.05$). Although an attempt was made to control for socio-economic variables by examining the data by occupational group, the authors comment that as the soft water areas both within South Wales and in England and Wales are predominantly located in less prosperous areas, the correction they made may not have been sufficient. This study also was limited by the information on water composition which was taken from routine water engineers' reports and therefore consists of a mixture of source, supply, and tap water analyses made at different times. These data are not detailed enough to accurately describe the water distribution systems, especially in South Wales, where they are especially complex.

Fielding and Smithells (1971) compared secular trends in the prevalence of anencephalus in Liverpool and St Helens from 1963 to 1970 during which time the water supply to St Helens was artificially softened. No secular change in prevalence was observed either in St Helens or Liverpool. The authors concluded that soft water is not associated with a higher risk of anencephalus in the short term, and so if the geographical relationship between anencephalus prevalence and soft water is causal, it must act before rather than during pregnancy. However, the hardness in St Helens was changed from a level of 250 mg to 125 mg per litre, which is still relatively hard water. This alteration may not be large enough to affect neural-tube defect prevalence rates. Moreover, the numbers of births in St Helens are too small to reliably assess any change because the prevalence rates vary from 2 to 4 per 1000 births in three years studied before softening, and from 0.5 to 5 in the five years after softening. A case–control study of 30 consecutive anencephalic births and 60 controls matched by city area, month of birth, maternal age and parity, and paternal social class was performed in Glasgow (Wilson, Watson, and Richards 1973). Samples of tap water were taken from the homes of the mothers and analysed for pH, calcium, magnesium, lead copper, zinc, and iron concentrations. No differences in the mean concentrations of these minerals between cases and controls were found.

An associaton between water hardness and infant mortality in the county boroughs of England and Wales was described by Crawford, Gardner, and Sedgwick (1972). They used a multiple regression model to estimate the independent associations of infant mortality with water calcium, latitude, and a 'social factor score' derived from nine indices of social conditions which included social class and population density. The regression coefficient for calcium was negative and significant, and examination of data from four time-periods spanning 1911 to 1964 showed that over this time the association with calcium became stronger and that with the social-factor score became weaker. They interpreted the findings as indicating that inter-borough differences in water quality became relatively more important as social differences became smaller. The strongest correlation with calcium concentration was a negative association with neonatal mortality rates; a weaker although significant negative association was found with post-neonatal mortality rates, and a non-significant negative assocation was seen with the stillbirth rates. These findings are relevant to the question of an association between neural-tube defect prevalence and water quality as there may be a non-specific association with several causes of perinatal and infant deaths. The South Wales situation was further explored by Morton, Elwood, P. C., and Abernethy (1976). They compared the prevalence rates from all central nervous system defects for the 48 local authority areas in South Wales with the concentrations of 12 elements estimated by atomic absorption spectrophotometry on samples taken from randomly chosen households in each area. They found significant negative associations between prevalence and calcium, copper and barium concentrations, and a significant positive association with aluminium. Multiple regression analyses suggested that the major associations were with copper and barium concentrations. The observation by Lakadawala and Widdowson (1977) of a significant negative association between the concentrations of copper and the prevalence rates of neural-tube defects in 48 areas of South Wales was followed up by Wald and Hambridge (1977). Their study of nine women who had anencephalic infants and 36 control women who had healthy infants found no difference between the mean maternal serum copper levels which were 184 μg/100 ml and 185 μg/100 ml respectively.

Zinc deficiency may produce abortion and congenital malformations, including anencephalus in rats (Hurley and Swenerton 1966; Sever, L. E. 1975) and this has been suggested as the basis for associations of anencephalus with poor maternal nutrition. Clinical zinc deficiency in man has been observed in Iran and Egypt (*Lancet* 1975) where the prevalence of anencephalus may be high (Appendix A.1). However, no more direct association with zinc deficiency in man has been reported.

Canadian Surveys

The British studies demonstrated a negative correlation between area prevalence rates for central nervous system defects and either water hardness or calcium concentrations. We also investigated the striking geographical variations in the prevalence of these defects in Canada with regard to drinking-water composition. Although there is an east-to-west decline in rates across Canada rather than the north-to-south trend as seen in England, it is interesting that these geographical trends in both countries appear to be specific to central nervous system defects (Stocks 1970; Elwood, J. M. and Rogers 1975). In Canada, we had the advantages of a very large geographical area, and a weaker correlation between soft-water areas and areas of low socio-economic status than in Great Britain. One survey examining the relationship between anencephalus mortality and drinking-water composition has been completed (Elwood, J. M. 1977) and a larger survey is in progress. The first study began in 1972. With the co-operation of Statistics Canada we compiled numbers of deaths and mortality rates attributed to anencephalus, spina bifida, hydrocephalus, all other congenital abnormalities, and total stillbirths and infant deaths for cities with populations of over 50 000 for each year from 1950 to 1969. Population size for each city selected was based on the 1966 Census estimates. Some were excluded because of major administrative boundary changes between 1950 and 1969, and London, Ontario, was excluded as its water supply had been changed during that time. For the 36 remaining cities, we obtained estimates of pH and of the concentrations of calcium, magnesium, lithium, copper, and zinc from the Ottawa research team headed by Dr L. C. Neri. This group is studying water composition in Canada in relation to cardiovascular disease and the University of Ottawa laboratory is the World Health Organization reference centre for drinking-water composition. For our work, we used information collected in a survey of 526 communities between 1970 and 1972 (Neri, Johansen, and Talbot 1977). Water samples were obtained from several residential dwellings in each city and analysed in a single laboratory. Calcium, magnesium, copper, and zinc concentrations were estimated by atomic spectrophotometry, and lithium concentration by flame emission. The concentrations were expressed in parts per million by weight (mg per litre). The standard deviations of measurements of calcium and magnesium were around 0.1 p.p.m. and those of other elements 0.03 p.p.m.; lower limits of detection are approximately twice the standard deviation. Sampling was carried out several times during the year to allow for seasonal changes and the taps were run for several minutes prior to collection to avoid obtaining water which had been stored in domestic pipes overnight. The houses sampled were not randomly selected. Within-city variations in water composition were very small. Mean income levels in 1951, 1961, and 1971, 30-year annual average rainfall estimates, population size, and geographical longitude and latitude were obtained for each city from standard sources.

Our results indicated that for these 36 cities, the anencephalus mortality rates over the 1950 to 1969 period ranged from 0.61 to 2.12 per thousand total births (mean 1.30) and the total hardness ranged from 0.4 to 409 p.p.m. The anencephalus rates showed significant negative correlation coefficients with mean income, magnesium concentrations, longitude, and latitude and a positive correlation with rainfall. However these environmental variables are strongly interrelated, which makes the evaluation of these associations most difficult. In these data, calcium, magnesium, and lithium concentrations are highly positively intercorrelated, as are longitude and latitude, while rainfall is negatively correlated with pH, income, and magnesium. We further analysed the data using a linear multiple regression model which assumes that the inter-city differences in anencephalus mortality depend on the additive effect of linear terms. This is expressed as:

$$y = \alpha + \beta_1 x_1 + \beta_2 x_2 \ldots . + \beta_k x_k + \varepsilon,$$

where y is the dependent variable (the mean anencephalus mortality rate 1950–1969), x_i is an independent variable, ε an error term, α the intercept, and β a regression coefficient. A least-squares method was used to estimate the α and β terms. As the variance of a mortality rate is inversely proportional to the numbers of births on which it is based, each city's observation was weighted by the number of births in that city, and thus in inverse proportion to the variance, in these correlation and regression analyses. The regression analyses showed independent and significant negative associations of the anencephalus mortality rates with mean income, magnesium concentration, and longitude. The final equation accounted for 69 per cent of the between-city variations in the anencephalus mortality rates (Table 19.1). As the choice of a linear additive model is arbitrary, we re-analysed the data using various interaction terms and transformations of the original variables, but we did not find any other significant associations. The residual variations (observed rates minus those estimated from the equation) for the cities showed no associations with the other variables studied, and no pattern suggesting alternative hypotheses. As a further step, the model incorporating income, magnesium, and longitude was applied to an independent set of data relating to 14 towns in Ontario with populations of between 20 000 and 50 000 persons. The model fitted these data reasonably well (Elwood, J. M. 1977). By comparing cities rather than individuals, we have assumed that the water sampled is representative of that consumed. Some residents may use water from sources other than the municipal supply but this effect will be minor, and the selection of large municipal areas excluded fringe and semi-rural areas where this is more likely. Some women may have moved into the city after the time of exposure to the postulated water factor. These effects will bias our results only if mothers of infants with neural-tube defects have different patterns of water usage or migration compared with other mothers; otherwise the only effect of these errors will be to decrease the strength of the associations observed. The use of domestic water-softeners in areas of hard water also will decrease any observed association.

TABLE 19.1 *Results of regressing longitude, mean income in 1961, and mean magnesium concentration in drinking water on mortality rates attributed to various causes in 36 Canadian cities—data 1950–69*

	Standardized coefficients†			
Cause of death	Longitude	Mean income	Magnesium	$r^2 \times 100$‡
Anencephalus	−0.66**	−0.19*	−0.21*	83
Spina bifida	−0.54**	−0.26*	−0.08	50
Hydrocephalus	−0.60**	−0.13	−0.07	46
Other abnormalities	−0.33*	−0.24	−0.17	29
All other stillbirths§	−0.48**	−0.41**	0.21*	67
All other infant deaths§	−0.31*	−0.29*	−0.18	32

† Standardized regression coefficient; the value of βb when all variables are transformed to a standard distribution with mean 0 and variance 1. The relative size of the beta coefficient reflects the relative size of the effect of the variable.
‡ Multiple regression coefficient squared; estimates the proportion of inter-city variation in the dependent variable which can be attributed to the factors included.
§ Adjusted to exclude contribution of congenital abnormalities.
* $p<0.05$ ** $p<0.001$

Although the magnesium association is of great interest, there are several indications which make a direct causal relationship unlikely. The finding of a negative association of anencephalus rates with magnesium in Canada but with calcium in Great Britain (Lowe *et al*. 1971, Morton *et al*. 1976) suggests that neither is a direct cause of anencephalus. However, as the concentrations of calcium, magnesium, and lithium and total water hardness are strongly positively intercorrelated, the separation of their effects in a small sample is prone to error. The constancy of water composition over time means the large decrease in anencephalus mortality rates in Canada must have some other explanation. Applying the regression model separately to the data for the 36 cities for each of the four quinquennia from 1950 to 1969 shows that over time the associations with magnesium and with mean income strengthen while that with longitude becomes less. This is consistent with the secular trend being due to a reduction in other factors, some associated with longitude, which permits the magnesium association to become more evident. This trend is similar to that noted with the association between infant mortality and water hardness in Great Britain (Crawford *et al*. 1972). Furthermore, the association with magnesium in the data for the 36 cities is neither linear nor wholly specific. It is produced by a fairly consistent negative trend giving lower anencephalus mortality rates at 10–20 mg/l magnesium concentrations than at very low levels, but three of four cities with concentrations higher than 20 mg/l had high rates which suggest a non-linear relationship. The range of magnesium levels up to 20 mg/l corresponds approximately to a range of total hardness of 0 to 200 p.p.m., similar to the total range in England and Wales. For the Canadian cities the mortality rates from spina bifida, hydrocephalus, all other congenital abnormalities, and also the infant mortality rates have negative but non-significant associations with magnesium concentration. The stillbirth rates from all causes, and from all causes other than congenital abnormalities, also showed a significant negative correlation with magnesium concentration (Table 19.1). In assessing that study (Elwood, J. M. 1976, 1977) we noted these aberrant findings and thought it unlikely that the observed association reflected a direct causal mechanism. The difference in the daily intake of magnesium between mothers using water having 0 to 20 p.p.m. magnesium is probably less than 40 mg, which is small relative to the estimated total daily intake of around 300 to 400 mg (Davidson, Passmore, Brock, and Treswell 1975). It is possible that the mineral concentration of water in an area affects the mineral content of food grown in that area and food cooked using the water, but even so an aetiological mechanism involving other metals or compounds whose concentration varies with magnesium or calcium content appears more plausible. In this regard, the anomalous position of Vancouver is of interest. Vancouver is an exception to the hypothesis in that the magnesium concentration of the water is very low and is similar to that in cities on the east coast of Canada, but the anencephalus rate also is low. However, the water supply for Vancouver is largely derived from snow melt and short fast-flowing rivers rising in the nearby mountains, while the eastern soft-water cities are supplied from large slow-moving rivers such as the St Lawrence and St John, or from lake water as in the case of Halifax. Although both water sources have low concentrations of the minerals studied, their content of other elements and particularly of organic material probably is quite different. A further indirect mechanism may be by a joint effect of soft water and another exposure. For example, Fedrick (1974) has demonstrated a positive association between the frequency of anencephalus and tea-drinking which appears to be most marked in soft water areas. The observed relationship between low magnesium concentrations and increased anencephalus mortality may reflect either an increase in the incidence of malformation during early gestation, or a decreased rate of early foetal loss. The latter mechanism might explain the increased stillbirth rate from other causes.

The relationship between water composition and the occurrence of neural-tube defects is far from clear. Studies in Great Britain and Canada have shown lower prevalence rates in areas with 'hard' water, but the strongest associations are with calcium in Great Britain and with magnesium in Canada. It is interesting that a similar situation holds with respect to adult deaths from cardiovascular disease.

Clearly, more detailed water analyses and much better control for other known predictors of neural-tube defect prevalence are required. Our current Canadian work is designed to deal with both these problems. The complete findings are not yet available, but no simple relationship with a major water component such as calcium or magnesium has been seen so far and the final results may well be different from those of our previous Canadian study. For the present investigation, all fatal cases of anencephalus occurring in Canada (excluding the Yukon, North-West Territories, and Newfoundland) between 1969 and 1972 have been identified with the co-operation of Statistics Canada. There were 758 stillbirths, and 457 infant deaths; of the latter 436 (96 per cent) were successfully linked to their birth certificates by computerized record linkage techniques. A control series consisting of 10 000 livebirths was randomly selected from the total livebirths in the same area and time period. The water data to be used are from the Ottawa group's survey of calcium, magnesium, lithium, zinc, and copper as used previously, supplemented by an additional study in 1970 of 249 localities in which nickel and lead concentrations were estimated by atomic absorption spectrophotometry, and selenium, chromium, silver, cobalt, cadmium, molybdenum, and tin estimated by neutron activation analysis. Thus in this case–control study, information on maternal variables such as age, parity, and birthplace is obtained from stillbirth and birth certificates, as in the 14-cities study, and appropriate water data and other information relate to the mother's place of residence as given on the birth certificate. The current study will still leave many questions unanswered. Water composition is a relatively simple way of obtaining an approximate guide to only one aspect of nutritional status. Surveys using detailed dietary histories and analyses of food and water, as well as perhaps measuring concentrations in body fluids and tissues, will be needed to provide more definitive information. It is unlikely that sufficient support will be obtained to conduct such studies on a large scale in human populations unless more specific hypotheses are formulated.

20

Clustering in time and space

SEVERAL authors have commented on the occurrence of births of infants having neural-tube defects close to each other in time and in geographical location (Polman 1950; Pleydell 1960; Flynt 1970). Although the events are well described their interpretation is not straightforward because clusters of events will occur on the basis of chance alone. Early studies were purely descriptive. Pleydell (1960) for example, looked at one vector (space) by plotting the place of birth of 64 anencephalics born in Northamptonshire over the period 1944 to 1957 on a county map and also plotted subgroups of cases on a larger scale to show their spatial distribution within urban districts and individual streets. He concluded that the prevalence of anencephalus in urban districts was double that in rural districts and this together with other associations with social class and season might be explained on the basis of an infectious disease such as Asian influenza.

Infectious diseases are known to cluster in time and space owing to person-to-person spread of the causative agent with or without intermediate hosts. There have been attempts to describe epidemics by mathematical models (Bailey 1975) so that if certain statistical conditions are fulfilled by the observations made at the beginning of an epidemic (for example, the attack rate, the numbers of susceptible and non-susceptible individuals in the population, and so on) then the future size and other characteristics of the epidemic can be determined. If time–space clustering were found to fit epidemiological observations concerning birth defects, then this would be presumptive evidence of transmissible agents being a likely cause. Alternatively, clustering in time and space could be produced by a group of mothers being exposed to an aetiological agent of a non-infective nature, but which produced a common source epidemic analogous to an outbreak of food poisoning. Such sources could be environmental contaminants present in air, food, or water and arising from natural processes, industrial pollution, or other sources. Furthermore, a substance newly introduced into the community such as a drug or food additive could mimic the pattern of time–space clustering.

We may define time–space clustering as the occurrence of two or more cases close together in time and in geographical location. We emphasize, however, that this definition is neither completely precise or universal because there are different statistical methods applied and different definitions used, particularly for the time vector, in papers published to date. Regarding the time vector, the critical time of exposure may be defined as a period during preconception, the time of conception, or the time of probable initiation of the neural-tube malformation (around 28 days—Table 2.1). Obviously, the most commonly used reference point, namely the time of birth, is not biologically meaningful in any real sense and is adopted on the assumption that it is related consistently to the true critical time of exposure to the causative agent. Similarly, regarding the space vector, there are various choices such as the place of residence of the mother during the first month of pregnancy or other residential addresses before or during the gestational period. These locations may be identified using latitude and longitude co-ordinates on a map. The analytical methods also are not all the same. Knox's (1963) method, which is widely used, estimates the distances in time and space between all possible pairs of cases and compares these to those specified assuming a Poisson distribution. Other techniques are described by Mustacchi, David, and Fix (1967) and Mantel (1967). Because of the difficulties in determining, *a priori*, the time period which is of importance, the statistical methods may be applied using several critical periods and several definitions of closeness in time and in space, with appropriate precautions against finding nominally significant results on multiple tests.

The aims of these analyses are to detect space–time clustering (within the context of the definitions of space and time vectors laid down by the investigators) and to provide estimates of how the observations (occurrences of neural-tube defects in our context) deviate from an expected distribution. Apart from searches for clustering of neural-tube defects, other malformations examined include cleft lip and palate and tracheo-oesophageal fistula (Knox 1963, 1964) and Down's syndrome (Leck 1966*a*, Stark and Mantel 1967).

Trichopoulos, Desmond, Yen, and MacMahon (1971) analysed data on 1003 affected infants having anencephalus or spina bifida born in Rhode Island between 1936 and 1965. Their criteria of time and space were based on parental place of residence at the time of birth and the first day of the last menstrual period ascertained from hospital records. Only in one space–time category, bounded by 30 days and from 0.25 to 1.0 km, was there a significant excess of observed over expected pairs and they conclude their results are essentially negative. Fedrick and Wilson's (1971) Glasgow study used less precise space–time definitions relating to district of mother's residence and month of birth. They looked at the time–space distribution of births with neural-tube defects and of a 5 per cent random sample of all births in Glasgow over the same time period, 1964 to 1968, using the method of Ederer, Myers, and Mantel (1966). Analyses by both this technique and Knox's method demonstrated significant clustering for hydrocephalus but not for anencephalus or spina bifida. Siemiatycki and McDonald (1972) applied the methods of Knox (1963) and Mantel (1967) to 1017 cases of anencephalus and 1421 cases of spina bifida occurring in the province of Quebec excluding Montreal Island, using the mother's address at the time of the birth and the month of birth. Again their findings were negative while validation of the methodology by examining 44 cases of typhoid fever and 175 cases of salmonellosis which also were reported in the province of Quebec outside Montreal Island gave highly significant positive confirmation of time–space clustering.

Aylett, Roberts, and Lloyd (1974) examined a small Wiltshire town, Corsham, in which there were 979 births including 5 with anencephalus, 12 with spina bifida, and 1 with hydrocephalus during the period 1968 to 1972. This study was initiated because Aylett, a family doctor, thought this high frequency might possibly be associated with parental occupational exposure to chemicals used at a near-by large, artificial-rubber-making factory. These investigators matched each abnormal birth with five normal births by maternal age, parity, social class, and time of birth, and then analysed the spatial distribution of cases and controls by Knox's method. They found that significantly more pairs of cases than of controls occurred at distances of up to 2000 m. The limitation of this study is that it applies to a small area chosen because a cluster of births was suspected. Without studying a large number of similar areas not suspected to have clustering *a priori*, it is impossible to exclude a chance association being the explanation for this particular cluster. Thus, they also examined a large sample of infants with neural-tube defects born in Cardiff (Roberts, Laurence, and Lloyd 1975). Some 406 affected infants born between 1956 and 1971 were investigated for evidence of space–time clustering and 100 similarly affected infants together with a control group matched by maternal age, parity, social class, and birth date were investigated for evidence of spatial clustering. Five controls were matched to each index case. This study failed to detect any evidence of space–time clustering and so did not confirm the earlier observation in Corsham. A Manitoba survey examined 299 (liveborn and stillborn) cases of neural-tube defects (113 anencephalus, 93 spina bifida, 47 hydrocephalus, and 46 unspecified malformations) occurring in Greater Winnipeg from 1964 to 1968 and ascertained from several sources including hospital notes, death registrations, and the Manitoba Congenital Anomalies Registry (Choi *et al*. 1972). Using the analytic method of Ederer *et al*. (1966) they found significant clustering if the time vector, estimated by conception date, was either two months or four months but this group do not give details of any further analysis.

The evidence based on a small number of independent sets of data analysed so far suggests the distribution of cases of anencephalus and spina bifida is not similar to the pattern normally associated with an infectious disease and the occasional observation of a cluster may be explained on the basis of chance alone. Clinical descriptions of these rare clusters, however, should continue to be reported because further epidemiological enquiry will confirm or refute the presence of any real low-intensity epidemic. Causative agents need not necessarily be organisms but could be other environmental factors such as chemical factory processes (Aylett 1974; Edmonds *et al*. 1978) or agricultural sprays.

Sare and Forbes (1972) described two spina bifida infants, born within one month of each other, whose families lived on adjoining hilly country farms in New Zealand which for several years had been aerially sprayed with 2, 4, 5-trichlorophenoxyacetic acid. The commercial chemical preparation also contains an impurity, dioxin, used as a defoliant by the United States Armed Forces in Vietnam. The domestic water supply of these two houses was collected from rain falling on the roof. Lowry and Allen (1977) also comment on a possible association between aerial spraying with phenoxy herbicides and one case of spina bifida in the Gulf Islands, British Columbia. In both these case reports no definite link between aerial sprays and neural-tube defects was substantiated.

There are several major difficulties in any investigation for space–time clustering of birth defects. Full ascertainment of consecutive occurrences of affected infants in a defined population of births is essential otherwise ranking of cases, particularly in time order, will be erroneous if some are excluded by being unknown to the researcher. Exclusions are equally important in biasing the space vector as well. Definition of the time of exposure is not simple; information on the location of affected infants in space may be inexact especially in rural areas where only a townland address is provided and the residence of a case family cannot be ascertained without field visits. Methodologically, statistical techniques for analysing this type of data are still being developed. A more serious limitation is the indirectness of this approach to measuring epidemicity or degree of contagion manifest by a particular birth-defect cluster compared with the distribution expected from infectious disease theory. Tests of time–space clustering are but one way to test hypotheses that groups of these defects may occur in association with a common exposure. Space-time clustering studies make an implicit assumption that closeness defined by geographical location of residence implies a likelihood of common exposure. This may be acceptable for diseases affecting young children who may play around the home and neighbourhood and for diseases spread by food or water. On the other hand, this may not (and probably does not) apply for diseases spread by interpersonal contact or from environmental causes in the case of adults. In modern society, a mother's main personal and environmental exposures are not necessarily similar to those of her neighbours, whom she may never have met, but will be shared more closely by colleagues at work, kinship networks, and by individuals sharing common recreational interests. All these persons may live in areas located considerable distances away from the mother's own residence. Thus if an agent of low intensity is the cause of anencephalus and spina bifida, detailed studies of interpersonal contacts similar to those performed in the search for transmissiblity of Hodgkin's disease and certain leukemias (Vianna and Polan 1976) are required. These investigations are far from simple to conduct and also to analyse (Smith 1978). In addition, if a common environmental exposure is the hypothesis to be tested, studies of neural-tube defects related to parental occupation, recreational activities, and contacts with domesticated and other animals may be more fruitful than studies based only on the place of residence and the time of birth.

IX

Maternal factors

21

Maternal age and reproductive history

THE literature describing the relationship of maternal age and parity to the prevalence at birth of anencephalus and of spina bifida is very confusing. We shall attempt to summarize some of the previous work and describe the results of recent Canadian studies.

Many studies have described a U-shaped distribution of the prevalence rates of anencephalus or spina bifida with either maternal age or parity considered alone, with high risks in mothers under 20 years and in primiparae, and also in those over 35 years and those of high parity. The minimum rates are usually in mothers aged 20–4 years and of parity one. This type of distribution has been shown in Birmingham (Record and McKeown 1949), Scotland (Edwards 1958; Record 1961; Fedrick 1976*a*), England and Wales (Fedrick 1970), South Wales (Carter *et al.* 1968), London (Carter and Evans 1973), New York State (Milham and Gittelsohn 1965), Quebec (Horowitz and McDonald 1969), Rhode Island (Ingalls, Pugh, and MacMahon 1954), and Budapest (Czeizel and Révész 1970). Some other reports show a linear increase in risk with either age or parity considered alone. This is seen in Israel (Naggan 1971), Australia (Collmann and Stoller 1962), and Finland (Granroth, Haapakoski, and Hakama 1978). The finding of an increased risk only in young and low parity mothers has been reported in France (Frézal *et al.* 1964) and in Oxfordshire (Fedrick 1976).

Joint effects of age and of parity

As maternal age and parity are correlated, it is essential to describe the relationship of the prevalence of anencephalus and spina bifida to each factor taking into account effects of the second factor. Record and McKeown (1949) thus showed an increased risk in first births and in births after the fifth in Birmingham, but no maternal age effect within strata of parity. This type of relationship was described in Boston (Naggan and MacMahon 1967). Ingalls *et al.* (1954) showed independent U-shaped associations with parity and maternal age, and concluded that the parity effect was the greater. The studies of Fedrick (1970) in Great Britain, Record (1961), and Fedrick (1976*a*) on Scottish data, Horowitz and McDonald (1969) in Quebec, and Imaizumi (1974) in Japan, all give results broadly consistent with independent U-shaped associations with both age and parity, but in each study the results are somewhat different, as the association between anencephalus occurrence and one of the maternal variables is modified by the other. Thus to examine the effects of age standardized for parity or vice versa is still insufficient: the age–parity specific rates must be examined. Fedrick (1970) concluded that the increased risk in births to primiparae is greatest for young mothers, while the excess at high parities occurs mainly in older women. She suggested this bimodal pattern reflects two distinct high-risk groups, young low-parity mothers and older high-parity mothers, and that these two groups may have different aetiological factors. Fedrick's hypothesis is supported by Scottish data (Record 1961) which show the increased rate for young mothers to be present in first births only, while an increase rate for mothers over 30 years occurs at birth orders above parity three.

Naggan (1971) found in Israel, and in Jews in Boston (Naggan and MacMahon 1967) that the risk of anencephalus rises steadily with increasing parity, with no independent age effect, and no excess in primiparae. He suggested that this pattern may be typical of a low-prevalence region, with the excess risk in primiparae being due to a separate aetiological factor found only in high prevalence areas. The data of Granroth *et al.* (1978) support this by showing that in Finland, where the prevalence of anencephalus is only 0.32 per 1000, the risk rises with birth order and shows no age effect or excess in primiparae. In the low prevalence area of Singapore (Searle 1959) the risk also rises monotonically with increasing parity. In Japan (Imaizumi 1974) this holds for mothers aged between 25 and 34 years; in younger mothers the risk falls with increasing parity, supporting Fedrick's hypothesis, but the risk also falls with increasing parity in mothers over 35 years. In Quebec, Horowitz and McDonald (1969) found a U-shaped parity association in births to mothers under 25 years and a decreasing risk with increasing parity in older mothers.

Several other studies give results which do not confirm the explanations put forward by Fedrick or Naggan. However, interpretation is difficult as in general these studies are based on relatively small numbers and the estimates of age–parity specific prevalence rates are unstable. Collmann and Stoller (1962) report a U-shaped association with parity and an increased risk in mothers over 30 years in the low-prevalence area of Australia. Czeizel and Révész (1970), in their large Hungarian study where the prevalence rate is low, show the highest rate in primiparae and especially older primiparae. Studies from the high-prevalence areas of Dublin (Coffey and Jessop 1957), and Dundee (Walker and Smith 1961) demonstrate no excess risk in primiparae, and only a very small excess is seen in South Wales (Carter *et al.* 1968). In London there is a U-shaped association with maternal age and a steady decrease in risk with increasing parity (Carter and Evans 1973).

History of abortions in other pregnancies

It is generally accepted that mothers of infants with anencephalus or spina bifida have greater than expected rates of spontaneous abortion in other pregnancies. While this conclusion is supported by several studies, these are not easy to interpret as the data are usually based on retrospective interviews which might be expected to lead to relative overreporting by mothers of defective infants, and often no adequate control group of mothers is used.

Two valid studies are available. Record and McKeown (1950) conducted interviews on 742 mothers, representing 81 per cent of infants with central nervous system defects born in Birmingham from 1940 to 1947, and on mothers of a systematic sample of infants free of defects. The case mothers reported that 11.2 per cent of their other conceptions ended in abortion, compared with 7.5 per cent of previous conceptions of the control group. In the South Wales study, covering 1964 to 1966, 17 per cent of pregnancies prior to the birth of a child with anencephalus or spina bifida ended in abortion, compared to 11.6 per cent of pregnancies prior to any birth in the study population (Richards 1973). This study shows high prior abortion rates in association with several other types of congenital defects, but not with hydrocephalus. Several other studies have good information on the families of affected infants, but lack an adequate control series. For example, Williamson (1965) reports an abortion rate of 17 per cent in all other pregnancies of mothers of infants with neural-tube defects in Southampton; Richards *et al.* (1972) report 15.4 per cent in Glasgow, McDonald (1971*a*) found 15.6 per cent in Quebec, and Smithells, D'Arcy and McAllister (1968) 15.6 per cent in Liverpool. These rates are remarkably consistent, and are generally higher than the rates reported for total populations, which are given in the four studies as 15, 13, 12.1, and 11 per cent respectively. Other estimates of abortion risks to siblings of neural-tube defect infants are 20 per cent (Böök and Rayner 1950) and 8.3 per cent (Frézal *et al.* 1964) but these studies have serious methodological limitations. Other studies show that the proportion of mothers of infants with anencephalus or spina bifida who report any prior abortions is higher than that of comparison mothers (Coffey and Jessop 1957, Granroth *et al.* 1978, Fedrick 1976). Record and McKeown (1950) show higher abortion rates in the proximal two pregnancies prior to the birth of an infant with a central nervous system malformation (14.1 per cent) than in earlier conceptions (6.4 per cent) or in those after the affected birth (11.1 per cent); for their controls all pregnancies prior to the index birth had similar rates (mean 5.8 per cent), but those later had a higher rate (12.9 per cent). Smithells *et al.* (1968) report rates of 16.2 per cent in prior, and 12.7 per cent in subsequent pregnancies, while McDonald (1971*a*) showed no differences in the abortion rate either by sequential pregnancy order or by the order of the pregnancy in relation to that of the affected birth. Clarke *et al.* (1975) combined data from several British studies and demonstrated a higher risk of spontaneous abortion in the pregnancy immediately preceding the birth of a child with anencephalus or spina bifida than in the subsequent pregnancy, and Gardiner *et al.* (1978) suggest on the basis of a small prospective study that pregnancies subsequent to a spontaneous abortion may have a higher rate of several midline defects, including those of the neural tube. The issue of spontaneous abortion is further discussed in Sections 22 and 27.

Canadian 14-city study

Our study of anencephalus in 14 Canadian cities has produced some new insights into the associations of anencephalus occurrence with maternal age and reproductive experience. This has been made possible by the practice of recording separately maternal histories with respect to previous livebirths, stillbirths, and deaths of earlier born children. The relevant questions on the birth certificate refer to the 'number of children previously born to this mother—(a) liveborn and (b) stillborn—after 28 weeks' gestation'. A separate question asks the number of liveborn children since deceased. The sum of previous livebirths and stillbirths is taken as 'total parity'.

Our results in their simplest form show U-type distributions of the anencephalus mortality rate with both maternal age and total parity similar to those seen in many other studies (Table 21.1). The risk of anencephalus is highest for women aged under 20 years and over 35 years although the differences in risk by maternal age are not large. There is a stronger relationship of risk to the total parity of the mother, the minimum risk being with one previous birth and higher risks are associated with primiparity or high parity. If only previous livebirths are counted, the excess risk at high birth-orders is less marked but the above-average risk at the first pregnancy persists. Large increases in risk are seen in women who have had a previous stillbirth or a previous childhood death. Paternal age also was examined but no definite relationship with risk was evident.

However, this simple tabulation is insufficient as the high rate in mothers of high total parity could be due to parity itself, or to these mothers differing from lower-parity mothers with respect to other factors such as age, previous stillbirth history, or ethnic group. In this study, we were able to control for differences with respect to these and other variables by using a multivariate model. The removal of the confounding effects of other factors makes little difference to the association with maternal age (Fig. 21.1 and Table 21.2). The relative risk for older mothers is reduced slightly, and a weak U-type relationship remains which is not statistically significant (Elwood, J. M., Raman, and Mousseau 1978). In contrast, the association of risk with the number of previous livebirths is considerably altered. In the unadjusted pattern there is a U-type relationship, but after controlling confounding a simpler inverse relationship of relative risk to the number of previous livebirths is seen, which is statistically significant. Thus the high unadjusted or crude risk in women with three or more previous livebirths compared to those having one or two previous livebirths is produced by confounding by another factor or factors. The marked increase in risk in women with a previous history of a stillbirth or of a child death persists after confounder control and both associations are highly significant. The control of confounding slightly reduces the strength of the association with previous stillbirths but increases the association with previous child deaths. The risk in women who have had two previous child deaths is higher than in those who have had one; no such 'dose–response' effect is seen in relation to the number of previous stillbirths.

TABLE 21.1 *Unadjusted risk-ratios for anencephalus associated with subclasses of mother's age, father's age, and previous reproductive history*

Factor	Subclass	Number of cases	Number of controls	Unadjusted risk-ratio
Mother's age	⩽19	164	513	1.19
	20–4	428	1587	1.00 (R)
	25–9	377	1368	1.02
	30–4	226	946	0.89
	35–9	152	453	1.24*
	40+	37	131	1.10
	Unknown	7	2	
Father's age	⩽19	18	75	0.80
	20–4	291	975	1.00 (R)
	25–9	378	1435	0.88
	30–4	281	1086	0.87
	35–9	172	650	0.87
	40+	139	441	1.06
	Unknown	112	338	1.11
Total number of previous births (live and still)	0	574	1826	1.00 (R)
	1	299	1281	0.74**
	2	218	863	0.80*
	3	130	465	0.89
	4	68	276	0.78
	5+	102	289	1.12
Number of previous livebirths	0	602	1853	1.00 (R)
	1	315	1288	0.75**
	2	200	854	0.72**
	3	121	465	0.80*
	4	71	267	0.82
	5+	82	273	0.92
Number of previous stillbirths	0	1250	4867	1.00(R)
	1	125	113	4.31**
	2+	16	20	3.11**
Number of previous child deaths†	0	1190	4740	1.00 (R)
	1	170	235	2.88**
	2+	31	25	4.94**

† Indicates death of a previous liveborn infant prior to the birth of the anencephalic propositus. Statistical significance is based on a chi-square test with one degree of freedom analysing the association of case–control status between the referent subclass (R) and each of the other subclasses.

* $p=0.05$, ** $p<0.001$.

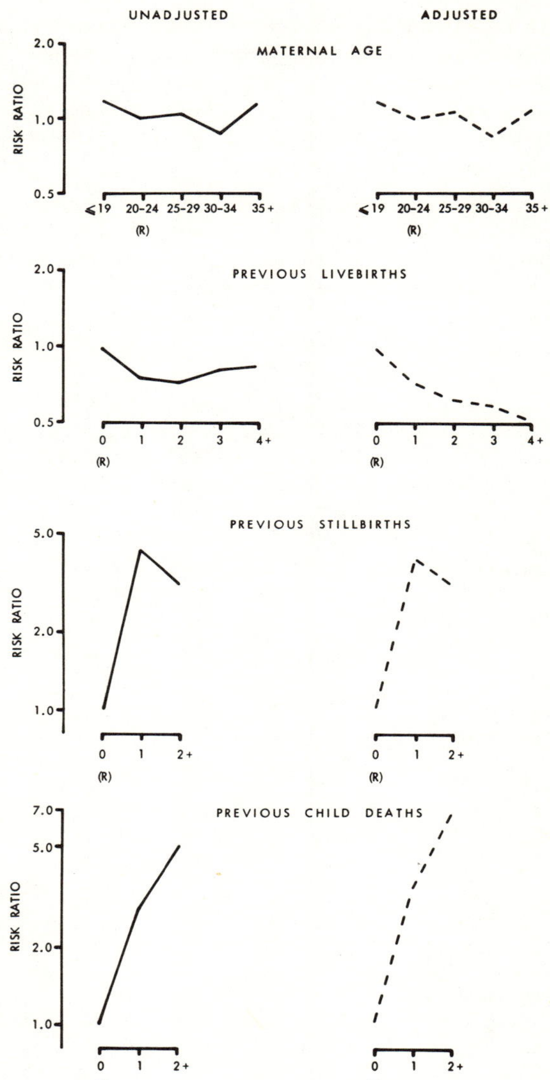

FIG. 21.1. Risk ratios (risk of an anencephalic stillbirth or infant death relative to the risk of 1.0 in the referent category (R) of mothers) by maternal age and reproductive history. *Left*: unadjusted ratios; *right*: ratios adjusted for all other study variables—Canadian 14-city study.

The large increased risk associated with a previous stillbirth or a previous child death explains the high crude risk seen in high parity mothers. The U-type association of the unadjusted anencephalus risk with total parity is clearly demonstrated in the Canadian data, as is the inverse association seen after controlling confounding by all other study variables (Fig. 21.2). If only women who have no history of stillbirths or child deaths are considered, this unidirectional inverse relationship is evident even in the unadjusted data, and control of confounding by the other study variables makes little difference. Thus the removal of the confounding effects of stillbirth and child death history, either by a multivariate method or by restricting the analysis to mothers with no such history, demonstrates that the effect of an increasing number of livebirths alone is to decrease risk. The crude and adjusted risks for mothers who have had no stillbirths or child deaths are very similar showing that no other factors have major confounding effects. This we suggest is the explanation of the frequently observed U-type relationship of

TABLE 21.2 *Unadjusted and adjusted† risks of anencephalus associated with subclasses of maternal age and the numbers of previous livebirths, stillbirths, and child deaths*

Factor and subclass		Number of cases	Number of controls	Mortality rate per 1000	Crude risk-ratio	Adjusted risk-ratio
Maternal age	≤19	164	513	1.34	1.19	1.18
	20–4	425	1586	1.12	1.0 (R)	1.0 (R)
	25–9	376	1368	1.15	1.03	1.03
	30–4	225	946	1.00	0.89	0.84
	35+	182	584	1.31	1.16	1.06
Number of	0	601	1852	1.36	1.0 (R)	1.0 (R)
previous	1	315	1287	1.03	0.75	0.72
livebirths	2	199	854	0.98	0.72	0.62
	3	121	465	1.09	0.80	0.59
	4+	148	540	1.15	0.84	0.51
Number of	0	1249	4860	1.08	1.0 (R)	1.0 (R)
previous	1	125	113	4.63	4.30	4.03
stillbirths	2+	16	20	3.35	3.11	3.22
Number of	0	1189	4733	1.05	1.0 (R)	1.0 (R)
previous	1	170	234	3.04	2.89	3.45
child deaths	2+	31	25	5.19	4.94	6.92

† Adjusted risk-ratio (standardized mortality ratio, Miettinen 1972), after controlling for the joint confounding effects of all ten other factors included in the 14-city study, by stratification on a multivariate risk score (Appendix A.3, Elwood, J. M. *et al.* 1978).
(R) = referent level.
Tests for linear trend in adjusted risk-ratios (Mantel 1963):

Maternal age		N.S.
Previous livebirths	$Z = -7.7$	$p<0.001$
Previous stillbirths	$Z = 10.0$	$p<0.001$
Previous child deaths	$Z = 12.8$	$p<0.001$

the prevalence at birth of anencephalus with total parity. The effect of previous livebirths themselves is to reduce risk. However, because among high-parity women there are a considerable proportion who have had previous stillbirths or child deaths, the high risks conferred by these factors increase the prevalence rate of the whole group. The expected prevalence rates for each total parity group in the 14-city study were calculated on the basis of the expected numbers of women with previous stillbirths or child deaths (given by the control group) and the unconfounded estimates are the risks associated with each number of previous livebirths, and with a history of stillbirth or of child death. These expected rates are close to those observed if a multiplicative model is used (Elwood, J. M. *et al.* 1978).

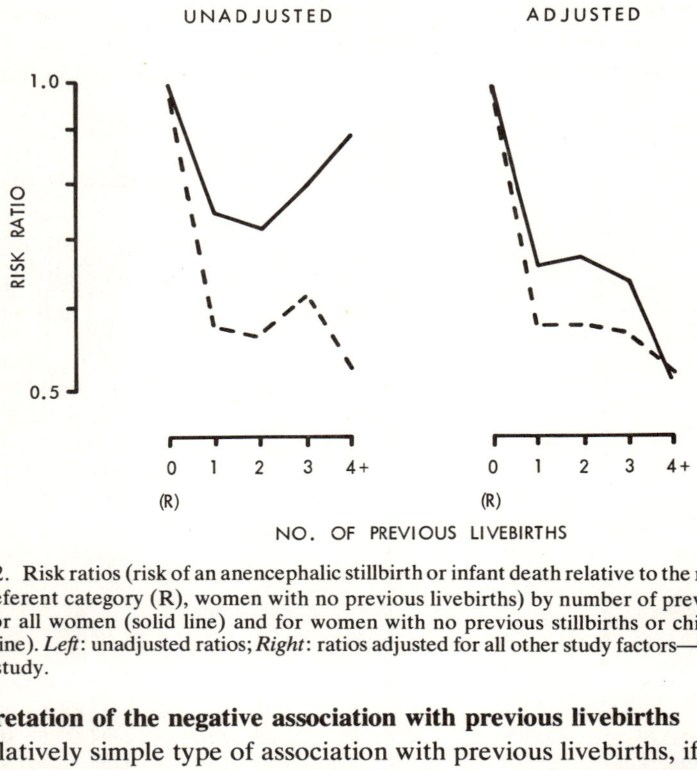

FIG. 21.2. Risk ratios (risk of an anencephalic stillbirth or infant death relative to the risk of 1.0 in the referent category (R), women with no previous livebirths) by number of previous livebirths for all women (solid line) and for women with no previous stillbirths or child deaths (dotted line). *Left*: unadjusted ratios; *Right*: ratios adjusted for all other study factors—Canadian 14-city study.

Interpretation of the negative association with previous livebirths

The relatively simple type of association with previous livebirths, if applicable generally, may provide an explanation for the confusing multiplicity of types of association in earlier work. Although no other similar analysis has been carried out, several other studies are relevant. James (1968) examined the risk of stillbirths in sibships included in the Kauai pregnancy study (Yerushalmy, Bierman, Kemp, Connor, and French 1956). Scrutiny of stillbirth rates from all causes, based on populations at one point in time, showed a U-type association with birth order rather similar to that recorded for anencephalus. However, study of completed sibships implied that the probability of undertaking another pregnancy was greater after a stillbirth than after a livebirth and James suggested there is a negative association between stillbirth risk and birth order within sibships; the increased stillbirth rate in the population at high birth-orders is due to the over-representation of stillbirth-prone women. He has extended this approach to studies of neural-tube defect sibships (James 1969). The ratio of anencephalus stillbirths to all stillbirths declines with increasing parity in extensive data from both Scotland and England and Wales. This suggests there is a strong negative association of anencephalus risk with increasing parity, or that mothers of anencephalics are under-represented in high-parity groups because of voluntary birth limitation or relative infertility. James used some sibship data from British Columbia to compare the numbers of births subsequent to a neural-tube defect with the numbers born subsequently to mothers who had had a stillbirth without a neural-tube defect. There was little evidence of reproductive limitation after a neural-tube defect birth and so his major conclusion was that within sibships there is a negative association of anencephalus risk with either birth order or maternal age; he did not attempt to separate these two factors. This work predicts that the risk of a neural-tube defect in pregnancies after the birth of a propositus (the recurrence risk) is lower than that in earlier pregnancies (the precurrence risk) while available studies suggest these risks are similar (Section 25). However, the birth order associations of second affected infants, and all affected infants, need not necessarily be the same.

Janerich's (1972, 1972*a*, *b*) analyses of the association of the prevalence rates of anencephalus and of spina bifida with maternal age demonstrate that the U-shaped relationship seen in cross-sectional data reflects a negative linear trend within birth cohorts (see below). This study is similar to the sibship studies described in that secular trends over time are controlled by the method of analysis. The Canadian data give similar results to those of Janerich when analysed in the same way, without control for other factors. On the other hand, in the Canadian data the cross-sectional U-type associations and the negative trends within cohorts for anencephalus risk by maternal age are both indirect associations and the direct association is with the number of previous livebirths rather than with maternal age. Thus there is some support for a negative association between the risk of a neural-tube defect and birth order in other studies which attempt to control for secular trends or for differences in fertility.

British Columbia sibship study

We have been able to confirm the results of the 14-city study by an extensive study of sibships in British Columbia (Elwood, J. M. and McBride 1979). From 390 796 sets of records representing marriages in British Columbia during the period from 1946 to 1970, and the linked subsequent births, we identified 414 sibships in which at least one birth affected by anencephalus or spina bifida had been observed. We selected 1362 comparison sibships in which no neural-tube defects had occurred, matched on the occurrence of the marriage and the first birth between 1946 and 1970 and by having a sufficiently high record linkage weight. With this material linked in sibships we were able to analyse the data by birth order and sibship size and to show that for a given sibship size the risk of a first neural-tube defect decreases sharply with birth order whereas for a given birth order the risk increases with sibship size (Fig. 21.3 and Table 21.3). Thus it appears that for one sibship, that is, one mother, her risk of bearing a child with a neural-tube defect decreases with birth order and is unaffected by her age. This finding is consistent with the other Canadian work and the study of James (1969).

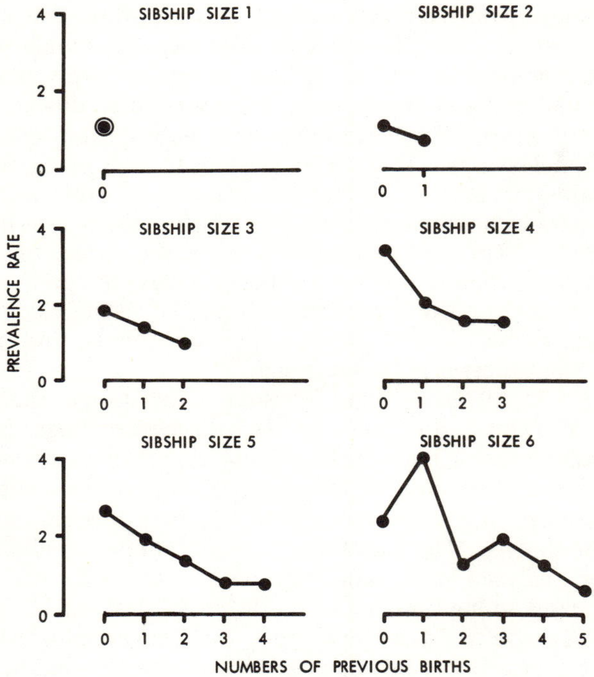

FIG. 21.3. Prevalence rates per 1000 total births for anencephalus and spina bifida combined by number of previous births and sibship size—British Columbia (Elwood, J. M. and McBride 1979).

However, mothers of affected infants have more pregnancies than other mothers. In British Columbia, these mothers demonstrate shorter inter-pregnancy intervals even before the birth of the first affected infant than do comparison mothers, as well as having more pregnancies after an affected birth (Fig. 21.4). Thus their greater reproduction is not solely a consequence of having had an affected birth, but precedes it. This suggests these mothers are either biologically more fertile or undertake more pregnancies because of other factors such as social class or ethnic or religious differences. Because of their greater frequency of reproduction, the population of high-parity mothers includes a greater proportion of these women and this contributes to the rise in prevalence rates seen in higher parities in population data.

The greater reproduction of mothers of infants with neural-tube defects likely reflects higher biological fertility. Although in the British Columbia study we have no direct social-class information, there was no difference between affected and unaffected sibships in terms of maternal age at first birth, which should be a reasonable indicator of sociological influences on reproduction. Unfortunately, the other studies relating to fertility suffer from similar limitations. Record and McKeown (1950) found the intervals between marriage or a previous birth and conceptions were shorter in mothers of neural-tube defect infants than in control mothers, both for the affected birth and for siblings. The mean family size in the affected families was larger. However, no control was made for socio-economic factors. Data

TABLE 21.3 *Numbers of neural-tube defect births, unaffected siblings and comparison births, and prevalence rates per 1000 births by sibship size and birth rank—British Columbia sibship study*

Sibship size	Birth rank	Affected births	Unaffected siblings	Births in comparison sibships	Prevalence per 1000	Standard error
1	1	47	0	414	1.16	0.06
2	1	51	36	472	1.11	0.05
	2	36	0	468	0.79	0.04
3	1	50	64	284	1.80	0.11
	2	37	27	283	1.34	0.08
	3	27	0	279	0.99	0.06
4	1	39	59	116	3.42	0.32
	2	23	35	116	2.03	0.19
	3	18	17	117	1.57	0.14
	4	17	0	111	1.57	0.15
5	1	14	25	54	2.64	0.36
	2	10	15	55	1.86	0.25
	3	7	8	53	1.35	0.18
	4	4	4	54	0.76	0.10
	5	4	0	54	0.76	0.10
6	1	4	14	17	2.39	0.58
	2	6	8	15	4.07	1.04
	3	2	5	16	1.28	0.32
	4	3	3	16	1.92	0.48
	5	2	1	16	1.28	0.32
	6	1	0	16	0.64	0.16

Data refer to prevalence rates for first affected births in a sibship: thus births subsequent to an affected birth are excluded. (After Elwood, J. M. and McBride 1979.)

from the British Perinatal Mortality Survey of 1958 show no significant differences between the period preceding a birth affected by anencephalus and the period for comparison births (James 1973; Fedrick and Adelstein 1973). Implications with regard to fertility also have been made on more indirect grounds. The lower risk of anencephalus in illegitimate births has been regarded as suggestive of an association with lower fertility (James 1973). Data on twinning has been variously interpreted. There is considerable evidence that mothers of twins are more fertile than other women (Allen and Schachter 1971; Milham 1964, Wyshak and White 1969), and therefore an association between twinning and neural-tube defect occurrence might be expected (Elwood, J. M. 1974*a*). This is discussed further in Section 24.

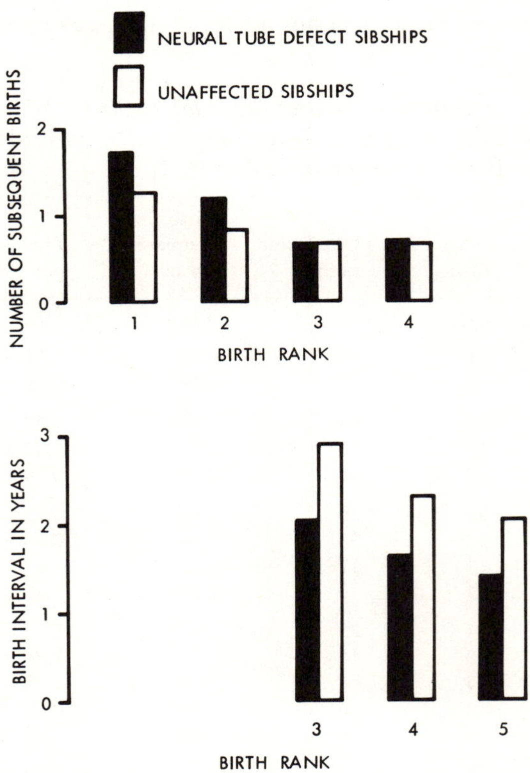

FIG. 21.4. Comparisons of fertility in sibships containing a birth with a neural-tube defect and in comparison sibships. *Top*: mean number of subsequent births by birth rank of the index case. *Bottom*: Mean interval between previous births, excluding the interval immediately prior to the index birth, by birth rank of the index case—British Columbia (Elwood, J. M. and McBride 1979).

Interpretation of the positive associations with previous stillbirths and child deaths

The strongest associations of risk in the 14-city study were seen in relation to a history of a previous stillbirth or a previous child death, with relative risks after confounder control of 3.8 and 3.5 respectively. These associations are the product of several influences. First, they are due in part to the occurrence of neural-tube defects in earlier siblings of the anencephalic index cases; but this effect does not fully explain the association observed. The 5000 control mothers had 7281 previous pregnancies, of which 452 (6.2 per cent) resulted in a stillbirth or infant death. The excess expected in the mothers of anencephalics due to previous children with neural-tube defects would be a maximum of 5 per cent on the basis of reported risks to siblings, giving a total risk of 11.2 per cent. A lower estimate of a 2.4 per cent excess as part of a total of 8.6 per cent would be given by the recent Canadian estimates of recurrence risk (McBride 1977). The observed risk was 408 in 2040 previous pregnancies which is 20 per cent.

The study did not include an estimate of socio-economic status and it is likely that women in the less prosperous social groups have a higher risk of anencephalus and also have more stillbirths and child deaths than other women. A positive association with 'child deaths', which as noted above includes all deaths of liveborn children up to the time of the birth of the index case, would be produced if mothers of anencephalics had longer interpregnancy intervals or more previous pregnancies. However, the latter factor was controlled and our sibship study shows the interpregnancy intervals in anencephalus sibships are shorter than those in unaffected sibships. Spontaneous abortions are more frequent than expected in mothers of anencephalics and appear to be most frequent in pregnancies before the birth of the affected infant. It seems likely that some causes may be common to spontaneous abortions and to stillbirths.

An important issue is whether the increased risk of anencephalus is related to the event of a previous stillbirth or child death or is related to the predisposition to such an event. Clarke *et al*. (1975) suggest that neural-tube defects may arise from an interaction between a foetus and a cell rest remaining from a previous pregnancy; they postulate such a rest is more likely to occur after a spontaneous abortion than after a livebirth. Also, if it is more likely after a stillbirth, this could provide a mechanism for the stillbirth association seen. The higher occurrence rate of anencephalus at later birth orders would be explained by a greater proportion of such mothers having had a stillbirth. The association with a previous child death is more difficult to explain directly by this model; however many of these may have been abnormal infants and the association may be due in part to socio-economic factors. The main support for Clarke *et al*.'s hypothesis is the evidence they present for a maximal rate of spontaneous abortion in the pregnancy immediately preceding the birth of an affected infant. The finding of a high risk in first births is against the hypothesis, as the authors themselves note and the

Canadian data suggest this primiparity association is stronger than previously thought. An alternative is that the real association is a predisposition to stillbirths, spontaneous abortions, and child deaths which may be related to social, nutritional, hormonal, or other features. In this case the explanation of the higher rate of anencephalus at high total parities depends on the increased representation of such women due to higher fertility, either biological or voluntary in origin.

Parity as an effect modifier

We have discussed so far the crude effects of risk factors in the 14-city study and the effects after controlling the confounding effects of other variables. We also searched for interactive effects between factors by computing prevalence rates for mothers categorized in terms of two variables, for example maternal age and parity. The multivariate method employed allows the computation of such rates adjusted for the confounding effects of all other study factors (Appendix A.3). It was seen that although maternal age had no apparent effect on anencephalus risk for all mothers combined, for first births the average risk decreased with maternal age while for later births the risk increased (Fig. 21.5). Although neither trend is statistically significant, the pattern is similar to that described in Great Britain by Fedrick (1970).

Each study variable was examined to detect other interactions with parity, and there was evidence of effect modification for maternal age and for three other factors: year of birth, season of birth, and legitimacy (Fig. 21.5). In each case the difference in effect was between first and later births with no apparent differences within categories of parity greater than one. For year and season, the difference is of degree: both in first and later births there is a decrease over time and a higher mortality rate in winter births but the variations are much greater for first births. Anencephalus risk is related positively to illegitimacies in first births, but negatively in later births. The other important risk factors studied, namely city of residence, ethnic group and history of a previous stillbirth, appear to affect first births and later births similarly. The prevalence rate of anencephalus is much higher in first than in subsequent births, and the sex distribution differs between first and later births (Section 14).

Analysis by maternal birth cohort

The relationship of the prevalence of neural-tube defects to maternal age and reproductive history is further complicated by a possible association with the birth year of the mother. In a cross-sectional analysis of population data, the prevalence rates at one time period are compared between mothers of different ages who, by being born at different times, have experienced different events at various stages of life. We can identify 'cohorts' of women defined by year or quinquennium of birth and follow them through time. This method of analysing data within cohorts defined by year or period of birth has been widely applied with respect to adult chronic diseases, as

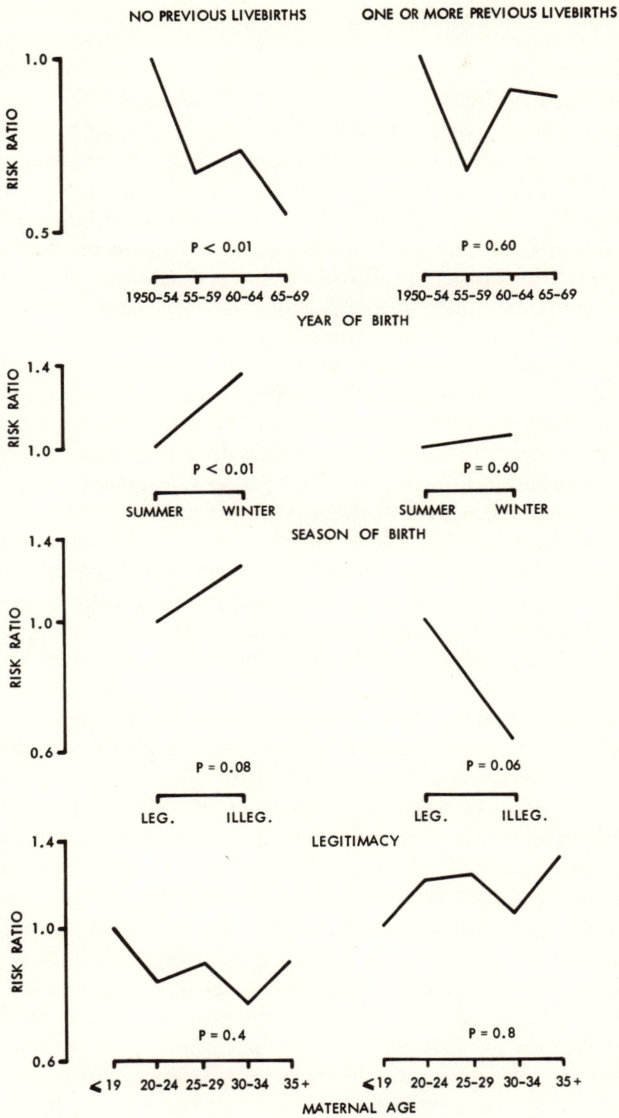

FIG. 21.5. Risk ratios (risk of an anencephalic stillbirth or infant death relative to the risk of 1.0 in the referent category (R) of women) by year of birth, season of birth, legitimacy, and maternal age for women with no previous livebirths (*left*) and for women with one or more previous livebirths (*right*). All risk ratios are adjusted for all other study factors and the *p* values shown are based on a linear trend test in the case of year of birth and maternal age—Canadian 14-city study.

described by Case (1956), but rarely has been used in studies of birth defects.

We have shown that secular variations in the prevalence at birth, both by year and by season, are more pronounced in first births than in later births in Canada; this has also been seen in Scotland (Edwards 1958) and in Rhode Island (Ingalls *et al*. 1954). Several investigators have studied the interaction of secular trends and associations with maternal age, parity, and social class. Janerich (1972, 1972*a*, *b*) examined the maternal age distribution of anencephalus and spina bifida in New York State from 1945 to 1967. The fall in prevalence of the order of 45 per cent was more marked in births to younger than to older mothers. Within cohorts defined by quinquennium of birth, the prevalence rates of neural-tube defects showed a decline with increasing maternal age, without the rise at higher maternal ages seen when a cross-sectional analysis was used. Janerich also considered the lifetime risk of bearing an affected infant as a function of the mother's year of birth; he found the lifetime risk decreased in successive cohorts born after 1906–10. Although this is interpreted as consistent with a high risk in mothers born during the depression (Janerich 1972), he also suggests (1972*b*) that as the highest risk is in mothers born in 1906–10, a possible mechanism is infection with influenza during early puberty associated with the 1919–21 pandemic which may have led to ovarian damage in a susceptible group of young girls. However, MacMahon and Yen (1971*a*) demonstrated that throughout the period from 1920 to 1944, the mean age of mothers of neural-tube defect infants was fairly constant and did not increase as predicted by Janerich's hypothesis.

Baird (1974) studied the perinatal mortality rate attributed to all central nervous system defects in Aberdeen, Scotland. He found the secular trends from 1950 to 1968 varied with maternal parity. A peak occurred in the rate for primiparae in 1951, for second births in 1954, and progressively later for higher birth-orders. Baird interprets this as a cohort effect with the high-risk groups beginning their childbearing life around 1948–52. He also claims that the data show variations with social class consistent with a later peak in the more prosperous groups due to a later age at childbearing. However, Baird only presents numbers of affected infants, without corresponding denominators, so any further interpretation is not possible. However, further data related to stillbirths from anencephalus in the whole of Scotland are given. These show that the secular trends in the stillbirth rates from anencephalus are different for different subgroups of mothers defined by age or parity. The maximum rates occur in later years in the older or high-parity groups, and the pattern supports the concept of a high-risk group of mothers being born in the period 1928 to 1934. This group, born during the economic depression, may have suffered relatively more chronic malnutrition in early childhood than later or earlier birth cohorts. In support of this, the excess of anencephalic births in this cohort is most marked in the lower social classes. Baird does not present these data in a fashion permitting analysis of the anencephalus prevalence and maternal age relationship, so

Janerich's proposition of a decreasing risk with increasing maternal age within cohorts cannot be tested directly. However, Baird's logic is similar. Emanuel and Sever (1973) also have considered a birth cohort mechanism. They suggest the 1930–4 peak in neural-tube defect prevalence in New England was related to mothers born in the early 1900s, a period characterized by 'massive immigration . . . and a major depression beginning in 1907'. They suggest that the absence of a major epidemic of neural-tube defects after the Second World War in the United States was due to efficient food distribution by the government preventing any major childhood malnutrition during the depression of the 1930s. Anderson, Baird, and Thomson (1958) commented that within the lower socio-economic groups the risk of neural-tube defects was maximal in births to mothers of short stature, which may indicate nutritional deprivation in early life.

As we mention, if the data from the 14-city study are analysed by birth cohort and maternal age the results are similar to those of Janerich. In the Canadian data the effect of maternal age itself is small and the rate in a particular maternal age subgroup is determined largely by the parity distribution of that subgroup. Therefore to see if there is a birth cohort effect, parity-specific rates, standardized for all other factors, were computed for each maternal quinquennium of birth (Table 21.4). There is some indication of a high rate in first births to mothers in the 1925 and 1930 birth cohorts, and in all birth orders in offspring of women from the 1915 cohort. However, the standard errors of these rates are substantial and the differences between rates by birth cohorts are not significant. The high prevalence rates in the 1925 and 1930 maternal birth cohorts in Canada are consistent with the hypotheses of maternal deprivation associated with child bearing during the depression years although the data are insufficient to lend much support.

TABLE 21.4 *Standardized† anencephalus mortality rates per 1000 livebirths, and standard errors, by parity and birth cohort*

Median year of birth	Number of previous livebirths					Parity-standardized rates
	0	1	2	3	4+	
1915	—	1.86 (0.82)	1.82 (0.46)	1.53 (0.40)	0.99 (0.21)	—
1920	1.79 (0.42)	1.01 (0.16)	1.09 (0.13)	0.98 (0.14)	0.80 (0.12)	1.29 (0.16)
1925	2.12 (0.34)	1.61 (0.33)	0.83 (0.08)	1.26 (0.15)	0.75 (0.09)	1.54 (0.11)
1930	2.03 (0.38)	1.16 (0.13)	1.12 (0.13)	0.75 (0.08)	0.84 (0.07)	1.40 (0.08)
1935	1.56 (0.09)	1.00 (0.09)	0.90 (0.10)	0.82 (0.11)	0.97 (0.13)	1.17 (0.07)
1940	1.54 (0.17)	1.08 (0.16)	1.17 (0.18)	0.67 (0.11)	0.93 (0.36)	1.21 (0.06)
1945	1.59 (0.39)	1.40 (0.35)	—	—	—	
1950	1.19 (0.16)	0.89 (0.32)	—	—	—	

† Standardized over strata of a risk score based on eight factors: city of residence, month of birth, legitimacy, previous stillbirths, previous infant deaths, maternal ethnic origin, kind of birth, and place of delivery.
— Insufficient data (less than 5 cases or 20 controls)

The concept of an 'intergenerational' effect, a term suggested by Emanuel and Sever (1973), is an intriguing one and deserves further consideration. Our data are insufficient to distinguish groups of mothers by ethnic origin and place of birth as well as by year of birth, but these factors would be expected to have some influence. A direct test of these intergenerational hypotheses would require a study of the early experiences of mothers of infants with neural-tube defects.

We conclude, therefore, that the relationships between maternal age and reproductive history and the occurrence of neural-tube defects are complex and involve differences in fertility and birth-cohort effects. Adequate explanations of the decrease in risk associated with an increase in the number of previous livebirths, and the increased risk in births to women with a history of stillbirths have not been provided. These relationships are important and further investigation may prove valuable. The suggestions of differences in aetiology between neural-tube defect occurrences in first births and in later births are also intriguing and may explain some of the inconsistencies of earlier studies.

22

Early foetal loss

AN important aspect of studies of anencephalus and spina bifida based on prevalence at birth is the degree to which this index reflects the true incidence and the extent to which the prevalence rate at birth is altered by affected foetuses being lost as spontaneous abortions prior to a gestational age when they would be recorded, currently 20 weeks or 28 weeks. In order to know how prevalence at birth reflects incidence, it is necessary to measure prevalence rates at different gestation times.

Creasy and Alberman (1976) studied a series of 2658 spontaneous abortions occurring in women hospitalized in London. A complete abortion or an intact sac was obtained in 1216 cases and of these 36 had some form of neural-tube defect giving a prevalence rate of 30 per 1000. Some 25 were examined cytogenetically and 10 were abnormal indicating that around 40 per cent of abortions having neural-tube defects represent types not analogous to those seen in stillborn or liveborn infants. After excluding such cases, Creasy and Alberman estimate the prevalence rate of anencephalus and spina bifida at 8 weeks of gestation at 5.3 per 1000. Their findings suggest 54 per cent of these abnormal foetuses spontaneously abort by 27 weeks, compared with a figure of 14 per cent for unaffected foetuses (Table 22.1). The prevalence rate then falls to 2.8 per 1000 corresponding to that reported in stillbirths and livebirths in London by Carter and Evans (1973). These estimates are among the best available but even so are open to sources of error. It must be assumed that the prevalence of defects is the same in the abortuses not examined as in those examined, and that those obtained through the several participating hospitals are representative of all abortions occurring in the community.

Nishimura's (1970) series of 2535 therapeutic abortions in Japan, of which 21 showed anencephalus or myeloschisis, estimates a prevalence of 5.9 per 1000. If we assume 40 per cent of affected embryos have chromosomal abnormalities, and use a life-table method analogous to that used by Creasy and Alberman the prevalence rate of anencephalus and spina bifida in early pregnancy is estimated as 3.5 per 1000, similar to that seen in London. The observed prevalence at birth of these defects in Japan is between 0.85 per 1000 (Neel 1958) and 0.5 per 1000 (Imaizumi 1974), thus the estimated early loss rate must be from 79 per cent to 87 per cent compared with 54 per cent in London. The similarity of the estimates of prevalence in early pregnancy suggests the difference in prevalence rates at birth between the two areas might be due to differing rates of foetal loss.

Also intriguing is the near equality of anencephalus and myeloschisis in early abortuses (10 and 11 cases respectively) in Japan while in stillbirths and livebirths there are about 3 cases of anencephalus to every one spina bifida, contrasting with the nearly equal ratio in most Caucasian populations. However, there are so many areas of doubt, particularly with regard to the representativeness of such specimens, that any conclusions are tentative.

TABLE 22.1 *Estimated prevalence of anencephalus and spina bifida (ASB) malformations at different stages of gestation for cohort counted (notionally) at eight weeks*

Stage of gestation (beginning of week)	Estimated number of surviving pregnancies of cohort counted at week 8	Estimated number of conceptuses with ASB in cohort	Estimated prevalence of ASB in surviving pregnancies of cohort (per 1000)
8	1000.00	5.29	5.29
12	930.10	3.78	4.06
16	888.45	2.86	3.22
20	876.62	2.62	2.99
24	868.83	2.56	2.95
27	864.73	2.46	2.84

From Creasy and Alberman (1976).

Investigation of complete population-based series of spontaneous abortions would be the best method of deciding which, if any, of the epidemiological features shown by the prevalence rates at birth of anencephalus and spina bifida are due to variations in rates of early foetal loss rather than to variations in incidence rates. The logistic problems of such studies are probably insurmountable and much less direct studies have been attempted. It is clear that differences in the rates of early foetal loss may produce large changes in prevalence rates at birth.

Roberts and Lloyd (1973) suggested geographical differences in the prevalence at birth of neural-tube defects in areas of South Wales might be due to differing rates of spontaneous abortion. They divided the eight major areas of South Wales into two groups according to the neural-tube defect prevalence rates and then studied the rates of previous spontaneous abortion reported by mothers resident in these two areas. For both mothers of infants having neural-tube defects and mothers of unaffected singleton infants, prior abortion rates were lower in women resident in the area with the higher prevalence rate at birth of neural-tube defects, and this difference was independent of parity, maternal age, and social class. However the difference was not very large; of mothers having unaffected infants, 13.0 per cent of those in the high prevalence area and 14.9 per cent of those in the low prevalence area reported having had a previous spontaneous abortion. The difference was greater for mothers of affected infants, 13.9 per cent and 19.6 per cent for high- and low-prevalence areas respectively. If we assume a higher rate of foetal loss for affected pregnancies then the data are consistent with the hypothesis that the incidence rate is the same in both geographical regions but the higher prevalence at birth in one area is due to a lower ratio of the foetal loss rate for neural-tube defects relative to the foetal loss rate for unaffected pregnancies. Fedrick and Adelstein (1976) also tested this hypothesis using material from England, Scotland, and Wales collected for the British Perinatal Mortality survey. They divided the data in two geographical areas with differing prevalence rates at birth of neural-tube defects and showed that mothers living in the area of higher prevalence had lower rates of prior spontaneous abortions.

Although there is some evidence that geographical variations in prevalence at birth may reflect differences in early foetal loss rates, it seems unlikely that this hypothesis explains all the epidemiological features of neural-tube defects as has been argued by Roberts and Powell (1975). The rates of spontaneous abortion by social class in South Wales were similar despite differences in the prevalence at birth of anencephalus and spina bifida. In Birmingham the seasonal trend in spontaneous abortion rates in neural-tube fraternities showed a spring peak, similar to that seen for anencephalus (Leck and Record 1966) while the seasonal variation in total spontaneous abortions in Quebec is also similar, rather than opposite, to the trend in anencephalus rates when both are expressed in terms of conception dates (McDonald 1971; Elwood, J. M. 1975). Spontaneous abortion rates in neural-tube defect sibships do not vary with birth order (McDonald 1971*a*) although prevalence rates at birth of neural tube defects show a strong decrease with respect to this factor (James 1968; Elwood. J. M. and McBride 1979). Thus these associations with three important factors namely, social class, season, and birth order, are not explained by the foetal loss hypothesis. Furthermore, mothers of neural-tube infants are not characterized by low early foetal loss rates but have above average numbers of spontaneous abortions as compared to other mothers.

X

Multiple pregnancy

23

Occurrence of anencephalus and spina bifida in twins

In any congenital malformation due to an abnormal intrauterine environment, it would be expected that if one member of a dizygotic twin pair is affected, the other would be affected more often than a non-twin sibling, because of the common environment. In any genetically controlled abnormality, monozygotic twins would be expected to show concordance more frequently than dizygotic twins, because of the greater similarity in their genetic composition. The prevalence at birth of neural-tube defects in full siblings of affected cases is between 2 per cent and 10 per cent (Section 25). Thus for almost any environmental or genetic model it would be expected that at least 2 per cent to 10 per cent of twin pairs would show concordance, and that a higher concordance rate would be found in monozygotic pairs if there were a genetic aetiology. However, lower figures could be produced if concordant twin pairs were more likely to be lost as early foetal deaths; in this case the total number of twin pairs observed in a population of mothers of anencephalics would be less than that expected assuming normal twinning rates.

Early reports recorded the non-concordance of twin pairs for anencephalus (Litt and Strauss 1935), even in two cases of conjoined twins (Mudaliar 1930; Stevenson *et al.* 1966). Josephson and Waller (1933) were the first to report concordance in a set of presumably identical twins. Most later studies show a similar lack of concordant twin pairs, although isolated reports of concordant twin pairs (six quoted by Yen and MacMahon 1968) and even concordant triplets (Scott and Patterson 1966) or triplets with two members affected (Carter *et al.* 1967) have been described.

Yen and MacMahon (1968) reviewed the question of the relative importance of genetic and environmental factors in anencephalus and spina bifida. From their own data from Boston and Providence, and six other consecutive series published at that time (Record and McKeown 1951; Dumoulin and Gordon 1959; Frézal *et al.* 1964; Williamson 1965; Böök and Rayner 1950; Carter *et al.* 1967), they showed that none of the 108 twin pairs described in which at least one infant was affected with either anencephalus or spina bifida had shown concordance. This lack of concordant pairs could be produced if there were a high early foetal loss rate of concordant twin pairs, in which case the total numbers of twin pairs in the series would be lower than the numbers predicted on the basis of population twinning rates. If the loss rate of monozygotic pairs were particularly high, the proportion of unlike-sex twin pairs in the series of affected births would be higher than that in the general population. Their calculations showed no evidence of any great loss rate of twins or any shift from the usual proportion of like-sex pairs, so they concluded that the low concordance rate and the normality of the proportion of like-sex pairs in discordant twins were not easily explicable by a genetic hypothesis. Instead, they emphasized the necessary role of environmental factors, as evidenced by variations in the prevalence rate over short time periods and by social class, and pointed out that the familial aggregation also can be accounted for solely by environmental influences.

Information on the occurrence of neural-tube defects in twin pairs is of importance in separating genetic and environmental issues, and more information is available now than at the time of Yen and MacMahon's study in 1968. We have summarized the information available in the literature which forms the basis of our discussion (Tables 23.1, 23.2, and 23.3). Recent summaries have also been made by Rogers and Weatherall (1976) and by James (1978), and the disparities between these reviews and our own reflect difficulties in interpreting many of the papers. Also, we intentionally exclude some studies as they are likely to have incomplete ascertainment; this applies to several very small studies and to the large studies of Hay and Wehrung (1970) and Barr and Stevenson (1961), whose data include livebirths only and exclude stillbirths.

Reports on anencephalus and spina bifida in twins

The collated data (Table 23.4) demonstrate a different pattern from that apparent at the time of Yen and MacMahon's study. The concordance rate, defined as the ratio of concordant pairs to total twin pairs, for anencephalus is 4.1 per cent and for spina bifida is 5.1 per cent; the difference is small and not significant. Considering both defects, the overall concordance rate is 5.4 per cent; it is higher because the seven anencephalus–spina bifida pairs are considered as concordant. For anencephalus and for spina bifida separately, the concordance rates are higher for like-sex twin pairs than for unlike-sex pairs. For both defects, 7.6 per cent of like-sex pairs show concordance compared to 2.8 per cent of unlike-sex pairs ($t = 2.7, p<0.01$). If we assume that dizygotic twins are equally likely to be of like sex or of unlike sex, the estimated concordance rate for dizygotic pairs is 2.8 per cent and for monozygotic pairs is 11.3 per cent. However, while this assumption holds for twin pairs in general (Weinberg 1901; Bulmer 1970), it may not apply to the current series of twin pairs with neural-tube defects, and the large number of pairs whose sexes are unknown are a source of error in any estimates. No large series of affected twin pairs where zygosity has been satisfactorily determined is available.

The concordance rate among twin pairs of unlike sex is 2.8 per cent for both defects. This contrasts with the sibling risks of around 5 per cent reported by most British studies. If the twin concordance rate is in fact lower than the sibling risk this would be most easily explained by the early loss of concordant dizygotic sets, although other mechanisms such as foetus–foetus interaction could be responsible. However, we cannot be certain that the risk is genuinely less. The 95 per cent upper confidence limit of the concordance rate is 5.2 per cent, close to the generally accepted full-sibling risk, and the recent studies showing low full-sibling risks of around 2 per cent (Janerich and Piper 1978; McBride 1979) make any firm conclusion questionable.

Occurrence of twins in series of births having anencephalus and spina bifida

If the risk of early foetal loss were higher for concordant than for discordant twin pairs with neural-tube defects, two effects would result. First, the total number of twin pairs in a series of cases of neural-tube defects would be lower than in a similar series of normal births and secondly, as concordance rates are higher for like-sex pairs, the proportion of these in series of affected twins would be lower than expected.

The information from series where the total number of cases of anencephalus or spina bifida is known (Tables 23.1 and 23.3) shows that of 20 773 infants with neural-tube defects there were 402 twins, that is 1.9 per cent of affected infants were twins (Table 23.5). To evaluate this, we need to estimate the twinning rate for normal births. However, twinning rates vary between areas and show secular trends, particularly in recent years; they also vary by maternal age and to a lesser extent by parity (Bulmer 1970; James 1972; Elwood, J. M. 1973, 1978). These factors should be taken into account in calculating an expected twinning rate, but sufficient information is not available for all areas. We have calculated expected numbers of twins taking into account differences by area and time but we have not adjusted for any maternal age or parity effects on the relevant twinning rate. In data from the United States this omission lowers the expected twinning rate (Yen and MacMahon 1968). The total expected number of twins is 432 compared to an observed number of 402 (Table 23.5). Thus on the basis of this estimate, the total number of twins in series of anencephalus and spina bifida cases is slightly lower than expected and the early foetal loss rates of affected twin pairs may be in excess of the losses of normal twin pairs but better data are required on this point.

Of the 600 twin pairs ascertained whose sex composition is known, 419, or 69.8 per cent, were like-sex pairs (Table 23.4). A high foetal loss rate of monozygotic pairs would produce a reduction in this proportion as compared to twins in the general population. The expected proportion of like sex pairs can also be calculated from the sources used to provide twinning rates. Monozygotic twinning rates in almost all countries lie between 3.5 and 4.0 per 1000 maternities (Bulmer 1970), and using these figures yields an expected proportion of like-sex pairs of between 67 and 69 per cent. There is therefore no evidence for a differential early foetal loss of like-sex pairs. Although this estimate also requires adjustment for maternal age and parity, it is likely that the change produced by such adjustment would be small.

The male proportion in anencephalus, but not in spina bifida, appears to

TABLE 23.1 *Selected reports of anencephalus in twins where the total number of anencephalics in the related population is known*

Reference	Total number of cases	Total number of sets	Discordant pairs: Like-sex Mm	Discordant pairs: Like-sex Ff	Discordant pairs: Unlike-sex Mf	Discordant pairs: Unlike-sex Fm	Discordant pairs: Not Stated	Discordant pairs: Total	Concordant pairs: Like sex	Concordant pairs: Unlike sex	Concordant pairs: Not Stated
British Isles											
Williamson 1965	29	2	0	2	0	0	0	2	0	0	0
Carter *et al.* 1968	247	6	2	3	0	1	0	6	0	0	0
Butler and Alberman 1969	503	12	4	4	1	2	1	12	0	0	0
Coffey and Jessop 1971	737	20	0	0	0	0	20†	20	0	0	0
Elwood J. H. and Nevin 1973	175	4	0	3†	0	1	0	4	0	0	0
Carter and Evans 1973	578	10	1	5	0	3	0	9	0	1	0
Fedrick 1976	177	7	2	5	0	0	0	7	0	0	0
Smithells *et al.* 1964	180	3	1†		0		2	3	0	0	0
Comerford 1965	150	1	0		0		0	0	0	0	1
Subtotal	2776	65	32		8		23	63	0	1	1
North America											
Yen and MacMahon 1968	782	14	4	5	3	1	1	14	0	0	0
Horowitz and McDonald 1969	1497	41	9	15	8	8	1	41	0	0	0
Cassady 1969	367	6	0	0	0	0	6	6	0	0	0
Solowy and Shepard 1971	23	1	0	1	0	0	0	1	0	0	0
McBride 1977	466	8	2	4	1	0	0	7	1 (MM)	0	0
Gittelsohn and Milham 1965	1504	43	24†		14		0	38	4	1	0
Subtotal	4639	113	64		35		8	107	5	1	0

Europe											
Böök and Rayner 1950	67	3	2	1	0	0	0	3	0	0	0
Frézal *et al*. 1964	402	7	3	2	1	0	1	7	0	0	0
Czeizel and Révész 1970	360	6	0	1	4	1	0	6	0	0	0
Granroth *et al*. 1978	199	8	0	0	0	0	7	7	1 (FF)	0	0
Subtotal	1028	24	9		6		8	23	1	0	0
Other areas											
Searle (Singapore) 1959	68	1	1	0	0	0	0	1	0	0	0
Stevenson *et al*. (Multicentre) 1966	436	11	6	3	0	2	0	11	0	0	0
Neel (Japan) 1958	41	1	1	0	0	0	0	1	0	0	0
Imaizumi (Japan) 1974	2661	38	0		0		38	38	0	0	0
Subtotal	3206	51	11		2		38	51	0	0	0
Grand total	11 649	253	116		51		77	244	6	2	1

† Co-twin having spina bifida.
M affected male m unaffected male
F affected female f unaffected female

TABLE 23.2 *Selected reports of anencephalus in twins where the total number of anencephalics in the related population is unknown*

Reference	Total number of sets	Discordant pairs						Concordant pairs	
		Mm	Ff	Mf	Fm	Not Stated	Total	Like sex	Unlike sex
British Isles									
Holland and Lane-Claypon 1926	1	0	0	0	0	1	1	0	0
Record and McKeown 1951	24	4	13	3	4	0	24	0	0
Wilson, J. K. 1955	2	1	0	0	0	1	2	0	0
Dumoulin and Gordon 1959	3	2	0	1	0	0	3	0	0
Pedlow 1961	1	0	1	0	0	0	1	0	0
Duncan *et al.* 1977	2	1	0	0	1	0	2	0	0
Smithells 1976*a*	3	3		0		0	3	0	
Subtotal	36	25		9		2	36	0	0
North America									
Monahan 1956	1	0	0	0	0	1	1	0	0
Alter 1962	1	0	0	0	0	0	0	1 (FF)	0
Fogel *et al.* 1965	1	1	0	0	0	0	1	0	0
Janerich and Piper 1978	31	10	10†	5	4	0	29	2 (FF)	0
Subtotal	34	21		9		1	31	3	0

Europe									
Simon 1932	1	0	0	0	0	1	1	0	0
Gruber 1934	3	0	0	0	1	1	2	1 (FF)	0
Hiilesmaa 1945	3	0	1	0	1	0	2	1	0
Verslege 1971	118§	84		29		0	113	4¶	1
Subtotal	125	85		30		2	118	6	1
Other area									
Field and Kerr (Australia) 1974	20	4	13‡	1	2	0	20	0	0
Total	215	148		51		5	205	9	1

† Co-twin having spina bifida; ‡ 2 such cases; ¶ Includes aplasia of the brain; § A further 5 anencephalic twinbirths are recorded (total of 123 from 1951 to 1968) but are excluded as they could not be classified.

M affected male m unaffected male
F affected female f unaffected female

TABLE 23.3 *Selected reports of spina bifida in twins where the total numbers of cases in the related populations are known and unknown*

Reference	Total number of cases	Total number of sets	Discordant pairs						Concordant pairs	
			Mm	Ff	Mf	Fm	Not Stated	Total	Like sex	Unlike sex
British Isles										
Carter *et al*. 1968	278	7	2	2	1	2	0	7	0	0
Butler and Alberman 1969	257	7	1	3	2	1	0	7	0	0
Elwood, J. H. and Nevin 1973	185	1	0	1†	0	0	0	1	0	0
Carter and Evans 1973	631	4	0	1	1	2	0	4	0	0
Smithells and Chinn 1965	258	5	0		0		5†	5	0	0
Subtotal	1609	24	10		9		5	24	0	0
North America										
Yen and MacMahon 1968	1009	16	4	10	1	0	1	16	0	0
Horowitz and McDonald 1969	2077	23	0	0	0	0	21	21	1	1
McBride 1977	597	7	2	2	1	2	0	7	0	0
Gittelsohn and Milham 1965	2025	43	24†		15		0	39	3 (MM)	1
Subtotal	5708	89	42		19		22	83	4	2
Europe										
Czeizel and Révész 1970	710	6	2	2	1	1	0	6	0	0
Granroth *et al*. 1978	239	4	0	0	0	0	4	4	0	0
Subtotal	949	10	4		2		4	10	0	0

Other areas										
Stevenson *et al*. (Multicentre) 1966	355	9	4	1	1	2	0	8	1 (FF)	0
Imaizumi (Japan) 1974	503	1	0		0		1	1	0	0
Subtotal	858	10	5		3		1	9	1	0
Total	9124	133	61		33		32	126	5	2
British Isles										
Record and McKeown 1951	Unknown	25	10	8	1	6	0	25	0	0
Dumoulin and Gordon 1959	Unknown	1	0	0	1	0	0	1	0	0
Coffey and Jessop 1971	Unknown	1	0	0	0	0	1†	1	0	0
Clarke *et al*. 1975	Unknown	3	1	0	1	1	0	3	0	0
Rogers 1976	Unknown	2	0	2	0	0	0	2	0	0
Lorber and Rogers 1977	Unknown	38	18		16		1	35	3	0
Subtotal		70	39		26		2	67	3	0
Other areas										
Janerich and Piper (US) 1978	Unknown	29	7	16†	2	3	0	28	1 (FF)	0
Myrianthopoulos (US) 1970	Unknown	3	1	1	1	0	0	3	0	0
Fogel *et al*. (US) 1965	Unknown	2	0	1	1	0	0	2	0	0
Field and Kerr (Australia) 1974	Unknown	17	2	7‡	3	3	0	15	1 (MM), 1 (FF)	0
Farrel (S. Africa) 1964	Unknown	1	0		1		0	1	0	0
Subtotal		52	35		14		0	49	3	0
Total		122	74		40		2	116	6	0

† Co-twin having anencephalus; ‡ 2 such cases.
M affected male m unaffected male
F affected female f unaffected female

TABLE 23.4 *Concordance rates for anencephalus and spina bifida in twins*

	Discordant pairs (number)	Concordant pairs (number)	Twin pairs (total number)	Concordance rate (per cent)
Anencephalus				
Like sex	264	15	279	5.4
Unlike sex	103	3	106	2.8
Unknown	82	1	83	1.2
Total	449	19	468	4.1
Spina bifida				
Like sex	135	11	146	7.5
Unlike sex	73	2	75	2.7
Unknown	34	0	34	0
Total	242	13	255	5.1
Both defects				
Like sex	387	32	419	7.6
Unlike sex	176	5	181	2.8
Unknown	114	2	116	1.7
Total	677	39	716	5.4

TABLE 23.5 *Total numbers of cases of anencephalus and spina bifida, numbers of twins affected and expected numbers of twins based on population twinning rates, from selected studies*

Neural-tube defect study	Total number of cases	Total number of twins	Expected number of twins	Twinning study
British Isles				
Smithells *et al.* 1964	180	3	4.1	James 1972
Comerford 1965	150	2	3.5	
Smithells and Chinn 1965	258	5	5.9	
Williamson 1965	29	2	0.7	
Carter *et al.* 1968	525	13	12.1	
Butler and Alberman 1969	760	19	18.7	
Coffey and Jessop 1971	737	20	23.0	Minogue 1974
Elwood, J. H. and Nevin 1973	360	5	8.3	James 1972
Carter and Evans 1973	1209	15	27.8	
Fedrick 1976	177	7	3.8	
Subtotal	4385	91	107.8	
North America				
Gittelsohn and Milham 1965	3529	95	74.1	Heuser 1968
Yen and MacMahon 1968	1791	30	37.0	Yen and MacMahon 1968
Horowitz and McDonald 1969	3574	66	75.8	Elwood, J. M. 1973
Cassady 1969	367	6	7.6	Hauser 1966
Solowy and Shepard 1971	23	1	0.5	
McBride 1977	1063	16	21.3	Elwood, J. M. 1973
Subtotal	10 347	214	216.2	
Europe				
Böök and Rayner 1950	67	3	1.9	Akesson *et al.* 1970
Frézal *et al.* 1964	402	7	8.7	Bulmer 1970
Czeizel and Révész 1970	1070	12	22.5	Czeizel 1974
Granroth *et al.* 1978	438	13	12.9	Timonen and Carpen 1968
Subtotal	1977	35	45.9	
Other areas				
Neel 1958	41	1	0.5	Bulmer 1970
Searle 1959	68	1	1.5	
Stevenson *et al.* 1966	791	21	19.6	Stevenson *et al.* 1966
Imaizumi 1974	3164	39	40.5	Bulmer 1970
Subtotal	4064	62	62.1	
Total	20 773	402	432.0	

be higher for affected twins than for affected singletons (Table 23.6). Combining all series, 39 per cent of anencephalics and 43 per cent of spina bifida cases amongst twins were male; the former proportion is higher than that seen for entire series. However, of a total of 723 affected births in twins, we know the sex for only half the cases, largely because many papers distinguished only between like- and unlike-sex pairs.

TABLE 23.6 *Sex distribution of anencephalus and spina bifida in twins*

Series with known and unknown total number of cases†	Numbers of cases of anencephalus or spina bifida				
	Total number in twins	Male	Female	Unknown sex	Male Proportion
Anencephalus					
Known	253	59	77	117	0.42
Unknown	215	34	60	121	0.35
Total	468	93	137	238	0.39
Spina bifida					
Known	133	31	36	66	0.46
Unknown	122	33	50	39	0.40
Total	255	64	86	105	0.43

† Data from Tables 23.1, 23.2, and 23.3.

In summary, the concordance rate amongst unlike-sex twin pairs appears to be somewhat lower than the risk to full non-twin siblings; but because of limited numbers and variable estimates of the full-sibling risk, this is uncertain and the risks to co-twins of unlike sex and to full siblings may be similar. The concordance rate for like-sex twin pairs is higher than that for unlike-sex pairs, supporting a genetic aetiology. In series of infants with neural-tube defects, the number of twins is lower than expected compared with series of normal births but the proportion of like-sex pairs amongst these affected twins is similar to that seen in normal births. The male proportion amongst anencephalic twins is higher than the male proportion occurring in anencephalic singletons; however, a female predominance is observed in anencephalic twins as in series of affected singletons.

24

Other associations with multiple pregnancy

THERE are several observations and hypotheses based on possible associations between the occurrence of neural-tube defects and the occurrence of multiple pregnancies to the same women or in the same populations. These ideas are not yet fully developed but a brief outline of the reasoning and the observations on which they are based may be of interest. We can state seven distinct hypotheses.

First, neural-tube defects may arise only if the pregnancy is originally a twin conception (Knox 1970). In contrast, certain types of twins such as double monsters may arise from embryos with neural-tube defects (Rogers 1969). Thirdly, certain individual women may have a tendency to bear both twins and, at preceding or succeeding pregnancies, infants with neural-tube defects (Janerich 1975). Twinning and neural-tube defects may be produced by the same exogenous agents (Elwood, J. M. 1974). Twins and neural-tube defects may be associated because of similar relationships between the times of conception and ovulation (James 1976). In contrast, women at high risk of having an infant with a neural-tube defect may have a below-average twinning rate (Spiers 1973*a*). Lastly, we can state the null hypothesis that there is no association between the probability of having an infant with a neural-tube defect and the probability of having a multiple pregnancy for any individual woman.

The observations on which these hypotheses are based are limited and usually of an indirect nature. There is some correlation on a world scale between the prevalence at birth of neural-tube defects and dizygotic twinning rates; for example, both are much less frequent in Japan than in Western countries. Stevenson and colleagues (1966) in their international hospital-based study of birth defects in 24 countries, noted a significant association between the prevalence rates at birth of anencephalus and spina bifida and of dizygotic twins. However, this association is produced by two centres (Belfast and Alexandria) having high rates of both neural-tube defects and twinning and there is no association if data from these two centres are excluded and the remaining data from 22 centres are analysed (Schlesselman and Spiers 1975). Janerich (1974) points out that some groups show high twinning rates but low anencephalus rates, for example the black populations of both Africa and the United States, and the populations of Denmark and Israel. Dizygotic twinning is due to multiple ovulation associated with high maternal levels of pituitary gonadotrophin and the racial differences in twinning rates probably reflect genetic differences in gonadotrophin production (Milham 1964; Benirschke and Kim 1973).

Janerich (1974) hypothesizes that high gonadotrophin levels may be primary, giving a high dizygotic-twinning rate and a low neural-tube defect rate, or secondary. In the latter situation, the ovaries have a polygenetically inherited defect in sensitivity to gonadotrophin, and for some reason associated with this produce abnormal ova which develop into anencephalic foetuses. Because of the insensitivity, a secondary type of hypergonadotrophinism is produced giving the high twinning rate. Janerich claims this hypothesis can account for the concordance rates in monozygotic twin pairs being higher than those in dizygotic pairs while yet still being quite low relative to the rates expected from current genetic theory. He further suggests that as the gonadotrophin receptors are determined partially by maternal non-nuclear material, a pair of monozygotic twins sharing the same original cell membrane and cytoplasm will be more alike than a dizygotic pair of twins and yet will not be identical. This non-nuclear influence would also support the cytoplasmic inheritance hypothesis suggested by Nance (1969), although as we point out (Section 26) this pattern seems more likely to be produced by errors in ascertainment. Janerich (1975) notes that levels of chorionic gonadotrophin in maternal plasma and in amniotic fluid are higher if the foetus is female and considers it possible that a female might be more easily affected by a lack of gonadotrophin function caused by receptor insensitivity, which would lead to the observed excess of females with neural-tube defects. On this hypothesis, the higher prevalence rate of anencephalus and spina bifida in lower socio-economic groups may be due to infectious disease, or possibly more frequent pregnancies. Dizygotic twinning rates increase sharply with maternal age and parity (Bulmer 1958; Elwood, J. M. 1978) whereas neural-tube defect rates show a U-shaped pattern, or a decrease with age when a cohort analysis is used (Janerich 1972*a*). The difference in the patterns is explained by Janerich (1977) as being due to the increase of gonadotrophin production with age (Milham 1964) compensating for the genetic receptor abnormality, which will not change with age.

This hypothesis, like several others, suggests that the same mothers will be predisposed to bearing both twins and offspring with neural-tube defects. There is some evidence that these two phenomena occur more frequently in the same mothers than would be expected if the likelihood of twinning and the likelihood of neural-tube defects were independent. Details of the sibships of propositi with anencephalus or spina bifida have been published for three British studies (Williamson 1965; Carter *et al*. 1968; Carter and Evans 1973). In total, excluding the index cases, there were 3146 pregnancies reported in these sibships of which 58 were twin pregnancies, a rate of 18.4 per 1000 with 95 per cent confidence limits of 13.7 to 23.1 per 1000. The rate is thus higher than the expected total twinning rate which is around 11.5 per 1000 (James 1972). However, adjustments for age and parity should be made and further evaluation is needed.

More indirect evidence of an association between twinning and the occurrence of neural-tube defects is given by comparisons of population groups and studies of illegitimate births and of women taking ovulation stimulants (Elwood, J. M. 1974*a*, *b*). The positive correlation between twinning and neural-tube defects is not consistent. Prevalence rates of twin births are higher in the black than in the white population in the United States whereas the rates of neural-tube defects are lower in blacks. Despite the large geographical variation in anencephalus rates in Canada, there are no interprovincial differences in twinning rates (Elwood, J. M. 1976). Although both anencephalus and dizygotic twinning in Canada show seasonal variations, the highest prevalence at birth is in January to March for anencephalus and August to November for dizygotic twins (Elwood, J. M. 1975, 1978). The secular trends in anencephalus mortality and in twinning rates in Canada show some similarities, but no constant association (Section 27). Twinning rates increase strongly with increasing maternal age but less strongly with increasing parity (Bulmer 1970; Elwood, J. M. 1978) and this pattern in Canada is unchanged by birth cohort analysis; the associations are therefore different from those found in relation to neural-tube defects. Twinning, unlike neural-tube defects, is probably more frequent in the higher socio-economic groups (Myrianthopoulos 1970), although this trend is weak and some reports show no association (Campbell, Campbell, and MacGillivray 1974) or an inverse relationship (Smith 1966).

It thus appears that there is no consistent positive association between twinning rates and prevalence rates of neural-tube defects in populations, and although some positive associations have been noted, an interpretation of a negative association also has been made (Spiers 1973*a*). Some association between dizygotic twinning and neural-tube defects may arise as mothers who are of above average fertility may be predisposed to both conditions. Dizygotic twinning is more common in illegitimate births (Eriksson and Fellman 1967) and in those conceived in the first three months of marriage (Bulmer 1959), and mothers of dizygotic twins have more pregnancies than others (Wyshak and White 1969; Renkonen 1969). A study in California (Allen and Schachter 1971) showed that during the rise in the birth rate in 1946 following the return of servicemen after the war, the dizygotic twinning rate rose a few months before the rise in the total birth rate. These studies can be interpreted as suggesting a greater chance of twinning in women who become pregnant more easily. The introduction of widespread contraception in a population may reduce the contribution made by such a group of highly fertile women to the number of total births and the twinning rate would decline (Elwood, J. M. 1973*a*).

Evidence about the fertility of mothers of infants with neural-tube defects has been based on illegitimate births in some reports, with the assumption that mothers of illegitimate births are more fertile than other mothers. James (1973) suggested as several studies showed a lower risk of anencephalus and spina bifida in illegitimate births (Record and McKeown 1949; Edwards 1958; Record 1961), mothers of infants with neural-tube defects must be subfertile. At that time we felt that the evidence for a positive association with twinning, implying high fertility, was stronger than that supporting a low-fertility hypothesis (Elwood, J. M. 1974), and our sibship study in British Columbia (Section 21) provides better evidence that mothers of infants with anencephalus and spina bifida are more fertile than comparison mothers. These arguments are related to the occurrence of neural-tube defects in births to mothers who, because of subfertility, used clomiphene to stimulate ovulation. If such women do experience a higher than normal prevalence rate of these defects, and the data are insufficient to show this at present, it appears more likely that this is due to the drug rather than to the subfertility state (Section 15).

The hypothesis that neural-tube defects arise from fusion of twin embryos also predicts a positive association with twinning, although an environmental trigger factor is also involved (Knox 1970). Rogers (1969) demonstrated similarities in the epidemiology of conjoined twins (double monsters) and neural-tube defects, and suggested that a twin pair concordant for anencephalus or spina bifida might fuse to produce such a conjoined twin. We discuss these hypotheses elsewhere (Section 27).

James (1976) noted that among twin pairs including an anencephalic the proportion of like-sex pairs is higher than in unaffected pairs. By calculating expected numbers from population twinning rates, he suggested that in series of anencephalic births, there was a small deficit in the number of unlike-sex pairs and an excess of like-sex pairs, and that this excess implied that monozygotic twins have a higher prevalence rate of neural-tube defects than dizygotic twins or singletons, irrespective of the status of the co-twin. He quotes other evidence suggesting that fertilization late in the cycle, after the ovum has 'aged' by several days, produces a greater proportion of female embyros and of monozygotic twins, and he suggests a higher prevalence of neural-tube defects also results. His data showing an observed to expected ratio for like-sexed twins of 1.36 yields an estimate of the risk of anencephalus for a monozygotic twin of 1.7 times that of a dizygotic twin. James supports his estimate by information on the zygosity of 18 anencephalic twin pairs (Field and Kerr 1974), which show that 9 were monozygotic compared with an expected number of 7.

In our summary of the literature on this topic (Section 23), we concluded that the overall frequency of twins in series of births having anencephalus or spina bifida was similar to that in all births, and the proportion of twin sets which were of like sex (69.8 per cent) was similar to that of normal births. The data used by James relate only to anencephalus, and he found 73.1 per cent of affected twin pairs to be of like sex; our summary yields 72.5 per cent like sex for anencephalus and 66.1 per cent for spina bifida. Thus James's hypothesis may apply only to anencephalus. However, more and better data are required; for example, the main contribution to the excess of observed over expected like-sex twin sets in James's paper is made by the study of Hay and Wehrung (1970), which we have excluded as it includes liveborn anencephalic infants only.

The hypothesis of a close association between monozygotic twinning and neural-tube defects is supported by some animal data showing the production of both conditions by methods involving delays in fertilization (Stockard 1921), and by case reports of human foetuses with neural-tube defects and incomplete twinning (Riccardi and Bergmann 1977). However, more relevant are systematic human studies. Burns (1973) found no evidence of delayed fertilization in an analysis of conception times of spina bifida infants, estimated from birth-weight and gestation, and Kuhr (1977) found a less frequent history of mid-cycle abstinence contraception before pregnancies resulting in neural-tube defects than before other pregnancies in 117 mothers in Pennsylvania. However, none of these studies is definitive and further investigation is warranted. Cross (1968) carried out several studies at the Rotunda Hospital, Dublin, and considered the prevalence of anencephalus and other birth defects could be influenced by a preconceptional regimen restricting the time and frequency of sexual intercourse to predicted dates of ovulation. However, his reported results are insufficient for more definite evaluation.

The question of some association between the occurrence of neural-tube defects and of twinning is one of the most intriguing aspects of the epidemiology of anencephalus and spina bifida. Several of the hypotheses which have been based on such an association imply that the mechanism of the production of neural-tube defects may be much more complex than a simple toxic action of a teratogen.

XI

Familial aggregation

THE presence of more than one malformed infant in a family has always been of interest particularly when the same type of malformation which has occurred in one child recurs in a subsequent child. Although the great majority of families having an anencephalic or spina bifida infant will only experience one such affected pregnancy a small minority of around 5 per cent will have more than one affected offspring (Edwards and Balfour 1976).

25

Sibling risks

IN single families, Martin (1840) and Stevenson (1960) described six affected sibs; Iffy (1963) and Christakos and Simpson (1969) described families each having three anencephalic siblings while Horne (1958) reported a family in which four anencephalics were born, the last resulting from a union with a man other than the father of the first three. Spreng (1938) records the reproductive history of a mother and her four daughters. The mother and oldest daughter lost their first pregnancies as miscarriages at around three months, the second daughter gave birth to a spina bifida infant who died at 22 days from meningitis, and the two younger daughters each produced anencephalic offspring. Subsequent births, five in the case of the mother, three to the older daughter, one to the second daughter, and none to the others at the time of writing were all normal.

Generally previous pregnancy loss irrespective of cause is associated with subsequent reproductive compensation which is more marked following post-neonatal deaths than stillbirths or neonatal deaths (Vogel and Knox 1975; Fedrick and Adelstein 1977), and we described earlier (Section 21) that mothers of anencephalic infants in British Columbia had more pregnancies than a control group of mothers having unaffected infants.

The prevalence at birth of anencephalus or spina bifida in full siblings of a propositus having either defect in reported series varies from less than 1 per cent to nearly 10 per cent (Tables 25.1 and 25.2). If we first consider ascertainment through anencephalic index cases, the lowest figure is a full sibling risk of 0.9 per cent in Birmingham, England, and the highest is 9.6 per cent in the Oxford area (Table 25.1). The Birmingham rate is very low and probably reflects a considerable degree of under-ascertainment. The full sibling risk calculated from all available series averages 3.9 per cent. Secondly, considering full sibling risks of anencephalus and spina bifida in index cases having spina bifida, these range from 1.8 per cent in New York State (excluding New York City) to 6.1 per cent in South Wales (Table 25.2). The full sibling risk calculated from all available series averages 4.0 per cent. Thus, based on all available series, the full sibling risk associated with a spina bifida propositus (4.0 per cent) is very similar to that with an anencephalic propositus (3.9 per cent).

An important finding is that there are differences between different countries in the full sibling risks of anencephalus and spina bifida ascertained through index cases having either defect. The average sibling risk for index cases having spina bifida is 2.8 per cent in North America compared with 4.6 per cent in the United Kingdom. The European figure of 2.8 per cent is similar to that seen in North America. Furthermore, for index cases with anencephalus, the average sibling risk of a neural-tube defect is 4.4 per cent in the United Kingdom studies, 3.1 per cent in North American data, and 3.4 per cent in European studies. The higher sibling risks seen in the United Kingdom as compared to North America are statistically significant (Table 25.3). The North American series show that the earlier studies of Yen and MacMahon (1968) relate to the period from 1945 to 1965 and they exhibit sibling risks similar to those seen in the United Kingdom; it is the recent surveys of McBride (1977) and Janerich and Piper (1978) which show lower sibling risks. Interestingly, the areas and time period covered by

TABLE 25.1 *Prevalence of anencephalus and spina bifida in siblings of index cases having anencephalus*

		Full Siblings			
Anencephalus reference	Number of propositi	Number	Anence-phalus	Spina bifida	Per cent affected
United Kingdom					
Penrose 1946	21	57	2	2	7.02
Record and McKeown 1950	302	582	3	2	0.86
Williamson 1965	27	41	2	0	4.88
Smithells *et al.* 1968	100	887	26	13	4.40
Carter *et al.* 1968	361	708	16	13	4.10
Richards *et al.* 1972	146	454	18	8	5.73
Carter and Evans 1973	392	754	24	17	5.44
Fedrick 1976	177	115	9	2	9.57
Subtotal	1526	3598	100	57	4.36
Europe					
Böök and Rayner 1950	42	66	0	1	1.52
Polman 1950	73	180	8	5	7.22
Frézal *et al.* 1964	354	423	5	3	1.89
Czeizel and Révész 1970	151	186	3	4†	3.76
Subtotal	620	855	16	13	3.39
North America					
Yen and MacMahon 1968	480	573	14	12	4.54
McBride 1977	466	797	10	12	2.76
Janerich and Piper 1978	NS	434	—	8‡ —	1.84
Subtotal	946	1804	24	8‡ 24	3.10
Grand total	3092	6257	140	8‡ 94	3.87

NS = Not stated
† Includes one case of encephalocele
‡ Anencephalus or spina bifida, not specified.

TABLE 25.2 *Prevalence of anencephalus and spina bifida in siblings of index cases having spina bifida*

Spina bifida reference	Number of propositi	Full siblings: Number	Anencephalus		Spina bifida	Per cent affected
United Kingdom						
Penrose 1946	79	297	2		8	3.37
Record and McKeown 1950	300	654	7		10	2.60
Lorber 1965	539	1256	22		54	6.05
Williamson 1965	59	119	1		6	5.88
Carter *et al*. 1968	423	854	20		32	6.09
Smithells *et al*. 1968	152	903	20		11	3.43
Richards *et al*. 1972	172	450	6		19	5.56
Carter and Evans 1973	478	730	12		13	3.42
Subtotal	2202	5263	90		153	4.62
Europe						
Polman 1950	50	123	1		4	4.06
Czeizel and Révész 1970	249	334	0		9	2.69
Subtotal	299	457	1		13	2.84
North America						
Yen and MacMahon 1968	615	690	14		18	4.64
McBride 1977	452	1109	12		12	2.16
Janerich and Piper 1978	NS	603	—	11†	—	1.82
Subtotal	1067	2402	26	11†	30	2.79
Grand total	3568	8122	117	11†	196	3.99

† Spina bifida or anencephalus, not specified.

TABLE 25.3 *Differences between full sibling risks of anencephalus or spina bifida in index cases having either defect in the United Kingdom and North America*

Area	Index case—anencephalus: Siblings (number)	Affected (number)	Affected (per cent)	Index case—spina bifida: Siblings (number)	Affected (number)	Affected (per cent)
United Kingdom	3598	157	4.36	5263	243	4.62
North America	1804	56	3.10	2402	67	2.79

Anencephalus: $t = 2.37$; $p < 0.05$
Spina bifida: $t = 4.12$; $p < 0.001$
Data from Tables 25.1 and 25.2.

Yen and MacMahon's work had population prevalence rates of anencephalus and spina bifida of a similar order to those in most of the United Kingdom, whereas the recently reported low sibling risks apply to populations where the prevalence rates at birth also are low. Unfortunately, no estimates are available for families resident in Ireland where the prevalence of anencephalus and spina bifida is very high. Coffey (1974) states that of 737 cases of anencephalus from whom information was available, some 49 (6.6 per cent) had more than one anencephalic infant. These 49 women produced 279 pregnancies of whom only 118 were normal, the remainder ending as 37 abortions, 103 anencephalics, 11 infants with other central nervous system defects, 6 infants with other defects, and 4 stillbirths.

Genetic counselling, however, is usually based not on full sibling risks but on the recurrence risks in sibs born subsequent to a propositus. We have calculated these risks for areas of the United Kingdom and North America depending on whether the propositus has anencephalus or spina bifida (Table 25.4). The trends are similar to those described for full sibling risks and again the figures are higher for the United Kingdom than for North America. If the propositus has anencephalus the recurrence risk of anencephalus and spina bifida in subsequent sibs averages 5.2 per cent in the United Kingdom and 3.0 per cent in North America. If the propositus has spina bifida, the risks are 4.6 per cent in the United Kingdom and 2.8 per cent in North America. Several studies have compared risks to siblings born prior to and subsequent to the propositus (Table 25.5) Considering all studies listed in which siblings born prior and subsequent to the index case can be identified, there is clearly no difference in the prevalence of neural-tube defects in these two groups in the British studies considered together, nor have differences been observed in individual studies. In the two North American studies, the risks in later born siblings are lower, and the difference is at the conventional significance level ($t = 1.97, p = 0.05$). This discrepancy will require further clarification. Yen and MacMahon (1968), in a study in which data on the risk to previously born siblings are not available, demonstrated the recurrence risk in subsequent siblings declined with time in the same way as the population prevalence was declining and no difference between the risk in the next born and in the later children was found when this secular variation was taken into account. Percentage recurrence risks for siblings born in the years 1936–45, 1946–50, 1951–5, 1956–60, and 1961–7 were 8.6, 5.8, 3.2, 3.3, and 3.3 respectively. Richards *et al.* (1972) thought the risk to subsequent siblings was greater if the affected infant was first born (7.9 per cent) compared with a figure of 4.3 per cent after other propositi, an observation also made by Walker and Smith (1961).

The sibling risk is thus similar whether the propositus has either anencephalus or spina bifida. Siblings have a higher risk of either abnormality compared with the general population and while in some studies siblings exhibit the same abnormality as the propositus (Carter and Evans 1973), this is not a consistent finding within individual studies (MacMahon *et al.* 1953; Yen and MacMahon 1968). A summary of available series demon-

TABLE 25.4 *Recurrence rates of anencephalus and spina bifida in sibs born subsequent to propositi in the United Kingdom and North America*

Defect in Propositus Area & Reference	Subsequent siblings			
	Number	Anencephalus	Spina Bifida	Risk of ASB (per cent)
ANENCEPHALUS				
United Kingdom				
Williamson 1965	39	0	2	5.13
Smithells *et al*. 1968	126	6	3	7.14
Carter *et al*. 1968	234	4	7	4.70
Richards *et al*. 1972	154	8	2	6.49
Carter and Evans 1973	336	9	5	4.17
Subtotal	889	27	19	5.17
North America				
Yen and MacMahon 1968	573	14	12	4.54
McBride 1977	448	4	6	2.23
Janerich and Piper 1978	327	5†	—	1.53
Subtotal	1348	23	18	3.04
SPINA BIFIDA				
United Kingdom				
Williamson 1965	16	1	0	6.25
Smithells *et al*. 1968	187	1	5	3.21
Carter *et al*. 1968	305	4	11	4.92
Richards *et al*. 1972	136	1	5	4.41
Carter and Evans 1973	271	9	5	5.17
Subtotal	915	16	26	4.59
North America				
Yen and MacMahon 1968	690	14	18	4.64
McBride 1977	625	6	6	1.92
Janerich and Piper 1978	415	—	5†	1.20
Subtotal	1730	20	29	2.83
Grand total	4882	86	92	3.65

† Spina bifida or anencephalus, not specified.

TABLE 25.5 *Comparison of risks of neural-tube defects in siblings born subsequently and in those born prior to the index case*

Area and type of index case	Prior siblings: Total number	Prior siblings: Affected Number	Prior siblings: Affected Per cent	Subsequent siblings: Total number	Subsequent siblings: Affected Number	Subsequent siblings: Affected Per cent	Test of difference t value
United Kingdom†							
Anencephalus	1955	91	4.65	889	46	5.17	0.59
Spina bifida	2141	98	4.58	915	42	4.59	0.02
Total	4096	189	4.61	1804	88	4.88	0.44
North America‡							
Anencephalus	456	15	3.29	775	15	1.94	1.39
Spina bifida	672	18	2.68	1040	17	1.63	1.42
Total	1128	33	2.93	1815	32	1.76	1.97*

† From Williamson (1965), Smithells *et al.* (1968), Carter *et al.* (1968), Richards *et al.* (1972), and Carter and Evans (1973).
‡ From McBride (1977) and Janerich and Piper (1978). The study by Yen and MacMahon (1968) is excluded, as data on previous siblings are unavailable.
* Significant at 5 per cent ($p = 0.05$).

strates a trend for siblings to exhibit the same abnormality as seen in the index case (Table 25.6). This is evident within the United Kingdom studies and the European studies but is not seen in the reports from North America. The sibling risk does not appear to change according to the sex of the propositus. The South Wales survey found the recurrence risk of either anencephalus or spina bifida was 5.9 per cent for siblings of male propositi, and 4.8 per cent for siblings of female propositi, a non-significant difference (Carter *et al.* 1968). The frequency of neural-tube defects in Greater London was slightly but not significantly greater in siblings of male cases of spina bifida and of female cases having anencephalus; also there was no difference between the sex ratios of affected siblings and index cases (Carter and Evans 1973).

A common source of error in family studies is incomplete ascertainment. Thus from 18 per cent (Carter and Evans 1973) to 47 per cent (Smithells *et al.* 1968) of relatives of index cases were not traced owing to non-response, illegitimacy, or other reasons. The British Columbia study is exceptional because computer-record linkage of family groupings of birth and marriage records retrieved 98.9 per cent of the family members related to the index cases (McBride 1977). These files, however, exclude records of births occurring outside British Columbia and records of births prior to 1952 and after 1970. The full sibling risks of anencephalus and spina bifida, 2.8 per cent, 2.2 per cent, and 2.4 per cent if ascertained through anencephalus, spina bifida, and both defects in index cases respectively, are much lower than in the United Kingdom. This is particularly striking as about 60 per cent of British Columbians are of British origin and 25 per cent are from other parts of Western Europe. Although there were some differences in sibling risks, varying from 1.6 per cent in brothers of male anencephalics to 5.0 per cent in sisters of female anencephalics, McBride (1977) concludes that the risk is not significantly affected by the type of defect, sex of proband, or the sex of the sibs.

Half-siblings and cousins

Some early studies (Hindse-Nielsen 1938; Murphy 1940) reported higher prevalence rates of neural-tube defects in mother's siblings compared with father's siblings but as most family studies are based on interviews with mothers rather than fathers this bias may produce under-ascertainment on the paternal side. Carter *et al.* (1968) for example, found the highest rate in cousins was in children of the mother's sisters and only this group exhibited rates greater than the population prevalence figure. Although data are insufficient at present for any firm conclusions the frequency in first cousins appears similar to the population rate (Tables 25.7 and 25.8).

Four surveys include information on half-sibling risks (Yen and MacMahon 1968; Carter *et al.* 1968; Carter and Evans 1973; Janerich and Piper 1978). Combining these series gives 407 half-siblings of propositi having anencephalus or spina bifida of whom eight were affected. This rate of 2.0 per cent appears less than the full sibling risk reported by these studies but from the numbers available for this estimate, the 95 per cent confidence limits are 0.6 to 3.3.

TABLE 25.6 *Correspondence between the type of neural-tube defect in siblings and the type of defect in index cases*

Area	Index cases		Siblings with		Percentage of siblings with same defect as index case	Test of association (chi-square value)
	Defect	Number	Anencephalus (number)	Spina bifida (number)		
United Kingdom	Anencephalus	1526	100	57	64	27.2
	Spina bifida	2202	90	153	63	$p<0.001$
Europe	Anencephalus	620	16	13	55	9.1
	Spina bifida	299	1	13	93	$p<0.01$
North America	Anencephalus	946	24	24	50	0.10
	Spina bifida	1067	26	30	54	Not significant
Total	Anencephalus	3092	140	94	60	27.1
	Spina bifida	3568	117	196	63	$p<0.001$

TABLE 25.7 *Numbers of cases of anencephalus and spina bifida in relatives of index cases having the same defects*

Area	Index patients (number)	Co-twins	Full sibs	Half-sibs			First cousins		
				Maternal	Paternal	Total	Maternal	Paternal	Total
South Wales (Carter *et al*. 1968)	784	0/13	81/1562	0/34	0/18	0/52	19/2149	9/2229	28/4378
Greater London (Carter and Evans 1973)	870	1/14	66/1484	3/115	1/84	4/199	19/3728	12/3685	31/7413
Hungary (Czeizel and Révész 1970)	400	12/?†	37/520	—	—	—	3/1416	2/1398	5/2814
New England (Yen and MacMahon 1968)	1037	0/30	58/1263‡	—	—	3/23	—	—	—
New York State (Janerich and Piper 1978)	628	4/59	19/1041	1/82	0/51	1/133	—	—	—
British Columbia (McBride 1977)	784	1/15	46/1906	—	—	—	—	—	—

— No data.

† 15 pairs of twins are recorded in whom co-twins had 6 anencephalics, 6 spina bifidas, and 3 hydrocephalics (rate 1.9 per cent). The total number of twin pairs is not stated.

‡ Subsequent sibs only.

TABLE 25.8 *Risks (per cent) of anencephalus and spina bifida in relatives of index patients having either defect*

Area	Population Prevalence	Co-twins	Full sibs	Half sibs	First cousins
South Wales	0.75	0.0	5.2	0.0	0.6
London	0.29	7.1	4.4	2.0	0.4
Hungary	0.27	1.9	7.1	—	0.2
New England	0.29	0.0	4.6	13.0	—
New York State	0.13	6.8	1.8	0.8	—
British Columbia	0.15	—	2.4	—	—

— Not estimated

Recurrence risk after two affected children

Some studies show an increased risk in subsequent births where two children have already been affected. This has been estimated at between 10 per cent and 12 per cent (Carter and Roberts 1967; Blyth and Carter 1970; Yen and MacMahon 1968). Much higher figures of 50 per cent (Smithells *et al.* 1968) or 58 per cent (Lorber 1965) based on hospital studies are biased and reflect preferential referral of affected families to hospital units. Richards *et al.* (1972) in Glasgow found no increase in risk after two affected cases compared to after one affected case. The British Columbia study found seven families who had children born subsequent to the second affected case. Of 21 children, one of 12 females had anencephalus and none of 9 males had any neurological malformations (McBride 1978). This gives a recurrence risk after two affected of 4.8 per cent (the 95 per cent upper confidence limit is 13.9 per cent) which is less than half that observed in Great Britain.

Children of parents having spina bifida

A small number of studies have been made of the children of surviving patients with spina bifida (Carter 1974). Combining data from London (Carter and Evans 1973*a*), Sheffield (Lorber 1971*a*), and Münster (Tünte 1971) shows 106 parents with spina bifida had 212 children of whom seven had anencephalus or spina bifida. This is a risk of 3.3 per cent with 95 per cent confidence limits of 0.9 per cent and 5.7 per cent. Carter and Evans and Lorber give data for affected mothers and fathers separately; two of 52 children having a father with spina bifida and three of 131 with an affected mother had neural-tube defects. This evidence suggests the risk to offspring of propositi is similar to that of siblings and is independent of the sex of the affected parent.

Consanguinity

The prevalence of neural-tube defects where the parents are related has been shown to be increased in Alexandria and Bombay (Stevenson *et al.* 1966), Israel (Klingberg, Chemke, and Levin 1971), and Hungary (Czeizel and Révész 1970). However, the importance of this in determining differences in population prevalence is probably small, as the proportion of affected families in which consanguinity can be demonstrated is low (Penrose 1957; Naggan 1969; Record and McKeown 1950; Carter and Evans 1973). It may however be important in local areas. Masterson (1970) estimated a first-cousin marriage rate of about 1 in 720 for all Ireland by analysing ecclesiastical dispensations from the impediment of consanguinity in relation to 190 557 marriages between Roman Catholics during the period 1959–68. For the Republic of Ireland only, the estimate was one in 625. Consanguinity rates for Northern Ireland calculated by Kilpatrick, Mathers, and Stevenson (1955) for first-cousin matings ranged from 0.13 per cent to 1.39 per cent for County Londonerry in 1954. For cousin marriages of all types (C_1, C_2, C_3, C_4, Oxford Dictionary definitions) the percentages were between 0.30 and 3.30. Analysis of data for four countries showed a significantly lower proportion of full-cousin marriages (C_1) in Roman Catholics compared with Protestants, but a greater proportion of marriages between first cousins once removed (C_3). This is probably due to the differing views regarding cousin marriages taken by these two religious denominations.

26

Genetic models

CONGENITAL malformations may be considered one consequence of natural variation in man brought about by evolution as hypothesized by Darwin. An important aspect of the genetic question, therefore, is whether these defects segregate in a Mendelian fashion or else are part of the continuous biological variation of human characteristics. Critical decisions in practice depend on these different interpretations, the former suggesting a minimum of external or environmental influence and the latter the occurrence of genetic interaction in which identification of trigger mechanisms may lead to effective primary prevention. Carter (1977) examined birth frequencies of several monogenic disorders, the work of Stevenson (1959) in Northern Ireland, and Trimble and Doughty (1974) in British Columbia in order to assess the contributions of Mendelian conditions to the load of moderately serious and serious disease in the community. He concluded that a total of about 10 per 1000 livebirths are currently affected of whom 7.0 are by dominant, 2.5 by recessive, and 0.5 by X-linked inherited illnesses.

In order to determine if anencephalus and spina bifida have a genetic component, mathematical models based on different types of dominant, recessive, multifactorial, polygenic, or other modes of inheritance should be constructed and the goodness of fit of each model to the observations examined. Before these investigations are carried out a crucial question is the definition of these defects. If we consider anencephalus and spina bifida as aetiologically identical but differing only in terms of the timing of an embryological insult, then all data relating to both defects are fitted to the same model. On the other hand, if the two defects are considered to be similar but not identical aetiologically, observations relating to anencephalus and to spina bifida are tested independently. Furthermore, the view that spina bifida occulta may be an incomplete manifestation of spina bifida aperta must be borne in mind when determining which data are relevant to a particular model. There are fewer problems with respect to anencephalus as no incomplete variants are widely accepted. Frens, Ziter, and Bray (1977) described an eight-year-old with underlying bony skull defects and abnormal cerebral blood vessels as a possible forme fruste of anencephalus. The mother's first pregnancy ended as an early abortion, the second was the aforementioned child with multiple bony and soft tissue anomalies of the head, and the third pregnancy was a premature anencephalic stillbirth. The second child had a partial Horner's syndrome, a malformed cribiform plate, absent crista galli, sclerosis of the lesser sphenoid wings, malformed left pterygoid plates, and other abnormalities diagnosed by orbital and axial tomography; some resemble deformities seen in the skulls of human anencephalics (Marin-Padilla 1965).

Anencephalus and spina bifida may occur as a component of certain syndromes which segregate along Mendelian lines, in association with chromosomal abnormalities or as part of other syndromes whose mode of transmission and causation are unknown (Table 26.1). Families have been described where the father had a translocation (DeGrouchy, Brissaud, Repessé, and Lamy 1964) and where the mother together with her unaffected sibs had an enlarged satellite on one chromosome (Ellis and Penrose 1961). Despite these reports, the great majority of cases have normal chromosomes (Polani 1959; Warkany 1971).

Clinically, the problem of possible inheritance of anencephalus or spina bifida is illustrated by the pedigree described by Fuhrmann, Seeger, and Bohn (1971) which exhibits an apparent monogenic inheritance (Fig. 26.1).

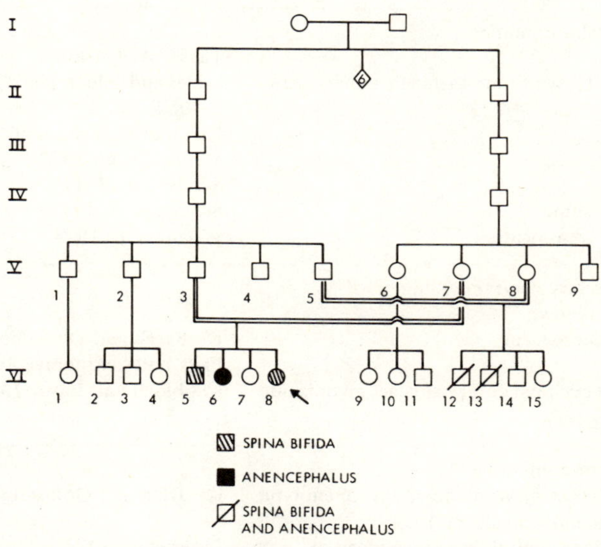

FIG. 26.1. Pedigree of German family compatible with monogenic inheritance of anencephalus and spina bifida. (After Fuhrmann *et al*. 1971 and courtesy of *Humangenetik*.)

Five out of eight children from two related German families had anencephalus and/or spina bifida. The fathers of both families were brothers who had married two sisters and were found by further investigation to be third-degree cousins to their wives. There were no malformations among more distant relatives. This particular pedigree is compatible with autosomal recessive inheritance of anencephalus and spina bifida.

TABLE 26.1 *Genetic syndromes associated with anencephalus and spina bifida*

Syndrome	Reference
Dominant	
Anterior sacral meningomyelocele and anal stenosis†	Say and Coldwell 1975
Median cleft face syndrome (may include anterior encephalocele)	De Myer 1967
Hereditary spondylolisthesis and spina bifida	Amuso and Mankin 1967
Recessive	
Meckel syndrome (may include occipital encephalocele or anencephalus)	Meckel 1822 Hsia *et al.* 1971; Opitz and Howe 1969 Fried *et al.* 1971
Robert's syndrome (includes anterior encephalocele)	Freeman *et al.* 1974
(Hard ± E) syndrome (includes encephalocele)	Pagon *et al.* 1978
Chromosomal abnormalities	
Trisomy 13	Taylor A. I. 1968
Trisomy 13–15 syndrome (arhinencephaly with encephalocele)	Miller and Selden 1967; Marshall *et al.* 1964
Trisomy 18	Passarge E. *et al.* 1966 Menashi *et al.* 1977
Triploidy	Simpson *et al.* 1972
Ring chromosome	Schmid *et al.* 1975*a*
Unbalanced translocation	Wright *et al.* 1974
Probable hereditary conditions—mode of transmission unknown	
Anterior encephalocele	De Klerk and De Villiers 1973 Flatz and Sukthomya 1970
Syndrome of occipital encephalocele, myopia and retinal dysplasia	Knobloch and Layer 1971
Syndromes—cause unknown	
Ankyloblepharon filiforme adnatum (phenotype includes meningomyelocele)	Kazarian and Goldstein 1977
Craniofacial and limb defects secondary to aberrant tissue bands (phenotype includes multiple encephaloceles)	Jones *et al.* 1974
Cloacal exstrophy (may include myelocystocele)	Marshall and Muecke 1962 Beckwith 1966
Sacrococcygeal teratoma (phenotype includes meningomyelocele)	Fraumeni *et al.* 1973
Occipital encephalocele, short-limb dwarfism, micrognathia	Dinno, Shearer, and Weisskopf 1976
Ivemark syndrome (absent spleen, cardiac defects, spina bifida and/or anencephalus	Van Went *et al.* 1977 Ivemark 1958
The OEIS complex (includes spinal defects)	Carey *et al.* 1978

† May be autosomal dominant or X-linked

Single-gene models

For a single-gene defect to be the major aetiological mechanism producing anencephalus or spina bifida, the gene frequency in the population would have to be maintained by a high frequency of spontaneous mutation. As observed genetic mutation rates are rarely more than one in 10 000, the prevalence rates of lethal single-gene conditions are of this order (Carter 1969). Also, the sibling risk would be much higher than the 3–6 per cent observed and this risk would not increase in families with two affected offspring. Thirdly, the consanguinity rate would be greater than that seen. Thus a single-gene mechanism is unlikely even though the observed risk to siblings could be explained by a single-gene effect having low penetrance. As mentioned, families are recorded in which a high proportion of members have been affected (Dunn and Salter 1944; Polman 1950). Although the existence of such families would be expected by chance alone, some types of anencephalus and spina bifida may have high recurrence rates. An autopsy series from Boston found 5 of 106 consecutively born infants with anencephalus or spina bifida were compatible with a diagnosis of Meckel's syndrome (Holmes *et al*. 1976). This recessive condition, comprising occipital encephalocele, microphthalmia, cleft lip and palate, polycystic kidneys, genital defects, polydactyly, and clubfoot has a 25 per cent recurrence rate (Hsai, Bratu and Herbordt 1971). Meckel (1822) described anatomical observations based on two affected sibs, one female and the other male. The female had microcephaly, a posterior exencephalocele, and dissection of the brain also revealed spina bifida of the first and second cervical vertebrae; the relationship of the brain to the encephalocele was not clear. The male sib showed similar abnormalities. Family histories were available for 103 out of the 106 infants in the series of Holmes *et al*. (1976). Considering all these 103 infants together the precurrence and recurrence sibling risks of similar defects as diagnosed in the index cases (stillborn and liveborn anencephalus, spina bifida or encephalocele) were 5.3 per cent (7 of 133 sibs) and 1.7 per cent (1 of 60 sibs) respectively. There were five index cases of the Meckel syndrome who had seven similarly affected sibs. If these five infants together with eight infants having other specific disorders are excluded, the precurrence and recurrence sibling risks calculated for the remaining infants were 0.8 per cent (1 of 119 sibs) and zero per cent (none of 51 siblings) respectively. The total sibling risk is 0.6 per cent, with an upper 95 per cent confidence limit of 1.7 per cent, suggesting that the sibling risks in this sample of anencephalus and spina bifida may be biased by the inclusion of these cases of Meckel's syndrome. In their review of the Meckel syndrome, Opitz and Howe (1969) point out milder forms may exist which resemble the Ullrich–Feichtiger syndrome (Ullrich 1951; Moszkowicz 1934), the D_1 trisomy syndrome and the Smith–Lemli–Opitz syndrome.

The heterogeneity of these rare conditions makes any clear distinction between them difficult. Clearly, more work is required to clarify malformation syndromes and the question of whether anencephalus and spina bifida are each a morphological homogeneous entity (Opitz, Herrmann, and Dieker 1969). Fried (1973) estimated a minimal prevalence of the Meckel syndrome among Jews in Israel, an ethnic group in which the condition may be more common than in others, as one in 50 000. In London, the risks to siblings of anencephalus propositi and of spina bifida propositi were similar (Carter and Evans 1973), although infants with encephalocele were grouped with spina bifida. This is rather against Holmes's argument, but as the Meckel syndrome may sometimes include microcephalus or anencephalus the data to date are insufficient to clarify this point (Welch 1976; Althouse and Kline 1976).

Cytoplasmic inheritance

A further hypothesis by Nance (1969) suggests cytoplasmic inheritance may be involved. Although nuclear genetic material splits equally when monozygotic twins are formed, the cytoplasm and therefore any extranuclear genetic material may be divided unequally, and discordance amongst monozygotic twins thus may occur. Cytoplasmic inheritance has been demonstrated in lower organisms, but not in higher animals or in man. The cytoplasm of the zygote is composed chiefly of maternal cytoplasm from the ovum and cytoplasmic traits are transmitted through the maternal line. Thus one piece of evidence supporting Nance's hypothesis is the apparently higher risk in maternal than in paternal relatives of propositi. The studies of Carter *et al*. (1968) and Carter and Evans (1973) both found increased risks in maternal cousins of infants with neural-tube defects, while the rates in paternal cousins were not greater than those in the general population. However, in both surveys the authors note the greater likelihood of obtaining information about affected infants from maternal relatives compared with relatives on the father's side of the family. They have since shown that the risk of a neural-tube defect in children of spina bifida survivors appears to be the same for affected fathers and affected mothers (Carter and Evans 1973*a*). Thus, the lack of demonstration of cytoplasmic inheritance in higher animals and the current epidemiological observations of anencephalus and spina bifida in man make Nance's hypothesis unlikely.

Multifactorial inheritance

Gruneberg (1952), studying developmental variations of the foramen ovale of the mouse, concluded genetic factors related to the formation of this cardiac defect, if present at less than a certain intensity, did not lead to the occurrence of the malformation. Such an effect forms the basis for one type of multifactorial model based on quasi-continuous variation; beyond the threshold level a defect is manifest while below it a defect is not present. Multiple genetic factors control the threshold level and may be triggered by agents in the environment. One of the best documented examples of this phenomenon relates to cleft palate (Fraser and Nora 1975). Fraser (1976) defines multifactorial inheritance as meaning 'determined by a combination of genetic and environmental factors' without reference to the nature of these genetic factors as distinct from polygenic inheritance implying 'a large number of genes, each with a small effect, acting additively'. When a smaller number of genes with more major effects are postulated to be involved as suggested by Morton (1967), Fraser uses the term 'plurilocal' meaning genetic variation more complex than predicted by a Mendelian model.

Edwards (1960) demonstrated that when a disease or disorder is fairly common and exhibits familial aggregation and if the concept of incomplete penetrance is accepted, the patterns of inheritance expected by a single gene hypothesis and by postulating multiple-gene effects may be indistinguishable even in extensive data. Thus observations of anencephalus and spina bifida are compatible with more than one mathematical model for polygenic or multifactorial inheritance. In the multifactorial model proposed by Edwards (1969), a normal distribution of both the general population of births and of affected cases is assumed, with the mean of the latter distribution shifted towards a threshold value beyond which the abnormality occurs (Fig 26.2). This model predicts that if the population prevalence is p then the prevalence in first degree relatives of propositi would be expected to be $\sqrt{p}$. For the second- and third-degree relatives the risks would be expected to be lower again of the order of $p^2/3$ and $p^4/5$ respectively (Edwards 1960; Carter 1965). Other predictions from this model are:

(1) The ratio of the risk to sibs compared with the population prevalence decreases as the population prevalence rate increases.

(2) The recurrence risk in sibs of families having two already affected children will be greater than the risk in subsequent sibs of families having one already affected child.

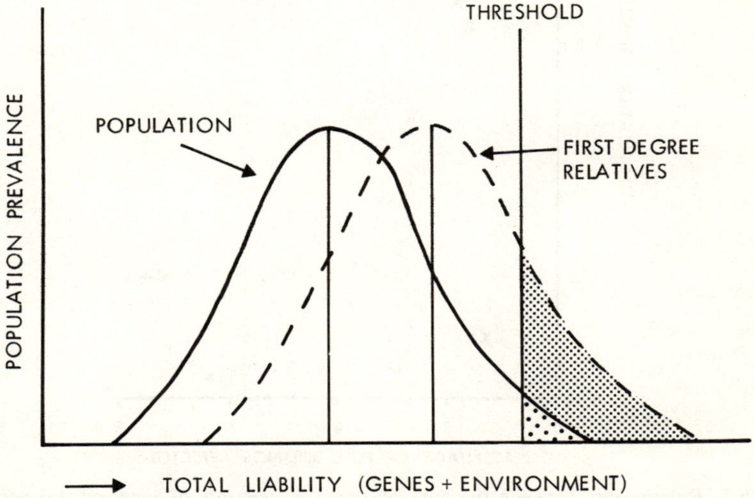

FIG. 26.2. Multifactorial model of inheritance. (After Carter 1969 and Edwards 1969 and courtesy of the Medical Department, The British Council.)

(3) More severe malformations will be associated with a higher sibling risk.

(4) Males having neural-tube defects will be associated with a higher sibship risk because, being less common, they represent more extreme deviations from the normal.

(5) A small increase in parental consanguinity will be expected.

Let us examine how well current observations fit this model of multifactorial inheritance.

The British data from London, Glasgow, and South Wales exhibit sibling risks which are 15.8, 10.0, and 6.8 times the respective population prevalence rates for both defects combined and the recurrence rate in sibs following two affected children is higher than that following one affected child (Carter and Roberts 1967). There is not, however, any definite association between population prevalence rates and full sibling risks if all

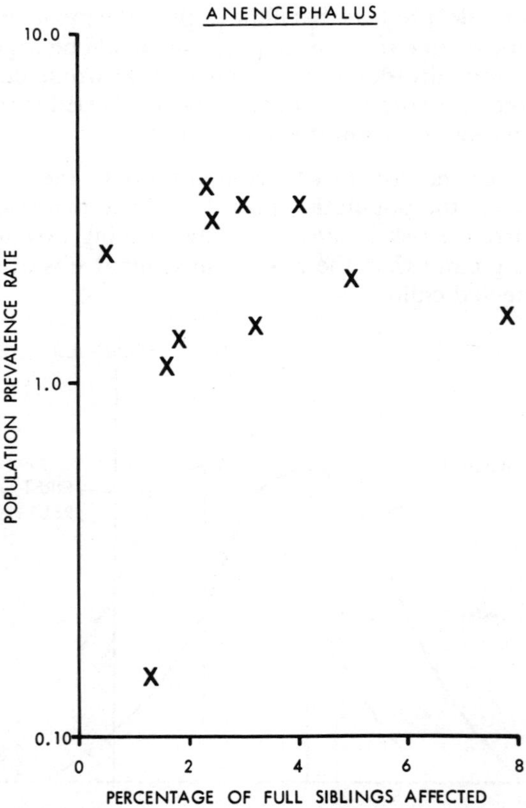

FIG. 26.3. Relationship between the population prevalence rate of anencephalus per 1000 total births and the percentage of full siblings affected by the same defect in eleven selected series.

available data are examined. Several correlations may be analysed depending on whether the population prevalence rate is based on anencephalus alone, spina bifida alone, or anencephalus and spina bifida combined and whether the full sibling risks considered also relate to one or both defects singly or together. The findings are similar for all possible combinations and we illustrate these associations by the following two examples. There are eleven series in Table 25.1 in which both the population prevalence and the risk of anencephalus in full siblings of index cases having anencephalus are known. The rank correlation between these two indices is not significant (coefficient $r = 0.31$; d.f. = 9; Fig. 26.3). Also, there are eight series in Table 25.2 in which the population prevalence of anencephalus and spina bifida combined and the risk of anencephalus in full siblings of index cases having spina bifida are known. Again the rank correlation between these two indices is not significant ($r=0.53$; d.f. = 6; Fig. 26.4). These coefficients, however, are in the direction predicted by the multifactorial hypothesis and

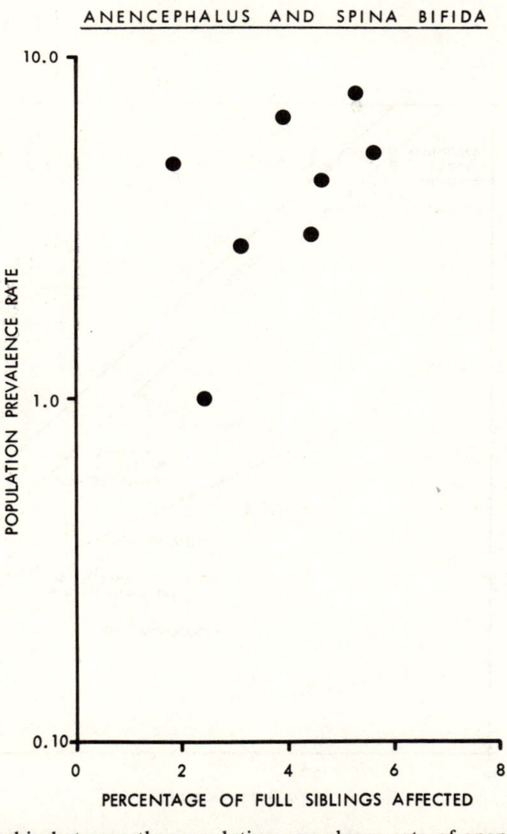

FIG. 26.4. Relationship between the population prevalence rate of anencephalus and spina bifida combined per 1000 total births and the percentage of full siblings affected by anencephalus in eight selected series.

further data are required to resolve this question. Newcombe (1964), using records from the British Columbia Population Study, looked at relationships between population frequency and the ratio of the prevalence in sibs to that in the community for a number of different diseases (Fig. 26.5). Two conclusions are apparent from these calculations. First, relationships for known Mendelian inherited characteristics such as albinism and achondroplasia are quite distinct from the relationships with respect to anencephalus and spina bifida. Secondly, although the latter fall in the area postulated as occurring due to multifactorial inheritance, so do a number of other conditions such as rheumatic fever and multiple sclerosis whose aetiologies are not thought to be mainly genetic. Mendelian inherited conditions form a discrete cluster in relation to the assumed multifactorial group.

The third postulate of higher sibling risks being associated with more severe defects is difficult to examine validly because anencephalus and spina bifida cannot be considered as different severities of the same condition as for example, unilateral and bilateral cleft lip can be. However, the sibling

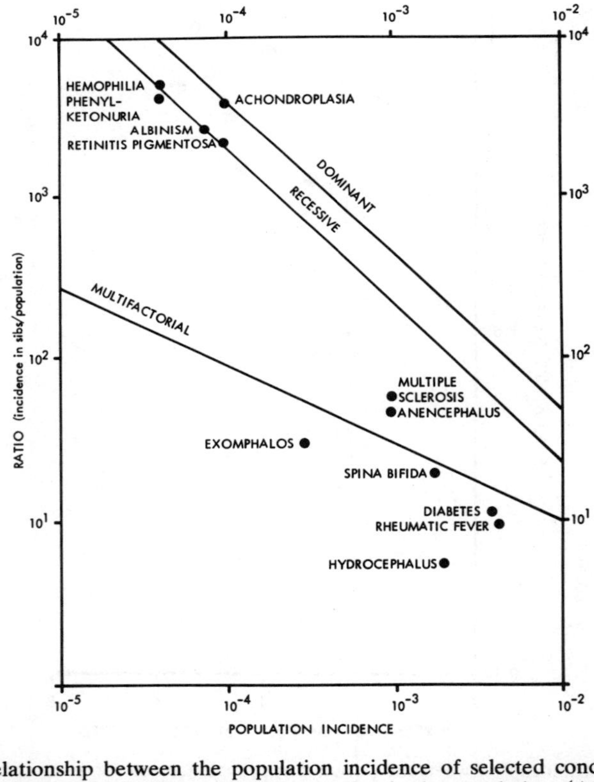

FIG. 26.5. Relationship between the population incidence of selected conditions and the corresponding ratio of the incidence in siblings to that in the population. (After Newcombe 1964.)

risks subsequent to anencephalic propositi and spina bifida propositi are similar. Also, risks appear independent of the sex of the propositus unless it is accepted that early foetal loss rates differ for male and female foetuses. Regarding parental consanguinity, there is some evidence of an increase in parents of anencephalus and spina bifida children compared with the frequency in the related community. Record and McKeown (1950) found three first-cousin and one second-cousin marriages among parents of 742 affected infants and one first-cousin marriage among parents of 742 controls. Cousin marriages were particularly common in Alexandria where a neural-tube defect prevalence rate of 14.2 per 1000 occurred among offspring of first-cousin or closer marriages (30 cases in 2109 births of consanguineous unions) compared with a rate of 5.7 per 1000 in offspring of unrelated marriages. Thus for high-risk areas, the prevalence of anencephalus and spina bifida is increased in children of consanguineous parents (Leck 1971).

Falconer (1965) described methods for estimating the heritability of a condition assuming a multifactorial mode of inheritance (Fig. 26.6). Heritability in this context is defined as the ratio of additive genetic variation to the total variance (Smith 1975). Thus environmental as well as genetic factors common to the family are counted as heritable. Estimates for anencephalus and spina bifida using this technique are 58 per cent, 61 per cent, 66 per cent, and 68 per cent for South Wales, British Columbia, Glasgow, and London respectively. Carter (1969) studied cases of cleft lip and palate obtaining heritability estimates of 76 per cent, 76 per cent, and 67 per cent for first-degree, second-degree, and third-degree relatives of index patients respectively. The similarity between these figures suggests very little influence of environment on the occurrence of these particular defects. However,

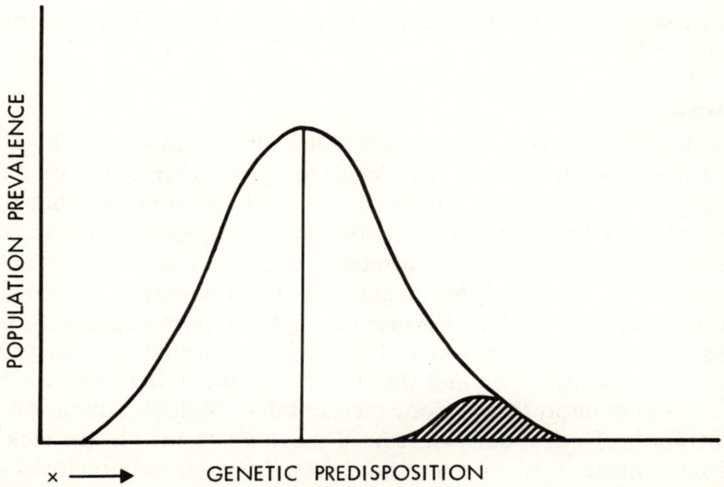

FIG. 26.6. Falconer's multifactorial model of inheritance—shaded area represents distribution of affected individuals. (After Falconer 1965 and courtesy of the *Annals of Human Genetics*.)

Falconer's method assumes normal distributions of liability in relatives and in the population which may not be the case (Fig 26.6). Even so, these calculations indicate additive genetic factors only are insufficient to account for the total variation in liability between individuals. Any interpretation of this measure of heritability is most difficult. If regressions of risks in relatives of varying degrees of the index patient can be made then these estimates may be more meaningful. One possible approach towards clarifying this difficult problem is the family set method applied by Schull, Harburg, Schork and Chakraborty (1977) in an attempt to determine the role of heredity in blood pressure (Tyroler 1977). Morton (1967) has suggested a further model in which the malformation is determined by small additive effects of many genes in most cases and by rare genes having a high recurrence risk in a minority. Some evidence for this view of morphologic heterogeneity are the numerous rare syndromes observed and other plurilocal and complex Mendelian models have been put forward. Reich, James, and Morris (1972) outlined a single locus having two alleles, each having incomplete penetrance; Chung, Ching, and Morton (1974) also outlined a model based on incomplete dominance and others have described various combinations of these possible types (Lange and Elslon 1975). Re-assessment of the various manifestations of anencephalus and spina bifida for possible diagnostic misinterpretation owing to heterogeneity within current classifications is indicated (McKusick 1969; McCormick 1971).

Yen and MacMahon (1968) point out the observed sibling risks and the increased risks in some families with two or more affected children are consistent with a causal role of an environmental agent to which certain families are more exposed than others. Their data show the risk in half-sibs to be as high as in full sibs although these estimates are based on small numbers. More convincing evidence of an environmental effect is the decline in sibling risk correlated with a declining population prevalence rate over the period from 1935 to 1967.

Conclusion

Firm evidence, therefore, clearly compatible or incompatible with a multifactorial mode of inheritance is lacking. Increased consanguinity and gradation of risk in different relatives of propositi are in favour, but the low association between sibling risk and population prevalence and the absence of a higher sibship risk related to affected males are against this hypothesis. Furthermore, the definite differences in the epidemiology of these defects in the United Kingdom and North America, evidence from migrant studies and the large variations in prevalence by time and place, argue against a predominant genetic aetiology. The fact that several mathematical models may fit the data does not imply that any one is acceptable. Biological plausibility and demonstration of an underlying causal mechanism for all are lacking. It should be remembered that a genetic aetiology for tuberculosis was so debated a generation or so ago and more recently a genetic basis was proposed for Kuru, now known to be a transmissible disease due to a slow virus (Gajdusek 1977; Harper 1977). The strongest evidence, in our view, for a genetic component contributing to the occurrence of anencephalus and spina bifida is not the goodness of fit of current data to any particular multifactorial or other mathematical model but the apparent increased risk in monozygotic compared with dyzygotic twins. Re-assessment of existing knowledge is valuable as seen by the analysis of Morton, Rao, Lang-Brown, MacLean, Bart, and Lew (1977) who examined pedigrees assembled by Penrose (1938) over 40 years ago relating to 1280 in-patients having mental deficiency and resident at the Royal Eastern Counties Institution, Colchester, England. By classifying these families into three types, biological (33 per cent), medical (7 per cent) and socio-familial (60 per cent), Morton and colleagues consider simple genetic mechanisms account for virtually all the biological category. Whether there is a baseline level of neural-tube defect prevalence produced by genetic factors with any excess due to environmental agents interfering with presumably basic molecular pathways, as suggested by Janerich and Piper (1978) is open to debate. After all, prevalence rates in some areas such as Finland and Sweden today are already only around 8 per cent of the frequencies in Ireland and rates in migrants from high-risk areas to North America are lower than in comparable non-migrant groups of the same ethnic stock.

27

Foetus–Foetus interaction

ROGERS (1969) presented an analysis of data relating to stillbirths attributed to anencephalus and to other causes in England and Wales from 1961 to 1966 in which he compared the distributions of each major group of stillbirths to that of anencephalus in terms of sex, maternal age, region, rural or urban residence, and year and season of birth. Only two conditions had similar distributions to anencephalus; spina bifida (except for a higher male proportion) and monster. The category monster had 103 cases, of which 50 were double monsters, having a male proportion of 30 per cent, compared to a male proportion of 28 per cent for anencephalus. This pointed to a possible common causation linking anencephalus with the occurrence of double monsters. In view of the lack of twin pairs concordant for anencephalus or spina bifida noted by Yen and MacMahon (1968), Rogers hypothesized that conjoined twins and double monsters arise by fusion of mono-amniotic twins, a concept also put forward by Robertson (1953), and that such fusion would be more likely if one or both twins have a neural-tube defect.

The following year Knox (1970) proposed another hypothesis that fusion of twins could produce a foetus with a neural-tube defect, rather than vice versa, and this also would explain the lack of twin pairs concordant for anencephalus or spina bifida. Such pairs would only occur from interaction between two members of a set of triplets. Knox suggests two sex-linked alleles are present which produce the excess of anencephalus in females and permit a selection bias in favour of heterozygotes leading to a stable gene frequency. The hypothesis involves an environmental 'trigger' so that the neural-tube defect incidence rate depends on the conception rate of twins, the trigger frequency, and the frequencies of the relevant sex-linked alleles. Knox (1974) tested a number of the epidemiological predictions arising from his hypothesis and noted the positive association between dizygotic twinning rates and the prevalence rates of neural-tube defects reported by Stevenson *et al.* (1966), and the secular decline in both indices in several countries. He showed positive associations between the female-to-male ratio and the prevalence rates of anencephalus in Great Britain by social class, region, season, and maternal age. These results support his hypothesis but are not conclusive. Knox then postulated that interaction may occur between the foetus and trophoblastic or other tissue persisting from an earlier pregnancy. If this were so, the interval before the affected pregnancy would be shorter than expected, as demonstrated by Record and McKeown (1950), and the sex distribution of the previously born infant should show a male excess, with the bias being greater if the affected infant was female. Unpublished data from the study by Record and McKeown (1950) support this because 95 of 155 (61 per cent) births immediately prior to an affected female infant were male and 63 of 118 (53 per cent) of those preceding an affected male were male. Knox concluded some two-thirds to three-quarters of cases of neural-tube defects may arise by foetus–foetus interaction during the affected pregnancy and the rest by interactions with tissues derived from the preceding pregnancy.

Other investigators have attempted to collaborate these findings with partial success. Durkin, Kaveggia, Pendleton, and Opitz (1976) reported a shift of the sex ratio of infants born prior to those with neural-tube defects consistent with the hypothesis, but no difference in pre-pregnancy intervals. In Canada, we examined the interrelationships of twinning rates, anencephalus rates, and the sex distribution of anencephalus (Elwood, J. M. 1976) in both time and space. Despite the very large differences in anencephalus mortality rates across Canada, this geographical trend is not consistently associated with changes in either the sex distribution of anencephalus or the twinning rate in all births. Secular trends are more supportive as twinning rates and anencephalus rates have fallen while the male proportion of anencephalics has risen. Whereas the fall in twinning rates has been consistent in all provinces, the trends in these other variables have varied greatly between provinces, and so there is no consistent relationship.

Rogers (1976) assessed further data relating anencephalus to twinning and concluded there was a higher concordance rate in like-sex twins (Rogers and Weatherall 1976). This work suggested monozygotic twins concordant for neural-tube defects will fuse to form double monsters, whereas dizygotic twins will fuse resulting in one survivor, the co-twin being represented by a teratoma or an area of skin cover which may have different chromosomal sex. While no specific supporting evidence is presented, some relevant observations are noted as for example, the high abnormality rate in monoamniotic twin pairs, the association of intraspinal teratoma with spina bifida and the rare occurrences of foetus *in fetu* (Du Plessis, Winship, and Kirstein 1974). This latter defect, the presence of a twin within another individual, seen by an axial skeleton and associated organogenesis usually presenting as an intra-abdominal mass (Willis 1962) is very rare with only 19 recorded cases in the medical literature at the time of the report from South Africa by Du Plessis and colleagues. The clinical reports of cases of anencephalus with incomplete twinning also are relevant to this hypothesis (Riccardi and Bergman 1971; Fontaine and Vankemmel 1978). Further evidence was put forward by Clarke *et al*. (1975). They re-analysed data from the survey by Carter *et al*. (1968) which show no disturbance of sex ratio in births immediately prior to that of a neural-tube infant. However, using data from several British studies they conclude miscarriages are most common immediately before the affected birth. They formulate a sequential interaction hypothesis somewhat similar to that of Knox (1974), but depending primarily on the occurrence of a previous spontaneous abortion. Residual trophoblastic material is postulated to be more likely to occur after an abortion than after a normal delivery and such material may be incorporated into the placenta of the next pregnancy leading to embryological abnormalities of which neural-tube defects may be one manifestation. The association between prevalence and social class may be secondary to a direct effect of an increased risk of spontaneous abortion. The abnormal sex distribution of anencephalus is explicable if trophoblastic rests are predominantly female, as are hydatidiform moles, and more severe interaction, leading to spontaneous abortion, occurs if the next pregnancy is male. This hypothesis predicts genetic mosaicism in the placentae of affected infants and sex differences in the cells of the skin patch over a spina bifida lesion compared with the sex of the host individual. Observations not explained by this hypothesis include the high rate of neural-tube defects in first births, and the negative association between anencephalus and spina bifida rates and spontaneous abortion in different geographical areas of South Wales (Roberts and Lloyd 1973). In Belfast some 25 per cent of mothers of infants with anencephalus or spina bifida have no previous pregnancy history in terms of known early foetal loss or other outcomes (Elwood, J. H. 1976*b*).

The 'rest' hypothesis as set out by Clarke *et al*. (1975) has been supported by the results of a small study by Gardiner *et al*. (1978). In this investigation the pregnancy outcomes of 289 women each of whose last pregnancy had ended in a spontaneous abortion, were compared to those of 284 women who had had a normal baby. The women were matched 'closely' on age and gravidity (that is, total number of pregnancies). Two index mothers and one control aborted again, and the pregnancy outcome was not ascertained for 31 index mothers and 29 comparison mothers. Of 256 births to index mothers, there were 17 having some type of birth defect, compared to four out of 254 controls; this is a statistically significant difference. Positional type deformities such as talipes and some abnormalities whose diagnosis is variable, for example clicking hips and heart murmurs were excluded. There were two neural-tube defects in the index group (one anencephalus and one spina bifida) and none in the controls. In addition six index infants and one control each had a sacrococcygeal dimple. The authors interpret the results as being consistent with the rest hypothesis, although this is now extended to include not only neural-tube defects but midline defects in general. This study, while interesting, is far from conclusive. Several methodological issues are unclear. Matching for total parity and maternal age is probably very important, in which case one requires more information than simply a statement of 'close' matching. Confounding by social class probably is considerable, given the strong associations between social class and the likelihood of both spontaneous abortions and neural-tube defects, yet no information on social class was available for 74 per cent of the women. The diagnoses of abnormality were based on routine examinations and reports. The physicians involved are stated to have been unaware of this study, yet they would know of the association between congenital defects and previous spontaneous abortions and also would probably have a knowledge of the earlier studies and hypotheses of this group of investigators as they all worked in the Liverpool area. While this might be unimportant for major defects, the diagnosis and recording of sacrococcygeal dimples certainly would vary with the skill and care of the examining physician. Some of the index mothers may have had the previous spontaneous abortions because these foetuses were affected by anencephalus or spina bifida and even the inclusion of a small number of such mothers would seriously bias the results. The authors clearly appreciate the limitations of this study, and their further investigations are awaited with interest.

Another relevant study is the work of Boué, Boué, Lazar, and Gueguen (1975). They followed up, by questionnaire methods, the subsequent pregnancies of 313 mothers who had had a spontaneous abortion earlier than at 12 weeks of gestation. This study is difficult to evaluate because of a lack of detail, but the authors report only six abnormalities (two cardiac, two hip dislocations, one clubfoot, and one umbilical hernia) which they say is no greater than expected. The results of this study would be consistent with those of Gardiner *et al*. (1978) if trophoblastic rests were unlikely to occur after foetal losses prior to 12 weeks of gestation.

This foetus–foetus interaction hypothesis, which has been specifically enunciated in more than one way, may be clarified by further research. As the Liverpool team point out, it may be possible to detect trophoblastic remnants by ultrasound or by finding that levels of human chorionic gonadotrophin, alpha-foetoprotein or other substances persist longer and at higher levels in the bloodstream of mothers who have had a spontaneous abortion compared with mothers delivered of normal infants. Rogers (1976) suggests trends in the prevalence at birth of intraspinal and pineal teratoma by time and place might be similar to those of anencephalus and spina bifida and that the tuft of hair sometimes found overlying a spina bifida lesion may in affected male infants carry female chromosomes.

XII

Prenatal diagnosis

PRENATAL diagnosis of foetal abnormality has received considerable impetus recently owing to the development of acceptable invasive procedures for investigating the foetus *in utero* and changes in abortion legislation permitting selective termination of pregnancy. This policy, in the light of the increasing relative proportion of early mortality now attributable to congenital defects, gives a method whereby the overall perinatal mortality rate in a population may be reduced. We earlier considered physical methods of diagnosis including clinical history, physical examination, X-rays, foetoscopy, and sonar scanning (Chapter IV) and we now examine methods of antenatal diagnosis. In particular the measurement of alpha-foetoprotein in amniotic fluid and maternal blood for purposes of detecting anencephalus and spina bifida to 20 weeks of gestation of pregnancy is discussed.

The work of Liley (1961) in New Zealand, demonstrating the value of estimating bilirubin concentrations in amniotic fluid of pregnancies complicated by Rhesus sensitization made amniocentesis a widely practised technique. Liley (1963) also noted a false peak in bilirubin optical density measurements at the 450-nm band associated with a pregnancy having hydramnios and a foetus with duodenal atresia. Bilirubin levels were found to be elevated in the amniotic fluid of full-term anencephalic foetuses (Cassady and Cailliteau 1967) and in a proportion of third-trimester pregnancies with anencephalus or spina bifida (Emery, Brock, Burt, and Eccleston 1974). Furthermore, high levels were reported in relation to pregnancies at 30 weeks of gestation or more having foetuses with ileal atresia (Grimes and Cassady 1970) and oesophageal atresia (Stewart and Taylor 1964). Bilirubin, however, is of relatively low molecular weight, has a rapid turnover and derives from both the maternal and foetal circulations hence its value as an index of foetal abnormality in early as distinct from late pregnancy is limited

Brock and Sutcliffe (1972) were the first to report elevated levels of alpha-foetoprotein in the amniotic fluid of pregnancies with anencephalus and spina bifida. They described 31 pregnancies leading to anencephalus (or anencephalus with spina bifida), three leading to spina bifida, and three leading to hydrocephalus (or hydrocephalus with spina bifida). In all the anencephalic cases amniotic fluid alpha-foetoprotein concentrations were well above the normal range between 25 and 35 weeks of gestation and in a single case of spina bifida examined at 13 weeks of gestation the alpha-foetoprotein concentration was four times the highest equivalent normal level. Observations that foetal cells are shed and biochemical substances leak into liquor amnii has meant samples obtained by amniocentesis can be investigated for possible associations between the cell and biochemical contents and a large number of foetal conditions. Theoretically, an efficent biochemical marker would be characterized by being exclusively of foetal origin, easily detected and measured and of high molecular-weight so that it would not cross the placenta in large amounts into the maternal blood. In addition it should be present during the first trimester only. Several substances contained in liquor amnii have been examined for these criteria (Brock 1976 and Table 28.1). In general, low-molecular-weight compounds such as bilirubin, certain amino acids (Emery, Burt, Nelson, and Scrimgeour 1970) and 5-hydroxyindolacetic acid (Emery, Eccleston, Scrimgeour, and Johnstone 1972) exhibit little quantitative difference when levels in normal amniotic fluid and in amniotic fluid from pregnancies associated with foetal abnormality are compared prior to 20 weeks of gestation although more distinction is evident towards the end of the pregnancy. Of the constituents of amniotic fluid examined so far, the most useful marker at present is alpha-foetoprotein.

TABLE 28.1 *Constituents of amniotic fluid examined for the prenatal diagnosis of anencephalus and spina bifida*

Constituent	Molecular weight	Reference
5-hydroxyindole acetic acid	191	Emery 1973
Bilirubin	585	Cassady and Cailliteau 1967
β-trace protein	31 000	Macri *et al.* 1974*a*
α-foetoprotein	64 000	Brock and Sutcliffe 1972
α_2-macroglobulin	850 000	Brock 1975
IgM	900 000	Cantuaria and Jones 1975
β-lipoprotein	2 400 000	Brock 1975
Foetal macrophages	—	Sutherland *et al.* 1973
Total proteins and γ-globulins	—	Higa *et al.* 1974
Products of fibrinogen degradation	—	Purdie *et al.* 1975
β-melanocyte-stimulating hormone	—	Smith, Shuster, *et al.* 1978

28

Alpha-Foetoprotein

ALPHA-FOETOPROTEIN, henceforth referred to by the abbreviation AFP, is present in foetal serum from the sixth week of gestation and is synthesized in the yolk sac and foetal liver (Gitlin and Boesman 1966). Various aspects of its function and occurrence have been reviewed by Adinolfi, Adinolfi, and Lessof (1975), Lau and Linkins (1976), and Pergament (1977). Initially it was investigated not in relation to antenatal diagnosis of birth defects but as a means of monitoring foetal development and as a model for studying cancer therapy directed against AFP-producing tumours. Alpha-foetoprotein was earlier thought to be related to a glycoprotein, fetuin, first described by Pedersen (1944) as being unique to the foetus, absent in the normal adult, but which may re-appear under conditions of carcinogenesis or other disease states. Pedersen isolated a globulin from the serum of calves not more than two weeks old and several authors have considered this substance, fetuin, as the bovine counterpart of other mammalian AFPs. Fetuin and human AFP, however, are quite distinct proteins (Lai, Peter, and Lorscheider 1978). Although it is now clear that AFP differs from fetuin, because of the difficulty of isolating and purifying AFP, synonyms previously used include alpha$_1$-foetoprotein, ESA globulin, alpha$_1$-embryo-specific protein, and protein F. Gitlin adopted the label alpha-foetoprotein; this was officially accepted by the International Agency for Research on Cancer at Lyon in 1959 (Gitlin and Boesman 1966; Abelev, Alpert, Hull, Masseyeff, de Nechaud, Tatarinov, and Uriel 1970) and an international standard for AFP is available from this agency.

There are several foeto-specific proteins which are synthesized during particular phases of embryogenesis of which AFP is only one. They then disappear or persist in minute amounts in normal adults. Human AFP is similar to AFP found in several animal species including the cat, dog, sheep, monkey, and armadillo (Masopust, Zizkovsky, and Kithier 1970; Gitlin and Boesman 1967). Gitlin (1973) suggests AFP may have been in existence in primitive animals such as the shark for around 400 million years. It was synthesized from the endoderm of the embryonic foregut and so arose from the gastro-intestinal tract. During the process of evolution, synthesis moved from the stomach to other endodermal structures, namely the liver and yolk sac. In the shark, AFP is produced mainly in the stomach while in birds AFP synthesis occurs in the yolk sac with no production in the liver. In man and higher mammals the main site of AFP synthesis is the liver, followed by the yolk sac, and only very small amounts originate in the gastro-intestinal tract.

During the first two months the human foetal liver and yolk sac produce roughly equal amounts of AFP, but as the yolk sac degenerates about 12 weeks after conception, the liver becomes the main site of synthesis. Foetal serum concentrations rise nearly 30 times between the sixth and ninth week and reach a peak of around 2000 to 3000 μg/ml at 14 weeks of gestation. The foetal serum level then progressively declines to between 10 and 80 μg/ml at birth. Although foetal serum concentrations fall from 14 weeks onwards, production by the liver, which releases an average of from 19 to 26 ng of AFP per minute (Kekomaki, Seppälä, Enholm, Schwartz, and Raivio 1971), reaches a maximum at 20 weeks and continues at this rate until 32 weeks of gestation. The observed decline in foetal serum levels, therefore, is due to the large increase in foetal and body fluid mass with an associated dilution effect rather than to any real decrease in hepatic synthesis of AFP. Owing to the fairly low molecular weight of AFP and its high concentration in the amniotic fluid, AFP spills over into the maternal bloodstream via the placental interface. When the foetal serum concentration is at a maximum around the fourteenth week of gestation, maternal serum levels become slightly raised above normal non-pregnant adult levels. There is, however, a very large difference in concentrations, maternal serum levels being estimated in nanograms and foetal levels in micrograms per millilitre. The serum AFP level in a normal adult is around 10 ng/ml. In neonates AFP is found in bile, faeces, urine, and cerebrospinal fluid, while during the second trimester it occurs in greatest concentration in foetal urine (Seppälä and Ruoslahti 1972). The major source of AFP in amniotic fluid is probably foetal urine. Synthesis on any scale seems to stop immediately after birth regardless of foetal maturity; the maternal serum concentration rapidly falls and by the end of the first month after delivery reaches a baseline level (Seppälä, Tallberg, and Enholm 1967). The level after delivery falls at the same rate whether the mother has been delivered of a pre-term or a full-term infant (Lardinois, Anaghostakis, Oritz, and Delisle 1972). Although AFP is virtually all of foetal origin it accounts for less than 0.5 per cent of the total protein present in amniotic fluid.

Nature of alpha-foetoprotein

There is some variation in the half-life of AFP as observed in the adult circulation according to clinical condition. It is longer, of the order of four to five days following delivery or abortion (Seppälä 1975), than that following surgery for hepatoma (3.7 days—Mukojima, Hattori, Nakayama *et al.* 1973), or after hepatectomy (two days or less—Alpert, Hershberg, Schurr, and Isselbacher 1971). The chemistry and molecular nature of AFP has been investigated by several workers (Brock 1974; Nishi and Hirai 1970; Ruoslahti and Seppälä 1971). It is a distinct chemical entity, probably a single polypeptide chain with a molecular weight of around 64 000; it is temperature stable between –20 °C and +37 °C, and contains hexose, hexosamine, sialic acid, nitrogen, and sulphur (Bergstrand and Czar 1956; Adinolfi, Adinolfi, and Cohen 1971; Nishi 1970). Alpha-foetoprotein produced by the normal foetal liver and by hepatomas is similar. Patients with hepatomas have serum AFP levels of 50 ng/ml or more (Alpert and Coston 1975) and children with malignant tumours sometimes may have grossly elevated levels exceeding 500 000 ng/ml (Mann *et al*. 1978) which are much higher levels than the amount detected in a normal adult of less than 10 ng/ml (Ruoslahti and Seppälä 1972). There may, however, be up to three variants of AFP, two of which are immunologically identical whilst the third does not precipitate a monospecific AFP antibody. AFP has been detected in foetal cerebrospinal fluid (Seppälä 1975), amniotic fluid, foetal urine (Linder and Seppälä 1968), and foetal and maternal blood (Masseyeff 1972). Human foetal blood is probably the best source and pooled cord blood is commonly used to obtain AFP for purification. Preparing pure AFP is difficult and the best methods appear to be immunochemical as reported by Nishi, Watanabe, Tsukada and Hirai (1971), Page (1973), and Ruoslahti and Seppälä (1971). Similarly, antibody production has been carried out using a variety of antigens including normal foetal serum and sera from patients with hepatoma or cirrhosis (Uriel, de Nechaud, Stanislawski-Birenwajg *et al*. 1968); also, different assay methods for estimating AFP levels have been adopted. As might be expected, problems of standardization have arisen and in comparing AFP values for normal amniotic fluid, Seppälä and Ruoslahti (1973) observed a twofold difference between their measurements and those of Brock and Sutcliffe (1972). Use of an impure or contaminated standard may be part of the explanation. A similar problem occurred in the United Kingdom Collaborative Study (1977). Adoption of a World Health Organization standard for international and multicentre comparisons has been proposed by Sizaret and Anderson (1976).

Diseases associated with production of alpha-foetoprotein

Although a pregnant woman having a hepatocellular cancer associated with an elevated AFP blood level in whom the diagnosis was missed has been reported (Purtilo, Clark and Williams 1975), most abnormally high values are associated with either adult diseases or abnormal foetal conditions. Of the former group, hepatomas are the the most common. AFP levels are higher in young compared with older patients (Masseyeff, Cassuto, Krebs *et al*. 1968) and in males compared with females (Alpert *et al*. 1971). Around 70 per cent of patients with primary liver cancer have elevated AFP levels (Abelev 1971). Alpert and Coston (1975) used AFP as a screening test to examine samples of patients with acute viral hepatitis, chronic active hepatitis, massive hepatic necrosis, and primary hepatoma; the percentages positive were 13, 23, 44, and 75 respectively. Negative results were obtained for acute or chronic nonviral hepatitis but the sensitivity of assays adopted probably influenced the proportion of positive cases. O'Connor, Tatarinov, Abelev, and Uriel (1970) studied the same diseases using two different methods for measuring AFP concentrations and found a 63 per cent positive rate using radioimmunoassay. Abnormal levels of AFP are found in the sera of patients with tumours containing embryonal elements and Abelev (1971) found 50 per cent of a series of patients having embryonal carcinomas had elevated serum AFP values. Other reports have associated high values with a number of different tumours and conditions (Table 28.2). Elevated AFP levels in hepatitis patients are usually transient. In the most severe cases associated with coma the presence of AFP in the serum is followed by clinical recovery (Karvountzis and Redeker 1974) suggesting AFP is related to hepatic regeneration.

Evidence suggesting adult patients with cystic fibrosis and some of their siblings have raised AFP concentrations (Chandra, Madhavankutty, and Way 1975) has not been substantiated by three further independent studies

TABLE 28.2 *Non-pregnant conditions examined for associated elevated levels of alpha-foetoprotein in blood*

Condition	Positive on AFP screening per cent	Reference
Tumours		
Primary liver cancer (hepatoma)	78	Abelev 1971
Teratoblastoma of testis	56	Mawas *et al*. 1969
Teratoblastoma of ovary, retroperitoneum, mediastinum	(if < 15 yrs old)	Hull *et al*. 1970
Teratocarcinoma (7 cases—3 sacrococcyx, 2 ovary, 2 testis)	100	Tsuchida *et al*. 1975
Yolk-sac derived solid tumours in children	100	Mann *et al*. 1978
Metastatic liver cancer	10	Bourreille *et al*. 1970
Carcinomas		
Stomach	—	Mehlman *et al*. 1971
Prostate	—	Kozower *et al*. 1971
Colon	—	Bernades *et al*. 1971
Pancreas	—	Masseyeff *et al*. 1968*a*
Non-neoplastic hepatic disease		
Acute viral hepatitis	13	Alpert and Coston 1975
Chronic active hepatitis	23	Kresno *et al*. 1970
Massive hepatic necrosis	44	Geoffroy *et al*. 1970
Haemochromatosis	—	Geoffroy *et al*. 1971
Other		
Subacute hereditary tyrosinemia (8 patients)	100	Belanger *et al*. 1973
Ataxia—telangiectasia (20 patients)	100	Waldmann and McIntire 1972

Around 50 conditions were examined by Masopust *et al*. (1968), Masseyeff *et al*. (1968), Buffé (1973), and Alpert and Coston (1975). Among those negative on AFP screening were: Biermer's disease, non-viral liver disease, various leukaemias (acute and chronic myeloid, acute lymphoid, chronic lymphocytic, chronic myeloid), lymphosarcoma, reticulosarcoma, myelomatosis, Hodgkin's disease, idiopathic bone marrow aplasia, Waldenstrom's disease, osteomyelosclerosis, haemoglobinosis C, thymoma, neuroblastoma, nephroblastoma, osteosarcoma, brain tumours, and liver angioma.

in the north of England (Wallwork, McFarlane, Hingley, and Ward 1975), Scotland (Brock, Manson, Raeburn, Bolton, and McCrae 1975), and Nottingham (Fitzsimmons, Smith, Hiller, and Wynne 1975). An apparent racial variation in maternal serum AFP values was observed in an analysis of samples from 20 Asian women and the same number of randomly selected Caucasian controls examined at 11 weeks of gestation and again at 16 weeks of gestation in Manchester; the Asian group had significantly lower maternal serum AFP values (Shapiro, Skinner, Phillips, and Whitfield 1975). No difference was found when blacks and Caucasians in the United States were compared (Macri, Weiss, Elligers, and Federgreen 1976).

Anencephalus and spina bifida

Early studies were unable to find any AFP in maternal blood owing to insensitive methods (Alpert and Zuckerman 1970) such as gel diffusion and it was only with the development of radioimmunoassay that amounts around the normal level of 10 ng/ml in non-pregnant adults became measurable. Improved techniques soon led to reports of AFP being present in maternal serum during normal pregnancy (Seppälä and Ruoslahti 1972; Ishiguro and Nishimura 1973) and to the observation of abnormally high levels in amniotic fluid of pregnancies associated with anencephalus and spina bifida (Brock and Sutcliffe 1972). Unlike the work mentioned in cancer research based on examination of blood and certain other body fluids, the first studies of neural-tube defects used analyses of samples of liquor amnii obtained by amniocentesis or sometimes from spontaneous and induced abortions delivered having an intact chorion and amniotic sac (Seller, Creasy, and Alberman 1974).

Amniotic fluid alpha-foetoprotein

Amniotic fluid AFP concentrations in normal pregnancy follow the same pattern as seen in foetal serum (Fig. 28.1). However, foetal serum concentrations are about 150 times those in the amniotic fluid at a corresponding gestation time (Brock 1974) and the maximal values in the liquor amnii, of around 40 μg/ml are present at 14 weeks of gestation (Brock 1976*a*). The normal AFP concentration is higher in the presence of a male than a female foetus (Brock 1978). One of the earliest reports from Edinburgh by Brock and Scrimgeour (1972) found a high level of AFP in the amniotic fluid of an anencephalic foetus at 18 weeks of gestation.

Demonstration of the value of measuring the concentration of AFP in amniotic fluid in early pregnancy as a marker for foetal abnormality was an important step which was soon confirmed (Allan, Ferguson-Smith, Donald *et al.* 1973; Lorber, Stewart, and Ward 1973; Nevin, Nesbitt, and Thompson 1973; Seller, Campbell, Coltart, and Singer 1973). Elevated levels commonly were observed in association with anencephalus and spina bifida prior to 20 weeks of gestation; these occurred most frequently in relation to anencephalus and extensive open myeloceles but were not found with closed spina bifida lesions where the defect was covered by skin or other tissues.

Laurence and Tew (1971) found that about 14 per cent of all neural-tube defects compatible with survival had closed lesions; some 6 per cent were encephaloceles often accompanied by severe brain anomalies, 4 per cent were myeloceles having thick epithelial coverings but which often have severe neurological handicap, and the remaining 4 per cent were meningoceles without spinal-cord damage. All pregnancies with neural-tube defects did not show abnormal AFP measurements and, for example Harris, Jennison, Barson *et al*. (1974) noted normal AFP levels in a case of open spina bifida examined at 33 weeks of gestation. Normal AFP values were reported in association with a case of iniencephalus (Nevin, Thompson, and Nesbitt 1974), a large occipital encephalocele covered with full-thickness skin at 16 weeks of gestation (Laurence, Turnbull, Harris *et al*. 1973), and a closed lumbar meningocele (Stewart, Ward, and Lorber 1975). It soon became clear that abnormally high AFP amniotic fluid levels are not specific for anencephalus and spina bifida, but may be elevated in association with other foetal abnormalities and pregnancy states. Predictably, the opposite condition exists, namely very low AFP levels possibly due to abnormality of the foetal liver or other conditions. Bennett, Grudzinskas, Gordon, and Turnbull (1978) have described this phenomenon based on ten patients who had depressed AFP levels at 14 to 15 weeks of gestation. Two had hydatidiform moles and the remaining eight anembryonic pregnancies or blighted ova.

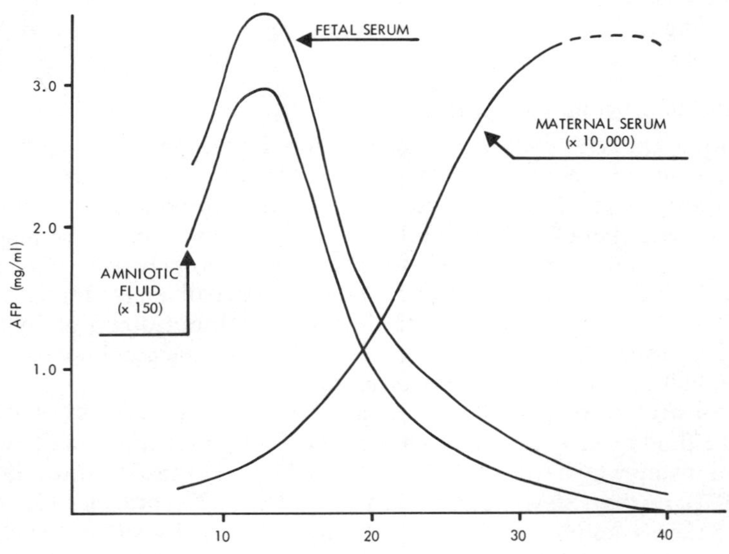

FIG. 28.1. Mean alpha-foetoprotein concentrations in foetal serum, amniotic fluid, and maternal serum at different gestation times. (After Brock 1976*a* and courtesy of *Obstetrical and Gynaecological Survey*.)

Several foetal abnormalities have now been examined for the presence of raised amniotic fluid AFP values (Table 28.3). Congenital nephrosis of the Finnish type (Kjessler, Johansson, Sherman *et al.* 1975), an autosomal recessive trait with an incidence of one per 10 000 births (Norio 1966) and uniformly fatal in early infancy, and missed abortion are confirmed as having abnormal AFP levels in nearly all instances. Exomphalos in a foetus of 33 weeks of gestation (de Bruijin and Huisjes 1975) and in one member of a triplet pregnancy at 16 weeks (Nevin and Armstrong 1975) had high values but estimates in two singleton pregnancies at 10 and 14 weeks respectively, each having a foetus with exomphalos, were normal (Brock and Sutcliffe 1973). High levels in assocation with the Turner syndrome (Seller *et al.* 1974) were found in fluid from intact sacs of spontaneous abortions in contrast to normal levels found in a case investigated by amniocentesis (Milunsky and Alpert 1974). The report of a 19-week foetus with the Meckel syndrome having a high AFP level may be atypical as this genetic condition does not always include an open neural-tube defect (Seller 1975).

TABLE 28.3 *Foetal conditions examined for associated elevated alpha-foetoprotein levels in amniotic fluid*

Foetal Condition	Reference
Early Pregnancy (<20 weeks)	
Anencephalus	Brock and Scrimgeour 1972
Spina bifida	Brock and Sutcliffe 1972
Congenital nephrosis	Kjessler *et al.* 1975
Spontaneous abortion†	Seller, Creasy, and Alberman 1974
Missed abortion and foetal death	Milunsky and Alpert 1974
Turner syndrome†	Seller, Creasy, and Alberman 1974
Meckel syndrome†	Seller 1975
Duodenal atresia	Weinberg, Milunsky, and Harrod 1975
Severe rhesus disease	Seppälä and Ruoslahti 1972
Skin and scalp defects	Whyley, Ward, and Hardy 1974
Late Pregnancy (>20 weeks)	
Hydrocephalus†	Seppälä and Unnerus 1974
Encephalocele†	Seppälä 1975
Exomphalos†	De Bruijn and Huisjes 1975; Kleijer *et al.* 1978
Oesophageal atresia†	Seppälä 1973
Sacrococcygeal teratoma	Schmid and Muhlethaler 1975
Pilonidal sinus	Jandial, Thorn, and Gibson 1976
Congenital skin defects	Leschot and Treffers 1975
	Fitzsimmons *et al.* 1976
Fallot's Tetralogy	Seppälä 1975
Respiratory distress syndrome	Seppälä 1975
Congenital absence of foetal urethra	Nevin *et al.* 1978

† These conditions are not invariably associated with high AFP values; conditions having high levels in early pregnancy will have high levels in late pregnancy.

Reports of high concentrations in late pregnancy associated with oesophageal atresia (Seppälä 1973), uncomplicated hydrocephalus (Seppälä and Unnerus 1974), and foetal distress (Seppälä and Ruoslahti 1973a) may not be consistent findings.

Contamination of an amniotic fluid sample by foetal blood during amniocentesis is a common source of a false positive result. Ward and Stewart (1974) estimated that a foetal bleed of 1 ml will give an abnormally high reading at 14 weeks of gestation and Doran, Allen, Pirani, and Shumak (1977) describe an experiment investigating effects of different amounts of foetal blood on the amniotic fluid AFP levels at various gestation times. They suggest screening samples for the presence of foetal red blood cells by the Kleihauer test. Brock (1976) considers examination for the presence of haemoglobin F using a highly specific commercial antiserum might be useful but Nørgaard-Pedersen (1978) suggests it may be easier to reconstitute the cell button to the original amniotic fluid volume with Drabkin's solution and measure the total haemoglobin concentration, as cyanmethaemoglobin at some 540 nm after dilution, and haemoglobin F (Nørgaard-Pederson and Lindholm 1972). Contamination of amniotic fluid by small amounts of maternal blood should make little contribution to the AFP level in amniotic fluid as the AFP level in maternal blood is relatively minute by comparison. Specimens obtained by amniocentesis also should be checked to distinguish amniotic fluid from urine (Duncan 1975) as the latter, which is similar in colour and appearance to liquor anmii, may be sampled if the needle is misdirected into the mother's bladder.

Brock (1976*b*) has postulated four possible mechanisms by which amniotic fluid AFP is increased by certain congenital malformations, assuming that the main route by which AFP passes into the amniotic fluid is by foetal urination, and degradation is principally by foetal swallowing and digestion. In the case of neural-tube defects leakage of the AFP occurs from foetal serum and cerebrospinal fluid whilst in exomphalos transudation from exposed blood vessels into the extruding viscera is suggested. Foetal proteinuria increases amniotic fluid AFP levels in nephrosis and impaired foetal swallowing or digestion may account for the elevated values found with anomalies of the gastro-intestinal tract such as duodenal atresia and oesophageal atresia. Formation of amniotic fluid in later pregnancy is mainly due to foetal urine as evidenced for example, by the oligohydramnios associated with absent kidneys or ureters in the foetus, but other sources including the respiratory tract may be important during the first trimester. Urine has been found in bladders of foetuses of 11 weeks of age (Abramavich 1968) and histological and radiographic evidence of renal function has been observed as early as the twelfth week of gestation (Fig 28.2).

Other constituents of amniotic fluid

A number of other constituents of amniotic fluid in addition to AFP have been examined as possible markers for the prenatal diagnosis of anencephalus and spina bifida (Table 28.1). As mentioned, the peak in the optical

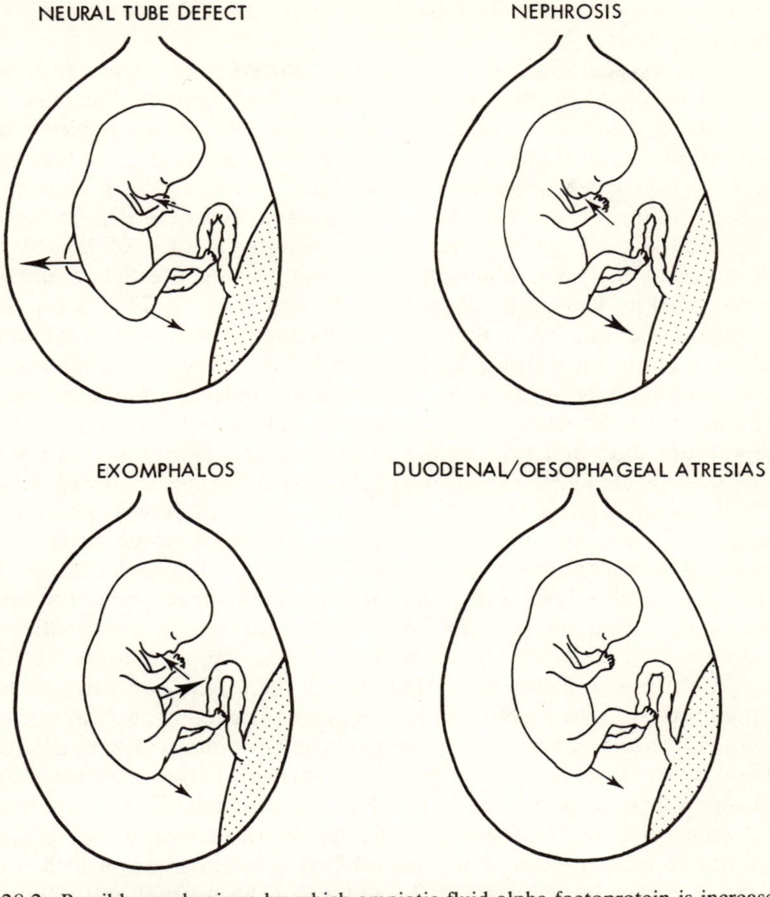

FIG. 28.2. Possible mechanisms by which amniotic fluid alpha-foetoprotein is increased by foetal malformation. (After Brock 1976*b* and courtesy of the *Lancet*.)

density of amniotic fluid bilirubin at 450 nm noted by Liley (1963) was further examined and observed in six out of seven pregnancies associated with anencephalus (Cassady and Cailliteau 1967), in four out of four cases studied by Lee and Wei (1970) and in 16 out of 17 cases of anencephalus by Emery *et al*. (1974). These estimates, however, were made during the period from 25 to 41 weeks of gestation. Why bilirubin levels in association with anencephalus are elevated is not clear. It may be partly due to the inability of such a malformed foetus to swallow properly leading to excess bilirubin being regurgitated into the amniotic fluid instead of being slowly degraded by passing through the alimentary tract. Low levels of other amniotic fluid constituents including oestriol, corticosteroids, 17-ketosteroids, and pregnanetriol and a significant reduction in 5-hydroxyindoleacetic acid during the last trimester of pregnancies having neural-tube defects and other conditions have been observed (Jeffcoate, Fliegner, Russell, Davis, and Wade 1965, Emery *et al*. 1972).

Macri, Weiss, Joshi and Evans (1974) reported that β–trace protein, a compound thought specific to cerebrospinal fluid, formed the basis of a qualitative test discriminating cases of anencephalus and spina bifida from normal infants. A study by Milunsky, Macri, Weiss, Alpert, McIsaac, and Joshi (1975) compared estimates of AFP and β–trace protein concentrations in 28 fluid samples from 10 pregnancies having neural-tube defects; they concluded AFP gave more reliable results. A case of the Meckel syndrome also has been diagnosed prenatally using these two markers (Chemke, Miskin, Rav-Acha, Porath, Sagiv, and Katz 1977). Olsson, Sherman, and Kjessler (1974), however, found β–trace protein in normal human serum. In a later study Brock and Olsson (1976) showed similar average β–trace protein concentrations in 19 amniotic fluids surrounding foetuses with neural tube defects and an equivalent number of matched controls. These authors state that the marked difference between their findings and those of Macri *et al* (1974, 1974*a*) may be due to differences in the specificity of the anteserum used to detect β–trace protein in each of two experiments. Brock and Olsson conclude β–trace protein is of no value in the early diagnosis of anencephalus and spina bifida. The high-molecular-weight proteins, a_2–globulin, IgM, and β–lipoprotein appear to be present in amniotic fluids from pregnancies associated with foetal neurological malformations and not in controls although further research is required (Brock 1976a). Canturia and Jones (1975) found high IgM concentrations in amniotic fluids from two spina bifida foetuses examined in early pregnancy. High concentrations of fibrinogen degradation products in amniotic fluid also were observed in late pregnancy. Comparisons between levels of AFP and fibrogen degradation fragment E (FgE) in amniotic fluid based on 214 normal controls and 27 pregnancies having foetuses with either an open neural-tube defect or exomphalos found FgE concentration of little value owing to considerable overlap of the values in the normal and abnormal groups (Gordon, Ratky, Leighton, Kitau, and Chard 1976). These authors show, by the use of exclusion chromatography of amniotic fluid samples, that normal pregnancies demonstrate FgE–reactive material comparable to the terminal degradation products of fibrinogen and this appears in the same region as AFP on the chromatogram. In fluids from neural-tube defect pregnancies a substance of higher molecular weight, corresponding to intact fibrinogen (molecular weight 340 000), was detected differing from fragment E which has a molecular weight of around 50 000.

Of the several markers other than AFP, the next most promising is high counts of foetal macrophages first noted in two cases of anencephalus by Sutherland, Brock, and Scrimgeour (1973). Further studies confirmed this observation (Nelson, Ruttiman, and Brock 1974), but the proportion of false positives was fairly high. Out of eight pregnancies examined before 22 weeks of gestation which had macrophage counts ranging between 82 to 6226, three were later shown to have anencephalus and two had spina bifida

(Sutherland, Brock, and Scrimgeour 1975). Gosden and Brock (1977) refined this test by looking at the morphology of cells rapidly adhering to polystyrene tubes in addition to making total cell counts. A semi-quantitative test of the cell content of anmiotic fluid has been devised by Bobrow, Evans, Noble, and Patel (1978). Freed (1977) speculated that the factor causing this adherence in abnormal amniotic fluid samples may be the high amount of AFP present. Even simple cell counts using glass slides, however, may be of value (Bryant and Hoehn 1977). Other discriminants, such as measuring lysozyme levels, an enzyme sythesized by macrophages and monocytic cells, are of little value (Seller and Adinolfi 1975).

Maternal serum alpha-foetoprotein

The development of more sensitive assay methods permitted detection of the very small amounts of AFP in maternal serum compared with the much higher concentrations in foetal serum and amniotic fluid (Gitlin 1975). Presence of a foetal immuno a–globulin in blood from a normal pregnant woman was reported by Bodman (1959). By using immunodiffusion, AFP was identified in around 50 per cent of normal women of 30 or more weeks of gestation (Foy, Kondi, and Linsell 1970). Maternal serum levels were found to rise progressively following the peak in amniotic fluid concentration at around 12 weeks of gestation and were virtually at baseline levels one week after delivery (Adinolfi *et al*. 1971). Maternal antibodies against AFP have not been detected to date (Seppälä and Ruoslahti 1972).

Reasons for elevated AFP levels in maternal serum include the various tumours and conditions discussed (Table 28.2). Also, if the concentration of AFP in amniotic fluid is sufficiently high a spillover effect will occur producing abnormally elevated levels in maternal serum. Several foetal conditions have been observed which produced high AFP values in both amniotic fluid and maternal serum, although the peak level in the former is in early pregnancy and in the latter is during the second half of the gestational period. Seppälä and Ruoslahti (1972, 1973) reported quite sharp rises in maternal serum AFP concentrations following threatened abortion, foetal distress, and intra-uterine death. Seven out of 126 women (5.6 per cent) who had spontaneous abortion had raised maternal serum AFP levels compared with 4 out of 247 controls (1.6 per cent) delivered of liveborn singletons in a survey from Oxford (Wald, Barber, Cuckle, Brock, and Stirrat 1977). This difference is statistically significant. No association between maternal serum AFP levels was discovered in relation to foetal weight, maternal age, and parity (Leek, Ruoss, Kitau, and Chard 1975) or a history of previous neural-tube defects (Wald, Barker, Peto, Brock, and Bonnar 1976), but some further surveys indicate a possible association between high AFP concentrations and low birth-weight (Wald, Cuckle, Stirrat, Bennett, and Turnbull 1977; Brock, Barron, Jelen, Watt, and Scrimgeour 1977).

The first report linking elevated maternal serum AFP levels with neural-tube defects was from the United Kingdom (Brock, Bolton, and Monaghan 1973). This was based on one case of anencephalus in which serum AFP values were estimated at 16 weeks and then 21 weeks of gestation. The pregnancy was terminated in view of the continued high AFP value. Conflicting evidence followed these publications, some suggesting no increased AFP blood levels (Seller, Singer, Coltart, and Campbell 1974) and others abnormal values only in the presence of anencephalus and open spina bifida lesions (Harris *et al.* 1974). Nevin *et al.* (1974) describe a case where an infant had an encephalocele, but no elevated AFP serum level was detected at 40 weeks of gestation; a second patient, whose pregnancy ended in a spontaneous abortion of a foetus with iniencephalus at 17 weeks of gestation, had a normal amniotic fluid AFP level of 17.0 ng/ml two weeks previously. However, better assay methods and further studies have demonstrated the usefulness of maternal serum AFP measurements in the diagnosis of neural-tube defects, as we discuss in Section 29.

Multiple pregnancy

The most important determinant of elevated maternal serum AFP concentration, excepting neurological malformation, is multiple pregnancy. Abnormally high levels occur both in the first half (Wald, Barker, Peto, Brock, and Bonnar 1975) and second half of the gestation period (Garoff and Seppälä 1973; Ishiguro 1973). Most twins, even if monozygotic, have separate amniotic sacs. For the purpose of amniocentesis, a twin in a separate sac is similar to a singleton pregnancy, but at the foeto-placental interface AFP produced by the two foetal livers enters the one maternal bloodstream producing high maternal serum concentrations. Between 2 and 6 per cent of twins have a common amniotic cavity (Bulmer 1970, Seller, Dumon, and Vanderheyden 1977). In these twins, high maternal serum AFP concentrations and a high concentration in the common amniotic sac would be expected.

This relationship, therefore, between the number of foetuses *in utero* and maternal serum AFP concentrations explains the observations by Wald, Cuckle, and Stirrat (1978) of higher maternal serum AFP concentrations in the second trimester in triplet pregnancies compared with twins, and higher levels again in quadruplet pregnancies compared with either triplets or twins. In a series of 100 twin pregnancies examined prior to 27 weeks of gestation, some 40 per cent had elevated serum AFP concentrations (Keilani, Clarke Kitau, and Chard 1978); none had any congenital defects except for one pregnancy which aborted at 20 weeks, the products of conception being a conjoined thoracophagus. A raised maternal serum AFP level in which the twin pregnancy consisted of a normal male weighing 2.9 kg and a foetus papyraceous has been reported (Letchworth, Gordon, and Leighton 1977). In a triplet pregnancy of a Belfast woman who already had one child with hydrocephalus, termination at 18 weeks revealed two amniotic sacs; one contained a normal male foetus and the second a normal male foetus together with another male foetus having an extensive omphalocoele. Alpha-foetoprotein levels in fluids from both sacs and in the maternal serum were highly elevated (Nevin and Armstrong 1975). A singleton pregnancy in which the foetus had multiple congenital abnormalities including an omphalocoele showing elevated AFP values from 20 to 30 weeks is described by Young and Crawford (1977). The association between high maternal serum AFP levels and low birth-weight in singletons without neural-tube defects (Brock *et al*. 1977; Wald *et al*. 1977), was further investigated on 102 unaffected twin pregnancies by Wald, Cuckle, Stirrat, and Turnbull (1978). A relationship between low birth-weight in twin pregnancies and elevated levels of maternal serum AFP was found.

Abnormal low levels of maternal serum alpha-foetoprotein

Lastly, regarding abnormally low levels of AFP in maternal serum, the Swedish study of an unselected series of women screened between 10 weeks and 25 weeks of gestation and having singleton pregnancies found 1 to 2 per cent of the samples had these concentrations (Johansson, Kjessler, Sherman, and Wallstrom 1977). Some 15 per cent of this group had negative pregnancy tests and either were not pregnant at all or a blighted ovum might have been reabsorbed. A further 28 per cent lost their pregnancies as spontaneous abortions during the ensuing 14 days and some of the remainder may have had trophoblastic disease which is associated with abnormally low serum AFP levels (Kjessler, Hemmingsson, Nilsson, and Johansson 1977).

29

Screening

MANY improvements in the state of the public health have been achieved by primary preventive medical procedures such as immunization or by improving sanitary conditions, housing, and nutrition. For many other conditions, however, primary prevention has not been successful either because the aetiology is unknown or if known, the appropriate preventive measures cannot be successfully applied. For these conditions, the role of medicine is to provide treatment services. As one component of this approach based on secondary prevention, screening may be used on the assumption that it is desirable to treat patients at an early rather than an advanced stage of disease or even before they complain of symptoms. Evolution of the principles of screening from work concerned with the primary prevention of infectious disease has a firm basis in microbiology because we know infections are spread by persons without symptoms. Thus screening for tuberculosis by mass radiography is a justifiable procedure if the prevalence of the disease is above a certain level in the community. Screening for non-communicable diseases does not carry the possibility of reducing risk to the community in general and so its value is often not easy to determine. Various criteria of acceptability for any given screening procedure have been outlined (Wilson and Jungner 1968; Holland 1974).

Definition

We define screening as the presumptive identification of unrecognized disease or abnormal conditions by applying tests which are relatively simple, inexpensive, and acceptable to apparently healthy individuals. The aim is to identify those who probably have the defined disease or condition and those who probably do not have this disease or condition. The procedure is not intended to be diagnostic and individuals with positive tests must be referred for further investigations and treatment.

How do these principles of screening relate to the question of identifying cases of anencephalus and spina bifida *in utero* by measuring maternal serum AFP levels on all pregnant women in the community? We shall examine this question using the available data which are mainly from retrospective and prospective surveys conducted in the United Kingdom and Sweden.

Retrospective surveys

The clinical observations relating elevated maternal serum AFP levels to pregnancies with anencephalus or spina bifida led to the formation of the

United Kingdom Collaborative Study Group who had their preliminary meeting in 1974 and published the first report in 1977. By late 1974 it was clear that effectively to screen large numbers of women in early pregnancy, attention would have to be paid to minimizing difficulties experienced by previous workers screening for other conditions in past years. These included definitions of the defects to be detected and in particular differences between open and closed neurological malformations. Other problems were lack of standardized laboratory methods and materials for assaying AFP, limitations of the preliminary studies owing to the small number of affected pregnancies examined, and the question of generalizing results based on women selected on the basis of attendance at a teaching hospital or genetic counselling clinic to the whole maternal population. It was appreciated that though the distributions of AFP values from pregnancies with and without foetuses having anencephalus and spina bifida were not totally distinct, measurement of AFP concentrations in maternal serum could be a useful screening test.

Some 19 groups participated in this multicentre study, the main criteria for inclusion of an AFP measurement being knowledge of the outcome of that particular pregnancy and a known gestation time when screened. The design was thus retrospective, as specimens were collected and frozen for several months until the pregnancy outcome was determined. After the completion of the pregnancy, the relevant frozen serum sample was identified and the AFP concentration measured. The analysis was based on 18 684 singleton pregnancies not associated with neural-tube defects, 146 having anencephalus, 142 having spina bifida alone, and 13 having encephaloceles, in which AFP levels were measured on maternal serum collected between 10 weeks and 24 weeks of gestation. Of the 142 spina bifidas, 108 had open lesions, 24 closed lesions, and 10 were unclassified. Scatter diagrams of maternal serum AFP levels measured on the first blood samples relating to the 146 singleton pregnancies with anencephalus and the 142 singleton pregnancies with spina bifida demonstrate a large range of values (Figs. 29.1 and 29.2). The discriminatory power of maternal serum AFP measurements appears much better after 16 weeks of gestation than before this time. At this gestation time almost all pregnancies with anencephalus have values above the 97th centile of the distribution of AFP levels of unaffected pregnancies. Most, but not all, open spina bifida cases are accompanied by similarly high values but closed spina bifida cases often have values similar to those of unaffected pregnancies. There was considerable between-centre variation in AFP measurements in unaffected pregnancies and therefore the measurement for each woman was compared to the median AFP value for all unaffected pregnancies examined at that centre, adjusted for gestation time, rather than using absolute values such as nanograms per millilitre. Multiples of the median AFP value were taken as cut-off points delineating normal from abnormal pregnancies with respect to assessing the value of AFP screening. This method was chosen because no AFP reference preparation had been generally accepted at the time when the study commenced. Use of ratios to the median rather than a particular centile as the cut-off point more easily permits pooling of data from the various centres and allows for variations over time in a particular laboratory due to their technical methods for measuring serum AFP concentrations. The results show better discrimination between affected and unaffected pregnancies at 16 weeks of gestation or later than before this time and indicate that 16 to 18 weeks is the best period in pregnancy to take a blood sample for screening for open spina bifida. Measurements made before 16 weeks of gestation are less efficient at detecting affected pregnancies while examination at later than 18 weeks of gestation gives a very limited time for further investigations and termination of pregnancy prior to 20 weeks if indicated.

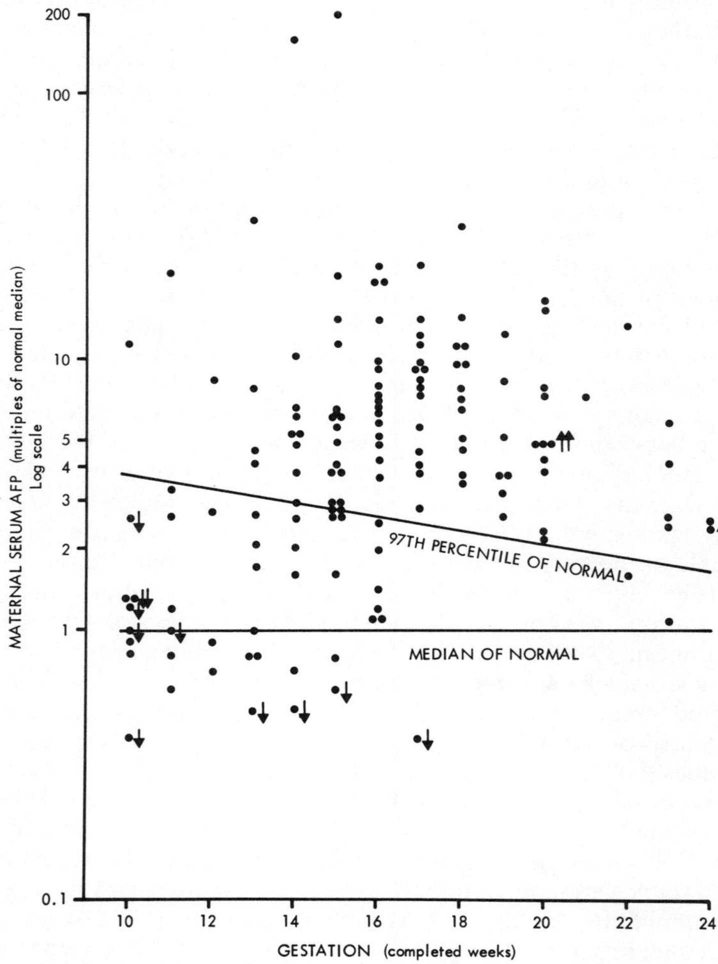

FIG. 29.1. First maternal serum alpha-foetoprotein value, expressed as multiple of the normal median, from 146 singleton pregnancies with anencephalus at different gestation times (Source as in Fig. 29.2).

Several cut-off points, corresponding to different multiples of the median, were considered. The study group suggest that for the British Isles, the optimum cut-off point to use is 2.5 times the median maternal serum AFP level in unaffected pregnancies. Some 3.3 per cent of unaffected singleton pregnancies and 26 per cent of unaffected twin pregnancies would have AFP levels above this cut-off point. Using this definition, the detection rates were 88 per cent for anencephalus, 79 per cent for open spina bifida and 38 per cent for closed or unclassified spina bifida. The proportion of pregnancies showing an elevated serum AFP level and which have neural-tube defects (the predictive value positive of the test) depends on the prevalence of neural-tube defects in the population. If we assume a prevalence rate for all

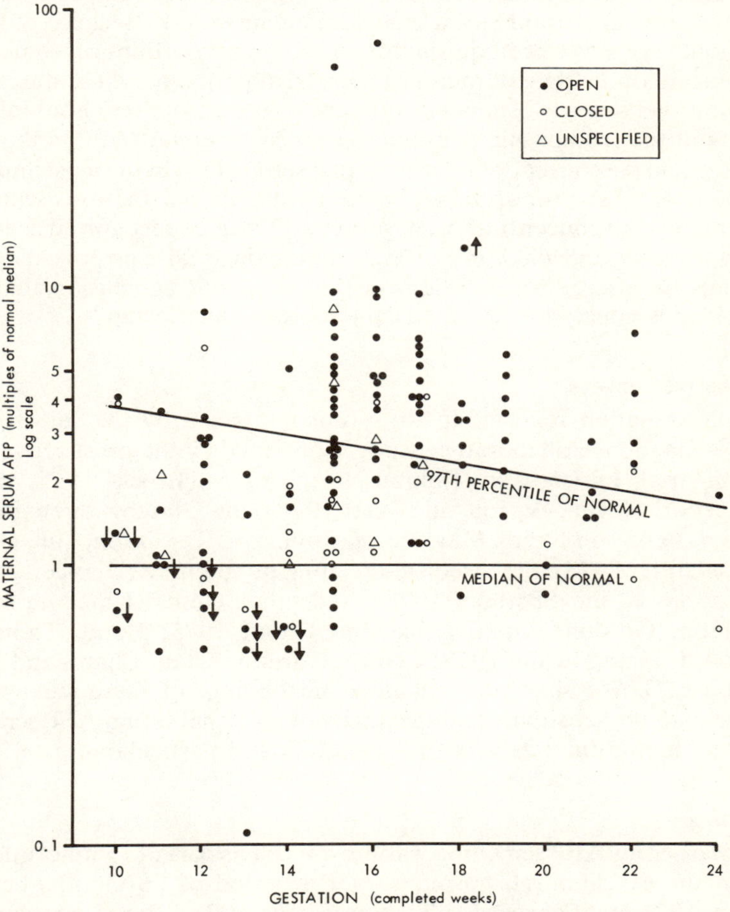

FIG. 29.2. First maternal serum alpha-foetoprotein value, expressed as multiple of the normal median, from 142 singleton pregnancies with spina bifida at different gestation times. (Courtesy of the UK Collaborative Study Group (Professor Polani, Chairman, Steering Group) and the *Lancet*.)

neural tube defects of 4 per 1000 total births, then 1 in 10 of pregnancies with a high maternal serum AFP level at 16 to 18 weeks of gestation will have a neural-tube defect and 1 in 21 will have an open spina bifida defect. The ratio of unaffected to affected pregnancies will increase as the prevalence in the population declines and is approximately inversely proportional to the population prevalence rate. Thus for the given detection rates and false positive rates in the United Kingdom Collaborative Study, using a cut-off point of 2.5 times the median, the ratio of all affected to unaffected pregnancies showing an elevated maternal serum AFP concentration is 21:1 if the prevalence rate of all neural-tube defects is 2 per 1000, 10:1 at 4 per 1000, and 5:1 at 8 per 1000 total births.

Owing to the experimental design and methods used in this retrospective study several important questions were unanswered. Because a known gestational age was a prerequisite for entry, the proportions of women who were unsure of the date of their last menstrual period or whose duration of gestation was wrongly estimated were unknown. Also, there is no information about the relationship between the concentration of AFP in the amniotic fluid and the concentration in maternal serum. One of the most important questions is what proportion of women with normal foetuses who have abnormally high concentrations of serum AFP can be recognized as normal by further tests, and what proportion will remain as false positive diagnoses and thus be offered an abortion on the erroneous conclusion that their pregnancy is affected when in fact the foetus is unaffected?

Prospective surveys

Some information relevant to the problems raised by the retrospective United Kingdom Collaborative Study is provided by the prospective intervention trial initiated in Edinburgh in 1975 (Brock 1978; Brock, Scrimgeour, Steven, Barron, and Watt 1978), the Glasgow screening programme (Ferguson-Smith, May, Vince, Robinson, Rawlinson, Tait, Gibson, and Radcliffe, 1978), the Swedish screening programme (Kjessler, Johansson, Lidbjörk, and Sherman 1977), and other United Kingdom surveys (Leighton, Gordon, Kitau, Leek, and Chard 1975; Bond, Thompson, Elwood, J. H., and Cran 1977; Clarke, Gordon, Kitau, Chard, and Letchworth 1977). We shall now examine the findings of these surveys with reference to the sensitivity and specificity of maternal serum AFP screening to detect neural-tube defects and spina bifida in particular.

Edinburgh

Maternal serum AFP screening was introduced as part of routine antenatal care at three Edinburgh hospitals over a period of 26 months between January 1975 and February 1977 (Brock *et al.* 1978). Blood samples were obtained from 6377 women representing 79 per cent of antenatal bookings and pregnancy outcome was determined in 96 per cent of these patients. The cut-off point separating normal from abnormal AFP values was defined as the 95th centile. Patients having raised levels had a repeat blood sample while those having AFP levels above the 99th centile were referred directly for ultrasonography. If the level in the second blood sample was below the 95th centile (we will refer to such levels as 'normal') no further action was taken; if the level was above the 95th centile, arrangements were made for ultrasonography and possible amniocentesis. Acceptance by the patient of the maternal serum AFP screening test was high, but some women had to make an extra antenatal attendance as their first prenatal visit was prior to 15 weeks. Women first booking after 20 weeks of gestation, those booking early but who miscarried prior to 15 weeks, and patients who found termination of pregnancy unacceptable were excluded from the study.

There were 339 women (5.3 per cent) who had a positive AFP result on the basis of the first blood test (Table 29.1). Of the 14 anencephalics occurring in the 6377 births screened, 13 were diagnosed and aborted and one had a normal serum AFP level. Of 10 open spina bifida cases, 7 were detected but only 5 were aborted, as two mothers refused abortion. All of 4 closed spina bifida lesions had normal serum AFP values. The detection rate for all neural-tube defects was 71 per cent, and for all spina bifida cases, 50 per cent. A further three defects were diagnosed by amniocentesis performed because of a prior birth having a neural-tube defect; we have not counted these in assessing the impact of maternal serum screening. Of the unaffected pregnancies, 319 had false positive serum AFP levels; 11 were due to twins, 13 to missed or threatened abortions, and most of the rest were excluded by a repeat serum AFP test and by checking the gestation of the pregnancy; 114 (36 per cent) proceeded to amniocentesis, one case of exomphalos was diagnosed, and one unaffected pregnancy was erroneously aborted because of a high amniotic fluid AFP level. This study demonstrates certain limitations which are also seen in other studies. The detection rate is high for anencephalus, but we would suggest that the antenatal diagnosis of anencephalus is of little benefit. The detection rate of all spina bifida lesions is the more relevant figure, and furthermore we suggest that to present only the detection rate of open lesions also is rather dubious. Although some closed spina bifida lesions may not be associated with mental or physical handicap, this proportion is very small and by contrast a relatively larger proportion of spina bifida infants with extensive open lesions are stillborn thus reducing the value of early diagnosis. The detection rate chosen by Brock *et al.* (1978) to be presented in their paper is 83 per cent; this is based only on open neural-tube defects (anencephalus and open spina bifida). However, we suggest a more relevant figure is 50 per cent, based on all spina bifida cases and excluding, as did the authors, the one case with a family history of neural-tube defect. A further useful summary is that testing 6377 women at between 15 to 20 weeks of gestation by measuring serum AFP levels allowed the selective abortion of five spina bifida cases, with two refusals and 13 anencephalics were also aborted. This screening programme also resulted in the abortion of one unaffected infant.

TABLE 29.1 *Summary of findings from maternal serum AFP screening programmes for detecting neural-tube defects in Scotland*

Data	Edinburgh	Glasgow Phase I	Glasgow Phase II
Length of study period (months)	26	12	12
Cut-off period (centile)	95th	99th	97th
Total number of pregnancies screened	6377	6122	11 585
Number with elevated AFP at first screening	339	103	202
Neural-tube defects diagnosed			
Anencephalus	13	13	27[5]
Open spina bifida	7[1]	6	8
Closed spina bifida	0	0	0
Neural-tube defects missed			
Anencephalus	1	3[2]	0
Open spina bifida	3	8[3]	7[6]
Closed spina bifida	4	6	14[7]
Neural-tube defects aborted			
Anencephalus	13	13[4]	26
Open spina bifida	5	6	8[8]
Closed spina bifida	0	0	0
Unaffected foetuses aborted	1	0	0
Number of false positive maternal serum AFP values at first test	319 (5.0%)	79 (1.3%)	161 (1.4%)
Number of amniocenteses on unaffected pregnancies	114	11	38
Other defects diagnosed (exomphalos)	1	1	1
Detection rate for all neural-tube defects (per cent)	71 (20/28)	53 (19/36)	63 (35/56)
Detection rate for spina bifida of all types (per cent)	50 (7/14)	30 (6/20)	28 (8/29)

[1] Includes 2 patients who refused abortion.
[2] Includes 2 patients who had normal serum AFP values; 1 had normal amniotic fluid AFP value being a twin sampled from the normal sac.
[3] Includes 4 patients who had normal first serum AFP values; 2 had repeat serum AFP values which were normal; 1 was misinterpreted owing to estimating gestational age incorrectly; 1 did not attend for follow-up after having a high serum AFP level at first test.
[4] Includes 4 cases diagnosed by ultrasonography without amniocentesis.
[5] Includes 1 patient who had refused abortion.
[6] Includes 3 women who had normal serum AFP first tests; 2 had serum AFP values wrongly regarded as normal owing to an error in interpretation (one case) and erroneous diagnosis of twins (one case); in 1 case amniocentesis failed; 1 case had a normal amniotic fluid AFP level.
[7] Includes 1 woman who had raised first serum AFP level but subsequent outcome is not stated in the paper; this case does not appear to have been aborted.
[8] Includes 1 affected pregnancy which aborted spontaneously prior to termination; this case is not counted.
Normal serum AFP value is defined as being less than the cut-off point defined in the related study.

Glasgow

In Glasgow, Ferguson-Smith and colleagues (1978) conducted a two-phase screening programme on 17 707 women from the west of Scotland. The first phase (May 1975 to June 1976) tested women at between 15 and 20 weeks of gestation and used the 99th centile as the cut-off point separating normal from abnormal maternal serum AFP values (Table 29.1).

In the 6122 pregnancies screened during phase one, 13 out of 16 anencephalics were detected; two had normal serum AFP levels and one with an elevated serum AFP value was a discordant twin in which the amniotic fluid was sampled from the normal sac. Some 6 of the 14 open spina bifidas, and none of the six closed spina bifidas, were detected. All 19 detected cases were aborted. Of the eight open lesions missed, four had normal serum AFP values, two had an initially high serum AFP level but the second serum AFP samples were assessed as normal (although in retrospect they were elevated), one did not attend for follow up, and one had, on retrospect, a high serum AFP value but the gestation time had been overestimated. We have counted such cases as false negatives because that was the result reached by the whole screening process, although in the report these cases are regarded as having been detected. Thus we calculate the detection rate for all neural-tube defects as 53 per cent, and for all spina bifida cases as 30 per cent. Only 79 (1.3 per cent) unaffected pregnancies had false positive serum AFP levels, and 68 of these were correctly diagnosed by a second blood test together with ultrasonography. Amniocenteses were carried out on only 13 pregnancies without neural-tube defects, of which 11 had normal results, one had examphalos and one a missed abortion.

In the phase-two study (July 1976 to June 1977) 11 585 pregnancies were screened at 16 to 20 weeks of gestation and the 97th centile used as the cut-off point. All of 27 anencephalics were diagnosed and 26 of these were aborted, one mother refusing abortion. Some 8 of the 15 open spina bifidas were detected; of the seven missed, three had normal serum AFP levels, one was misinterpreted, one erroneously diagnosed as twins, in one amniocentesis failed, and in one the amniotic fluid level was regarded as normal. We have excluded completely one spina bifida case which spontaneously aborted before amniocentesis was performed. None of the closed spina bifida cases appears to have been diagnosed, although one had a high initial serum AFP level. Thus the detection rates were 63 per cent for all neural-tube defects and 28 per cent for all spina bifida cases. Of 161 (1.4 per cent) unaffected pregnancies with positive serum AFP results, only 38 (24 per cent) proceeded to amniocentesis (compared with 36 per cent in Edinburgh), the rest being excluded by repeat serum AFP tests and ultrasound, and all amniocentesis results were normal, except in one case of exomphalos.

These Glasgow studies show that with careful repeat maternal serum AFP testing and ultrasound examinations, only a small proportion of pregnancies with false positive serum AFP levels need to proceed to amniocentesis, and that the risk of aborting a normal infant is very small. However, the detection rates, except for anencephalus, are quite low and in part this is a result of the careful follow up of an initial positive test. By successfully excluding false positive tests, some true positive first tests will be wrongly regarded as normal after follow up investigations. If the aim of a screening programme is to reduce the demands for long-term care of infants with spina bifida, these British prospective studies suggest that the impact of maternal serum AFP screening is likely to be limited. Detection rates for all spina bifida cases in the Edinburgh, Glasgow phase-one, and Glasgow phase-two studies were 50 per cent, 30 per cent, and 28 per cent respectively. It could be argued that the detection rates in terms of an initial first positive serum AFP level are higher, and that as more experience is gained in interpreting high and borderline AFP values, the detection rate will rise. On the other hand, at least two considerations suggest that these results are better than those which would be expected if all pregnancies in the population were screened. First, the studies include only women who attend and accept an initial AFP blood test at the required gestation time, thus ignoring a substantial source of reduction in efficiency. Secondly, if initial testing were to be carried out in small hospitals and in family practice, follow up of women with positive tests will be much more difficult and the opportunities for error much greater than in studies restricted, as these have been, to large teaching hospitals.

Sweden

The Swedish study (Kjessler *et al.* 1977) initiated in 1974 and covering 23 public antenatal care units is of interest in view of the low prevalence of neural-tube defects; the rates for anencephalus and spina bifida being 0.37 and 0.72 per 1000 births respectively (Appendix A.1). These are similar to the present frequencies in the western provinces of Canada, the western United States, Australia, South Africa, and much of Europe. Outcomes of some 7158 pregnancies have so far been reported and abnormally raised AFP levels were defined as values exceeding the arithmetic mean plus 3 standard deviations for the appropriate gestation (Johansson *et al.* 1977). Assay of AFP in maternal serum was made using a paper disc radioimmunoassay method (Johansson, Kjessler, and Sherman 1976; Johansson, Kjessler, Sherman, and Bennich 1977) with the whole blood samples being mailed to the laboratory without further additives. There were no serious administrative, organizational or laboratory problems and results were available within 24 hours after initiating the AFP assay; between 200 and 300 patient samples were processed per technician per day. Each sample was analysed twice; if the AFP level was abnormally high for the given estimated gestation time, the sample was re-tested and if still elevated the patient was requested to provide a second sample of blood. Additional control samples were obtained in some instances. Some 289 (4.0 per cent) of the 7158 samples obtained by original screening were abnormally raised of which 206 were subsequently shown to be associated with normal singleton pregnancies, 36 with multiple pregnancy, 17 with foetal wastage, 5 with neural-tube defects (three anencephalus, one open spina bifida, and one myeloschisis), and 25 with other types of congenital defects. The latter included one case of omphalocele and infants with other defects of the gastro-intestinal and cardiovascular systems for which no explanation for a raised maternal serum AFP value is apparent. There were two additional foetuses affected by neural-tube defects which did not have original raised AFP levels; one had anencephalus and one had an open spina bifida lesion. The detection rate was therefore 71 per cent (5 out of 7) for all types of neural-tube defects. Interestingly, no infants with closed spina bifida lesions were observed. Kjessler and colleagues comment that there was at least one instance where a completely normal infant was born subsequent to having serially elevated AFP values in both maternal serum and amniotic fluid.

Other surveys

A simple and yet important practical problem is what happens when maternal serum AFP screening is introduced into routine hospital prenatal care without any special modifications such as arranging repeat visits for early attenders or serial AFP measurements. This scheme was used in a pilot study of 1844 consecutive prenatal patients attending the Royal Maternity Hospital, Belfast, during the period from September 1975 to March 1976 (Bond *et al.* 1977). There were 28 pregnancies with an 'abnormal' outcome; three anencephalics, six spina bifidas (four with open defects and two with closed defects), and 19 associated with twins. Only four pregnancies with neural-tube defects were screened at between 15 and 19 weeks of gestation and two of these had serum AFP values above the 95th centile.

Another report of 5539 consecutive patients attending three maternity units in the City and Hackney District of London (Clarke *et al.* 1977) follows from earlier work by Leighton and colleagues (1975). This study found 54 per cent of women booked at or before 15 weeks of gestation and 26 per cent booked at between 16 and 22 weeks. Eighteen infants had neural-tube defects. Some seven anencephalics and one open spina bifida (whose mother had had an affected child previously) were diagnosed and aborted. Three other anencephalics had high serum AFP levels but the clinician in charge was not informed of these results as the study was only beginning. A further three anencephalics were missed because of late booking, one anencephalic and one open spina bifida were missed by errors in assessing gestation, one anencephalic was missed by having a normal serum AFP level at 15 weeks and no further test, and one open spina bifida had a high serum AFP level but a normal amniotic fluid AFP level and later spontaneously aborted at 27 weeks of gestation. Thus 10 out of 15 anencephalics and none of two spina bifidas were diagnosed, ignoring the one spina bifida with a family history, which gives a detection rate for neural-tube defects of all types of 59 per cent. As in the Swedish study, no closed spina bifida lesions were observed in this population. One pregnancy with hydrocephalus had a normal serum AFP value. Three other defects (exomphalos, gastroschisis, translocation of part of chromosome 18) were diagnosed by high serum AFP levels together with further investigations and were aborted.

Implications

Findings from these retrospective and prospective studies which have not all used the same screening definitions raise many problems. No screening test yet devised is completely efficient. With respect to anencephalus and spina bifida, acceptance of the usefulness of estimating maternal serum AFP levels depends on the proportion of false positives that is, unaffected pregnancies with serum AFP levels above the cut-off point, which require investigation. Of special concern is the risk that normal foetuses may be aborted on the basis of finding high AFP levels in the maternal serum together with false positive results of further investigations. False negatives, where foetal malformation is not picked up by screening and the pregnancy continues to term, resulting in an affected stillborn or liveborn infant as occurs with many cases at present, are associated with fewer ethical and legal problems, at least in the United Kingdom. In North America false negatives pose a greater problem if a pregnancy continues after having been fully investigated and results in the birth of a handicapped child, mainly owing to differences in legislation (Section 30). Even if there is general agreement on the cut-off point for the maternal serum AFP level separating normal from abnormal, this is only the first step in the screening process. The first blood sample should be taken at 16 weeks with a second sample at 17 weeks if the initial serum AFP level is abnormally high. Ultrasound examination should then be carried out principally to exclude multiple pregnancy; where the pregnancy is singleton amniocentesis is performed as a diagnostic test so that termination, if indicated, may be performed prior to 20 weeks of gestation. Alternatively, all women could have a serum AFP level determination and an ultrasound scan at 16 weeks. The latter is impractical at the moment in the United Kingdom as ultrasound tests are mainly confined to obstetric teaching centres where equipment and trained staff are available. Only in one city, Dundee, is every patient in that community attending for prenatal care routinely screened by sonar (Christie 1977) although, as we have described, certain teaching hospitals may now be examining all mothers attending particular clinics. These specialized units, however, provide antenatal care for only a minority of the 700 000 women delivered in the United Kingdom annually. In North America, ultrasonography but not maternal serum AFP estimation may be more readily available.

Given the sequence of maternal serum AFP determinations and ultrasonography, a number of patients would then require amniocentesis as a diagnostic test. Again false positive, false negative, and equivocal amniotic fluid AFP values have been reported due to various problems of laboratory methods and interpretation of the findings (Ward and Stewart 1974; Field and Kerr 1975; Laurence, Walker, Lloyd, and Griffiths 1975; Brock 1975*a*, Henry and Robinson 1977). A Norwegian study found a low correlation (r=0.17) between the AFP level in maternal serum and the AFP level in amniotic fluid based on 71 maternal-serum–amniotic-fluid pairs investigated at 15 to 17 weeks of gestation on unaffected pregnancies (Berg, Noer, Molne and Bjøro 1976). More disturbing are the human errors of confusing amniotic fluid and maternal urine due to misdirecting an amniocentesis needle into the bladder or by mixing up test specimens when they reach the laboratory (Kohn 1975). Also there is the problem of contamination of amniotic fluid specimens by foetal blood which may produce a false positive result (Section 28). In their analysis of 2495 amniotic fluid AFP assays in New England, Milunsky and Alpert (1976) describe receiving two samples on which the identifying numbers had inadvertently been mislabelled. One sample had a high AFP value; this pregnancy was terminated and an entirely normal foetus was found. The second sample showed a normal AFP value; this pregnancy proceeded to term and an anencephalic infant was born. Such errors are unacceptable but they may be impossible to avoid completely, especially in a screening programme handling large numbers of specimens in more than one laboratory. Also, further investigations, particularly amniocentesis are procedures not without risk.

Risks of amniocentesis

The foetus *in utero* at 16 weeks of gestation is surrounded by an average of 175 ml of amniotic fluid (Fuchs 1966). A small number of reports covering around 3500 infants born after second-trimester amniocentesis are available for assessing possible hazards of this procedure (National Institute of Child Health and Human Development 1976; Henrion 1976; Murken 1976; Scrimgeour 1976; Medical Research Council of Canada 1977; Henry, Peakman, and Robinson 1978). Variations in the frequency of different complications are most likely due to the stage of gestation at which amniocentesis is performed, the skill of the investigator, and the quality of the reporting. The findings of the two largest studies, one from the United States relating to 1040 case subjects and 992 controls and the other from Canada relating to 990 women, are similar. The Canadian data show 70 per cent of tests were successful at 16 weeks and the success rate increases with increasing gestation. Better results were obtained using a large needle (20 or 21 gauge) than a small needle (19 gauge) but multiple needle-insertions per amniocentesis were associated with more complications compared with one insertion only per test. The overall frequency of pregnancy complications was 17 per cent (211 complications and 1223 amniocenteses) but not all of these are attributable to the test procedure. Of those possibly causally related, bleeding or threatened abortion occurred in 24 cases (2 per cent), premature rupture of membranes and premature or false labour in 21 cases (1.7 per cent), and fluid leakage in six cases (0.5 per cent) giving a total complication rate from these causes of 4.2 per cent. The difference between this figure and 17 per cent is due to conditions such as toxaemia, oedema, hypertension, and urinary infection which are not specifically related to amniocentesis. The foetal loss rates in the United States study did not differ significantly in the subject group (3.5 per cent) compared to the controls

(3.2 per cent). However, Bennett (1978) has reported that foetal loss after second-trimester amniocentesis in women with raised maternal serum AFP levels may be of the order of 10 per cent, a high rate probably greater than the incidence of spontaneous abortion after this stage of gestation which may be about 4 per cent (Wald *et al.* 1977). Bennett's figure is not easy to interpret. If the true cause of foetal loss were a third factor such as concealed threatened abortion associated with both an elevated AFP level and the amniocentesis investigation, the foetal loss would appear to be related to this procedure when in fact the real association was with concealed threatened abortion. Scrimgeour (1976) estimates the chance of miscarriage being precipitated by the amniocentesis as about 1 in 200 and Philip and Bang (1978) attribute 0.3–0.7 per cent of all spontaneous abortions in a consecutive series of 1177 pregnant women examined by amniocentesis to this procedure. Trauma to the foetus may occur and there are reports of foetal loss with gangrene of an extremity secondary to amniocentesis (Lamb 1975), one case of ileocutaneous fistula (Rickwood 1977), and foetal skin lesions (Golbus, Conte, Schneider, and Epstein 1974). Karp and Hayden (1977) found four babies with puncture marks after 190 amniocenteses, a rate of 2 per cent, which is similar to the figure of 3 per cent in the paper by Golbus *et al.* (1974) on 100 amniocenteses. Another report describes destruction of an eye in a foetus following amniocentesis (Cross and Maumenee 1972) and there are reports of foetal cardiac taponade (Berner, Seisler, and Barlow 1972), laceration of the foetal spleen (Egley 1973), pneumothorax (Cook, Shott, and Andrews 1974), and arteriovenous fistula (Gottdiener, Ellison, and Lorenzo 1975). Careful localization of the placenta by ultrasound might reduce the incidence of blood-stained specimens of amniotic fluid by 90 per cent (*British Medical Journal* 1975). A working party of the Medical Research Council of the United Kingdom (1978) assessed the hazards of amniocentesis by comparing outcomes in 2428 women tested in the first 20 weeks of pregnancy with a control group of 2428 women who did not have amniocentesis, matched for age, parity, and obstetric history. This careful multicentre study estimated amniocentesis was associated with an increased foetal loss of about 1.0 to 1.5 per cent and certain types of infant morbidity including unexplained respiratory difficulties and congenital orthopaedic abnormalities such as talipes equino varus and congenital dislocation of the hip. They recommend the procedure should be conducted only in centres with ultrasonography available, that rhesus-D-negative women without antibodies should be given anti-D serum following amniocentesis and that the baby should be supervised for possible respiratory difficulties at delivery and examined shortly after birth for any congenital defects.

Cost effectiveness

If the evidence to date suggests maternal serum AFP screening for neural-tube defects might be worthwhile, would this programme be cost effective? Hagard, Carter, and Milne (1976) examined this question with reference to spina bifida in the Western Regional Hospital Board, Scotland, area in

1973. A benefit–cost index was derived based on several indices to take account of life expectancy and degree of handicap, hospital in-patient and out-patient care, physiotherapy, permanent care, education, and loss of maternal income. The economic benefit of preventing the birth of one liveborn spina bifida child was calculated using annual discount rates varying from 5 per cent to 15 per cent. Their analysis demonstrates the benefit–cost index is influenced mostly by the prevalence at birth of spina bifida in the population and by the sensitivity of the screening test (Fig. 29.3). Other items which significantly influence any provision are the costs of ultrasonography and reagents for AFP immunoassay. Breakdown of costings to screen 43 000 pregnancies (around 6 per cent of all births in the United Kingdom annually) indicated a capital outlay of around £68 000 over several years and recurrent annual sums of around £89 000 to the National Health Service and £24 000 to patients. Of the National Health Service costs, the largest two items as percentages of the total are publicity (£29 000) and expensive reagent and anti-serum (£44 000). Considering current economic inflation and the high costs involved in caring for spina bifida children (Lightowler

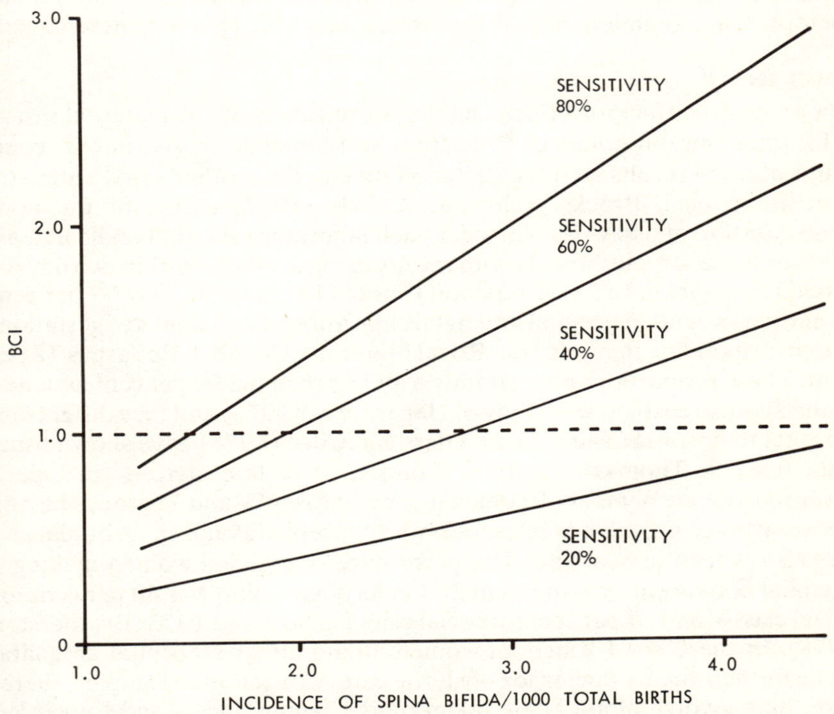

FIG. 29.3. Relationship between estimated benefit–cost index, sensitivity of maternal serum alpha-foetoprotein screening test, and the population prevalence rate at birth of spina bifida per 1000 total births. (After Hagard *et al.* 1976 and courtesy of the *British Journal of Preventive and Social Medicine*.)

1971), this screening programme is cost effective within the strict meaning and definitions of the study. An assessment by the Department of Health and Social Security of the cost-effectiveness of screening for neural-tube defects reached similar conclusions but again emphasized the economic element as only one of several aspects contributing towards any decision (Glass and Cove 1978). The Ontario study by Sheffield (1978) emphasizes the considerable costs of ultrasound scanning and cytogenetic examination of amniotic fluid in North America. If all amniotic fluid specimens irrespective of the presenting maternal conditions were to be cytogenetically screened the cost becomes virtually prohibitive. There is, however, considerable pressure in North America for such a comprehensive type of analysis of any specimens obtained because of the unclear legal position of the physician in this situation. Not to carry out all tests might be regarded as professional negligence. The British study by Hagard *et al.* (1976) estimated a cost per ultrasound examination of £3.3 but for Ontario the health insurance plan pays $43 (£21) for each test of which the professional component is $34 (Sheffield 1978). Henry, Peakman, and Robinson (1978), who work in Denver, Colorado, estimate the total cost of genetic counselling, ultrasound, amniocentesis, cell culture, chromosome analysis, and alpha-foetoprotein estimations is $350 (approximately £175) per patient screened.

Other factors

There are other factors influencing the organization of any maternal serum AFP screening programme. Collection and handling of specimens, communication of results, and the gestation time at the mother's first antenatal visit are critical. Brock, Wald, and Cuckle (1977) argue for the non-centralization of assays but consider each laboratory should handle at least 1000 or more samples weekly with results being available within two days of blood being taken. In Leicestershire, Clarke (1977) found only 55 per cent of mothers attended hospital antenatal clinics prior to 18 weeks of gestation; the corresponding figure for the Royal Maternity Hospital, Belfast, is 72 per cent. These proportions are certainly a lot less than the 90 per cent assumed in the Scottish cost–benefit study of Hagard *et al.* (1976) and they differ from hospital to hospital (Table 29.2). Glass and Cove (1978) have shown using data from St Thomas's Hospital, London, that 'late arrivers' include a disproportionate number of women in social classes IV and V, groups having above-average prevalence rates for both anencephalus and spina bifida, and this also is seen in Scotland. The percentage of married women making a prenatal booking after more than 20 weeks of gestation was 40 per cent for social class V and 27 per cent for social class I in Scotland 1973 (Brotherston 1978). In the United Kingdom women attend either a hospital antenatal clinic or their family doctor for obstetric care. Collection of samples, therefore, may involve blood being taken by the family doctor and forwarded together with a request card for AFP testing by post, special delivery, or other means to an assay laboratory; a parallel system based on hospital antenatal clinics would also be necessary. Office-based specialist or familydoctor prenatal care is the norm in North America, hence organization of AFP screening to cover much larger geographical areas and the numerous sources of medical care requires a different approach. The Oxford group currently notify and trace only patients who are found to have an abnormally elevated AFP level. These are then followed up by a paramedical member of the research group, via the doctor originating the test request or by a home visit with a view to arranging further blood tests, ultrasonography, and amniocentesis. Women having normal maternal serum AFP levels are not routinely informed of the result of the test although a procedure of giving the test results to all women screened is used in some other areas of the United Kingdom.

TABLE 29.2 *Cumulative distributions of antenatal clinic attendance rates from 16 to 20 weeks of gestation at three maternity hospitals in the United Kingdom*

Gestation (weeks)	St Thomas's (London) 1973 (per cent)	University College (London) 1975 (per cent)	Royal Maternity (Belfast) 1975 (per cent)
16 or less	60	72	67
17 or less	65	79	72
18 or less	69	85	77
19 or less	72	88	81
20 or less	75	90	85
Total number (all gestations)	2619	1000	1844

London data after Glass and Cove (1978).

Ultrasonography, as well as being an adjunct to AFP screening, may be used independently in the near future as an alternative method to AFP estimation in maternal serum or amniotic fluid for detecting anencephalus and spina bifida. Ultrasonic examination may become routine for all pregnancies for reasons other than the detection of foetal abnormality and this technique offers the only non-invasive method of visualizing the foetus *in utero*. X-rays and body scanners are unacceptable as they employ significant amounts of radiation. Campbell and colleagues (1972, 1975) have diagnosed cases of spina bifida prior to 20 weeks of gestation by ultrasound alone; in one case dizygotic twin foetuses discordant for spina bifida were correctly assessed at 17 weeks (Campbell, Grundy, and Singer 1976). Considering the mixture of technical and human errors likely with indirect diagnostic methods such as AFP and other laboratory indices, and the hazards of amniocentesis, further development of ultrasonography offers a possible alternative system. A survey is being conducted in South Wales to evaluate the relative merits of screening women prior to 20 weeks of gestation using maternal serum AFP measurements combined and not combined with ultrasonography. This is in addition to further studies by the United Kingdom Collaborative Study Group and other British teams. However the application of ultrasonography on a wide scale may be limited by the considerable degree of expertise needed by the physician performing the examination, and by the cost.

Views of society

Around 200 Members of Parliament from all parties signed a Commons motion in January 1978 urging immediate implementation of routine maternal serum AFP screening for all pregnant women. Hampson, the Member of Parliament behind this campaign, estimates the costs at one million pounds a year with an expected reduction in the prevalence rate at birth of spina bifida of 90 per cent if all cases detected were aborted (*Lancet* 1978). Both the Department of Health and the Royal College of Obstetricians and Gynaecologists are urging caution because of the hazards of amniocentesis and the extent of false positive results. The results of the prospective studies suggest that only 30 per cent rather than 90 per cent of cases of spina bifida would be diagnosed antenatally. Undoubtedly, the findings from work to date based on relatively small numbers and by groups working in centres of excellence are quite different and probably better than those that are likely to be obtained by screening all 700 000 births in the United Kingdom per year using all available family doctor and obstetric hospital services. The public and the politicians seem not to appreciate that maternal serum AFP measurement is only one step in the screening process and that ultrasonography and amniocentesis are procedures needing much skill and experience for their accurate conduct and interpretation. These attributes have been acquired by only a small minority of medical practitioners at the present time. Furthermore, the whole operation must be telescoped into a time period of two or three weeks if abortion is to be induced prior to 20 weeks of gestation. All these steps carry risks of harming the foetus either directly or indirectly due to false positive findings. Who will carry legal responsibility for all these various cases of misadventure? Furthermore, as Edwards (1978) has pointed out, spina bifida infants do not fit into neat distinct groups but may have small harmless lumps or irreversible incapacity of both brain and spinal cord. In the United States, with 3.1 million births annually, Pergament (1977) estimates if the 98th centile of the maternal serum AFP distribution were chosen as the upper limit of normal, a screening programme would lead to an additional 62 000 amniocenteses per year and might detect 1200 spina bifida foetuses. Without screening , approximately 50 per cent of these would die at or around the time of birth and perhaps 25 per cent would be ambulatory or free from severe handicap while the other 25 per cent would have varying degrees of major mental and physical deficit.

Screening for other foetal conditions

Before looking at legal and ethical problems, the question of prenatal screening for other congenital abnormalities should be mentioned. This applies virtually exclusively at present to amniotic fluid samples and not to maternal blood. If by means of a maternal serum AFP screening programme many amniotic fluid samples are obtained, a number of which are 'unnecessary' from the standpoint of diagnosing anencephalus and spina bifida, then examination for Down's syndrome, other chromosomal disorders, and inborn errors of metabolism should be considered. The service in the West of Scotland provided by Ferguson-Smith and colleagues (1976) tests all amniotic fluid samples irrespective of the initial indications for AFP levels and cells are cultured for foetal chromosome analysis. Over the period 1969–75 some 676 cases were studied, 41 cases of foetal abnormality detected and 36 of these were terminated. No false negatives and one false positive result with regard to amniotic fluid AFP estimations occurred. In relation to 589 chromosomal diagnoses there were no false positive results but three false negative results occurred associated with two male infants and one female infant, each having Down's syndrome. Indications for amniocentesis included a high maternal serum AFP level, a prior occurrence of Down's syndrome or other chromosomal abnormalities, and a pregnancy at maternal age exceeding 40 years or sometimes 38 years. The risk of chromosomal abnormality in the offspring of mothers aged 40 years or over is around 5.7 per cent. Ferguson-Smith (*British Medical Journal* 1977; *Scotsman* 1977) is reported as stating that the number of babies born with spina bifida in the Glasgow area, a community having an above average prevalence rate, has been reduced by two-thirds by prenatal screening tests combined with selective abortion. However, in the Edinburgh study (Brock *et al*. 1978), two women having pregnancies with spina bifida and whose serum AFP levels were abnormally elevated refused abortion and as we noted, one unaffected infant was mistakenly aborted.

Proposals for screening using cultures of foetal cells from amniotic fluids obtained by amniocentesis, to be followed if positive by pregnancy termination, were put forward by Stein, Susser, and Guterman (1973) to reduce the prevalence of Down's syndrome in New York City. These were heavily criticized (Edwards 1973; Steele 1973; Grunberg 1973) on the grounds of the medical risks involved by using amniocentesis as a screening test together with the associated legal and ethical problems. Apart from malformations associated with raised AFP levels and Down's syndrome, other chromosome abnormalities such as Klinefelter's syndrome and Turner's syndrome in which the chromosome complements most commonly are 47 XXY and 45 X respectively may be diagnosed prenatally. Whereas these are recognized clinical entities, certain chromosome complements do not present any clear-cut syndrome and are only apparent as a result of chromosome-screening surveys. Much debate has surrounded males with 47 XYY chromosomes since some evidence suggests a twentyfold greater prevalence rate of XYY individuals in mental–penal settings and a fourfold greater rate in exclusively penal settings than in the general community (Hook 1973, 1975). This apparent association between chromosomal constitution and criminality may be spurious and requires further elucidation

(Beckwith and King 1974; Beckwith 1975). X-linked disorders in which a specific diagnosis is not possible but where determination of the foetal sex is important, and several inborn errors of metabolism depending on assay of a specific enzyme or other biochemical marker, may also be detected by analysing amniotic fluid samples. Milunsky (1973) surveyed by postal questionnaire 41 centres in North America undertaking amniocentesis for prenatal diagnosis. Of 1663 pregnancies studied, 1368 (82 per cent) were examined because of a suspected chromosomal abnormality, 115 (7 per cent) because of a family history of an X-linked disorder, and 180 (11 per cent) because of a suspected metabolic disorder. Out of this total of 1663 pregnancies, tests were abnormal in 127 (7.6 per cent) and 102 foetuses were aborted. Absence of any AFP determinations is due to the early date of this survey in relation to the progress of this work in the United States and Canada as compared with the United Kingdom and Europe. At another level, national legislation in the United States was enacted in 1972 for post-natal genetic screening of sickle cell anaemia (Reilly 1975). Several states including Kansas, New Mexico, Ohio, and North Carolina have passed genetic-screening laws and automated screening systems are being developed assisted by Federal funds. Some 40 states have laws requiring newborns to be tested for phenylketonuria following the initial work in Massachusetts, and these methods have been extended to include other disorders such as galactosaemia, histidinaemia, homocystinuria, maple syrup urine disease, and tyrosinuria (Reilly 1975*a*, 1977). A National Amniocentesis Registry has been set up in the United States (Lowe 1978) which collects information similar to the central data bank in Kingston, Ontario, co-ordinating the amniocentesis results from 13 collaborating centres in Canada (Medical Research Council of Canada 1977).

Conclusion

An answer to the question as to whether screening for neural-tube defects by measuring serum AFP levels on all pregnant women in the community should be introduced is most difficult as it depends not only on the interpretation of the available medical evidence but also on wider legal and ethical issues (Section 30). Some discussion about the scientific observations *per se* is pertinent.

No screening programme has ever been introduced which did not have a number of both false positive and false negative results. False positives occur when unaffected foetuses are associated with abnormally elevated AFP levels in maternal serum and in amniotic fluid; the foetus may be completely normal or may have a disease or condition known not to produce high AFP concentrations. Termination of these pregnancies and of normal foetuses is an extremely serious matter. In Massachusetts three apparently normal foetuses were aborted because of elevated fluid AFP concentrations, according to Milunsky (1977), a false positive rate of 0.1 per cent. We noted the Swedish prospective survey (Kjessler *et al*. 1977) observed one pregnancy with a normal foetus where repeated AFP measurements in both maternal serum and amniotic fluid were abnormally high. Abortion was not recommended as an amniogram was normal. The special problem of a multiple pregnancy in which one foetus is affected and the other or others healthy presents a particular dilemma. Aberg, Mitelman, Cantz, and Gehler (1978) reported the selective birth of the unaffected twin in a 26-year-old woman. The co-twin was diagnosed as having Hurler's syndrome and her only other living child, a boy aged five years, also had this disease. The affected twin in the current pregnancy was aborted by cardiac puncture carried out under ultrasound examination; after two attempts the heart stopped. The dead foetus remained *in utero* from the time when the abortion was carried out at the 24th week of gestation until delivery at 33 weeks of gestation. The living foetus was born by caesarean section and the remnants of the dead foetus were delivered vaginally.

False negatives are also serious. These occur when the screening programme fails to detect a foetus with a neural-tube defect which is then apparent only after the infant is born. If we consider acceptability depends critically on the sensitivity and specificity of AFP testing as observed in clinical practice, cut-off points demarcating normal from abnormal maternal serum AFP levels would have to be clearly laid down. Current evidence indicates methods, such as serial rather than single serum AFP measurements with or without ultrasonography and amniocentesis, by which the proportions of false positives and false negatives may be minimized. However, we would point out that observations so far are biased because they relate to samples of women who are not representative of all expectant mothers in the population. The Swedish study is the nearest to a community survey but the British work serves only as an approximate guide to what would happen if AFP testing were performed as comprehensively as for example, prenatal haemoglobin measurements.

The reports from Edinburgh and Glasgow include cases of anencephalus in their calculations of detection rates. We seriously doubt whether this is acceptable. As we mention several times, anencephalus is a uniformly fatal condition and is not a burden on society as is spina bifida. If the costs of detection by AFP screening and selective termination were compared with the costs of allowing a mother with an anencephalic pregnancy to continue and have a spontaneous or induced delivery we would expect that the former would exceed the latter. As Davidson and Sheffield (1978) state, 'we run the risk of providing couples with answers for which they had no question'. Prenatal diagnosis of anencephalus, therefore, only replaces an affected stillbirth or perinatal death with an induced abortion. Furthermore, induced abortion and amniocentesis are associated with certain risks both to the mother and the foetus. It is clear that any population screening programme must be justifiable on the basis of its impact on spina bifida. We note the detection rates given in the studies considered are higher for anencephalus than for spina bifida. From the British prospective studies they appear to be between 30 per cent and 50 per cent for spina bifida of all types, being higher for open spina bifida cases and lower for closed spina bifida cases, on the present evidence. Even so, about 20 per cent (215 out of 945, Table 7.1) of all spina bifida infants are stillborn and for the purpose of evaluating screening are in the same category as anencephalus. A further smaller proportion of perhaps 5 per cent of spina bifida infants will not be seriously handicapped (Table 7.2).

The voluntary nature of each stage of the screening process needs to be emphasized as mentioned by the Bishop of Durham (Dunelm 1978) and others (Gould 1978; Haddow 1978). Even if written consent is obtained as is suggested for the California programme (Crandall, Lebherz, and Freihube 1978) this may not be legally valid. Also, Harris (1978) has stated with reference to the United Kingdom that some facilities may be inadequate for proper investigation of pregnancies where foetal abnormality is suspected. If any service such as maternal serum AFP screening is to be provided only the highest clinical and laboratory standards are acceptable.

30

Law and ethics

DESPITE biological observations of two critical times at the beginning of life, the time of conception and the time of birth, science alone cannot give a wholly satisfactory reply to the question, when does life begin? The embryonic human heart first beats 22 days after conception (Table 2.1). Foetal viability, however, traditionally has been medically defined with respect to the gestational age or sometimes the birth weight at which the foetus is likely to have an independent existence *ex utero*. Thus the international World Health Organization definition states that:

> perinatal deaths include foetuses born without signs of life at or after 28 weeks from the recorded date of the mother's last menstrual period and also infants born alive irrespective of gestational age who die within one week.

The International Conference on the Ninth Revision of the International Classification of diseases met in Geneva during September 1975 and recommended a new definition of perinatal mortality to include only those babies born weighing 1000 g or more at birth (Goldstein and Butler 1977). Present definitions of foetal viability of 28 weeks of gestation in the United Kingdom, 20 weeks in Canada and the United States, 35 cm physical length in Sweden, and 30 cm in Switzerland as discriminating between a stillbirth (synonymous with a late foetal death) and a livebirth are confusing (Lewis and Williams 1977). Under common law, three reference points, conception, quickening, and livebirth, have been applied to define foetal viability, but all are open to different interpretations. Out of 42 279 single (live and still) births born to women resident in Belfast 1962–6, some 1428 died during the perinatal period. Of the latter 226 (16 per cent) were at less than 28 weeks of gestation and 8 deaths occurred in singleton livebirths estimated to have been at less than 20 weeks of gestation at the time of birth (Elwood, J. H. and Thompson 1975). Usher (1977) reported the smallest survivor out of 272 445 livebirths in the Province of Quebec in 1970–2 was at 24 weeks of gestation and weighed 623 g at delivery; an infant weighing 450 g at delivery at 27 weeks of gestation (Lelek, Limanowski, and Hager-Malecka 1973) was alive and well when examined at three months of age (Avery 1975).

If any programme of maternal serum AFP screening is to reduce the prevalence at birth of anencephalus and spina bifida, then selective abortion would need to be accepted by the majority of women with these affected pregnancies. This policy, however, raises wider issues including the question of terminating pregnancies for other reasons and ethical considerations.

It would be a mistake to assume therapeutic abortion is less hazardous than normal delivery. The risk of maternal mortality was around 110 per 100 000 abortion operations (Hungerford 1971) compared with an overall maternal mortality rate of about 25 per 100 000 livebirths in England and Wales in 1969 even though the former rate may decline, as in Hungary, a few years after abortion is legalized (Henzl 1971; Czeizel and Bognar 1971). Furthermore, a high incidence of post-abortion complications has been reported by Hungerford (1971) and others (*Lancet* 1971); these include trauma, haemorrhage, post-operative sepsis, and possibly sterility.

Interpretation of the law is greatly influenced by court decisions dealing with specific cases and we will mention certain relevant experiences in the United Kingdom and North America which are based on the Anglo-American common-law tradition.

The law

Medical research into prenatal diagnosis of anencephalus and spina bifida in the United Kingdom at the moment is further advanced than in other countries. However legal aspects have been more critically examined in the United States and the reasons for the different scientific approaches to the same problem are bound up with differences in legislation. The Canadian situation is more akin to the United Kingdom but this may change owing to influences from the United States.

United Kingdom and Ireland

The main relevant legislation in the United Kingdom at present is the Abortion Act (1967) and the Congenital Disabilities (Civil Liability) Act (1976). Previously, relevant statutes were the Offences Against the Persons Act (1861) stating 'an attempt to procure an abortion is a felony punishable by imprisonment for life', and the Infant Life (Preservation) Act (1929) under which abortion induced for the sole purpose of preserving maternal life was not a criminal offence (Binney 1968). Precedents were set by judgment in individual cases, that concerning Rex v. Bourne (1938) being particularly influential in England. Bourne, a London obstetrician, performed an abortion on a 14-year-old girl raped by soldiers in the Guards barracks. They were arrested for assault and Bourne invited the police to charge him with the crime of procuring an abortion. Bourne was prosecuted under Section 58 of the Offences Against the Persons Act (1861). This Act made it an offence to perform an abortion 'unlawfully' while the Infant Life (Preservation) Act (1929) made the killing of unborn children an offence except if this was carried out in good faith for the purpose of preserving the life of the mother. Justice McNaghten's ruling in the Bourne case essentially depended on his interpretation of the word 'unlawful'. He implied that not all abortions were prohibited and by legislative analogy between child destruction and induced abortion considered the saving clause in the 1929 Act implied a similar content in the 1861 Act. He went on to propose a test of 'lawfulness' and held the onus was on the Crown to establish that the act of performing an abortion was not lawful. McNaghten's ruling reads:

> . . . if the doctor is of the opinion, on reasonable grounds and with adequate knowledge, that the probable consequence of the continuance (of the pregnancy) will be to make the woman a physical or mental wreck . . .

then the jury may take the view that the doctor is operating for the purpose of preserving the life of the woman. The Bourne decision was radical and unprecedented but was the foundation on which induced abortion was performed in England and Wales for the next 30 years. It was especially criticized for not distinguishing clearly enough between a danger to the life and a danger to the health of the mother. McNaghten's ruling probably could not have occurred in Scotland owing to differences in legislation (MacGillivray and Horobin 1973).

An Abortion Act (1967) came into effect in England and Wales in April 1968. Termination of pregnancy is permitted subject to three conditions namely that, the abortion must be performed by a registered medical practitioner, in a National Health Service hospital or place approved for the purpose by the Act, and the abortion must be certified by two registered medical practitioners as necessary on one or other of various grounds including that there is a substantial risk that the infant if born would suffer serious handicapping abnormalities. However, during the past ten years the Abortion Act has been challenged several times by Private Members' Bills presented at Westminster. Gryll's Bill (1974), aimed at stopping such abuses as touting, was not passed owing to Parliament being dissolved in February of that year. White's (1975) Bill, aimed at severely restricting the number of abortions induced was accepted in principle by the government as were the recommendations of the Select Committee on the Abortion (Amendment) Bill (1975), but they had not been fully debated by the end of the 1974–5 Parliamentary session. The Benyon Bill, similar to that of White, received a second reading in February 1977 and the Braine Abortion (Amendment) Bill also has been introduced (*Lancet* 1978*b*). The main purposes of the latter are to set an upper limit of 20 weeks of gestation for abortion, to have all pregnancy advisory bureaux charging fees licensed by the Secretary of State, and to ensure they have no financial connection with abortion clinics.

Around 35 000 abortions were induced in England and Wales in 1968; the number reached a maximum of 167 000 in 1973 and by 1976 was 128 000 giving a resident abortion rate of 17.3 per 100 livebirths. One in six viable foetuses are now being aborted. The proportion of abortions carried out under the National Health Service has declined from 65 per cent in 1968 to 49 per cent in 1976. Around 21 per cent of induced abortions carried out in Great Britain today are for women resident outside the United Kingdom, mainly from the predominantly Roman Catholic countries of France, Italy, Spain, and the Republic of Ireland. Despite these statistics, the induced abortion rate in Britain is low compared to the rates in other countries with more permissive legislation. The abortion rate per 100 livebirths in England

and Wales in 1973 was 16.8, but the figures for Sweden, New York City, and Hungary were 23.7 , 80.8, and 102.3 respectively. Within the United Kingdom the Abortion Act has not been applied uniformly throughout the country. For example, Aberdeen has had a very liberal policy even before 1968 (Thompson 1977) and some 98 per cent of induced abortions in Scotland were performed by the National Health Service in 1974; yet only 10 per cent of Birmingham residents having an abortion in 1975 did so under the National Health Service in their own Health Region. Prior to 1972 Northern Ireland had its own elected parliament which passed its own laws, admittedly often very similar to those enacted by Westminster. The Abortion Act (1967) was never passed by the Northern Ireland parliament hence substantial numbers of women obtain abortions in Great Britain. The number rose from 36 in 1968 to around 1000 in 1973 (Compton, Goldstrom, and Goldstrom 1974). Some selective abortions of foetuses having neural-tube defects and induced abortions for other reasons are carried out in Northern Ireland but these procedures are not on the scale practised in Great Britain. The Congenital Disabilities (Civil Liability) Act (1976) applies to England and Wales and Northern Ireland, but not to Scotland. This includes provision for a child born disabled as a result of antenatal injury to claim damages from those persons whose negligence caused the injury. An important point is that it applies only to liveborn children and does not confer any right in law on the foetus. It also replaces any existing common-law liability. In the Republic of Ireland, also a high prevalence area for anencephalus and spina bifida, abortion is illegal. Until recently, even the use of contraceptives was banned under the Criminal Law Amendment Act (1935) which translated the doctrine of the Roman Catholic Church into law prohibiting the sale, importation, and advertising of unnatural methods of contraception. A ruling by the Supreme Court in Dublin in 1973 in the McGee case considered the ban on importation unconstitutional and a violation of human rights, so today around 20 000 women in the Irish Republic are estimated to use the contraceptive pill (Wilson-Davis 1974, 1975).

Clive (1978) has discussed the position and differences between the present English and Scottish laws with reference to antenatal screening causing injury to the mother, death or non-fatal injury to the foetus, and failure to diagnose an affected foetus. He concludes the first raises no special legal problems but there are real legal risks associated with causing the death of a normal foetus and of non-fatal injury while the legal consequences of negligently failing to diagnose an affected foetus are difficult to assess. Clive also comments on the Kilbrandon Committee Report (1969) on the Marriage Law of Scotland which considered but did not recommend the introduction of compulsory pre-marital medical examinations. There is, however, compulsory screening for syphilis by appropriate blood tests of all persons prior to marriage in most states in the United States, and all newborn infants are legally required to have ophthalmic silver nitrate drops administered shortly after birth to prevent gonorrheal eye infections in some provinces of Canada (British Columbia Health Act 1971).

Canada

Prior to 1969, the Criminal Code of Canada (1953) included equivalent provisions to the two British Acts of 1861 and 1929. However the word 'unlawfully' which as interpreted by Justice McNaghten decided the verdict of the Bourne case, is not included in the relevant section dealing with abortion. Some Canadian lawyers argue that the Bourne decisions might be inapplicable even though most doctors seem to have assumed abortions which met the test in the Bourne case were permissible in Canada. Section 251 of the Criminal Code was amended in 1969 in order to make therapeutic abortion legal under four conditions: the abortion must be performed in good faith by a registered medical practitioner in an accredited or approved hospital, with the prior written consent of that hospital's therapeutic abortion committee, who certify that continuance of the pregnancy would or would be likely to endanger the mother's life or health. There is no specific Abortion Act in Canada and the present legislation is not very satisfactory. Decisions by abortion committees have varied considerably (Harris and Tupper 1977) and the Badgley Committee (1977) prepared a special report on the operation of the law. They found a situation rather similar to that in the United Kingdom. There is an average delay of eight weeks between the initial consultation by the woman with her physician and the performance of the abortion; for every five women obtaining an abortion within Canada, one travelled to the United States for this purpose (Thomas 1977). Around 30 000 legal abortions were performed during 1971 in Canada. The dissatisfaction was evidenced in the trial of Dr Morgentaler who was arrested in August 1973 at his Montreal clinic together with eleven patients, three nurses, and one receptionist; three vacuum suction apparatuses were removed from the premises (Maksymiuk 1974–5, Dickens 1976). Morgentaler had campaigned for years for reform of the abortion law. He operated a clinic and performed abortions which had not had prior approval by hospital therapeutic abortion committees. He was prosecuted for aborting a woman who had been unable to obtain a termination at those Montreal hospitals which carried out such procedures. Morgentaler's defence on the grounds of the 'necessity' of the abortion, an argument similar to that accepted in the Bourne case in England, was rejected and he was sentenced to 18 months' imprisonment in July 1974. The Supreme Court of Canada dismissed his subsequent appeal. Morgentaler served ten months of his sentence in various jails and his case is not yet closed (Dickens 1976).

United States

A number of specific disease-related bills have been put forward in the United States Congress in recent years and a bill, concerning all forms of genetic disease, the National Genetic Diseases Act, was examined by Congress in 1975. Because of the problems about foetal and human rights, the United States Congress imposed a moratorium on foetal research in 1974 and a commission was set up to study and report on these issues. They later recommended such research could resume only under strict review procedures. Important case precedents in the United States include the fiasco of the Edelin trial (Nathanson 1974) and the case of Roe v. Wade, together with a companion case, Doe v. Bolton.

Edelin, a chief resident obstetrician at Boston City Hospital, was found guilty of manslaughter after the death of a foetus during a legal abortion of a second trimester pregnancy. The original verdict carried a maximum sentence of 20 years in jail and it was only with considerable public support that his appeal was upheld. The prosecution in this trial alleged that Edelin was responsible for the death of a 'baby boy' who was viable and 'born alive'. As explained by Glantz (1975) great emphasis was placed on the gestational age of the foetus and every attempt was made to demonstrate that the foetus was 'killed' between the 24th and 28th weeks of pregnancy. In the Roe v. Wade case, the issue was whether a State has the constitutional power to interfere with the decision of a woman, in consultation with her physician, to have an abortion performed. The Supreme Court held that this decision was encompassed within the previously recognized fundamental right of privacy which could be infringed only if the State demonstrated a compelling State interest. Green (1975) raises several unresolved questions about this decision which dealt only with the right of the State to prohibit abortion; for example if this is so, does the foetus itself have a legal right not to be the victim of abortion? While this judgment held that a foetus prior to viability is not a person within the meaning of the law as presently interpreted, what happens if the foetus is on the borderline of viability? This American court, however, established a zone of privacy around the pregnant mother and her physician. The decision to abort during the first trimester lay within this zone and could not be disturbed by the State. But concerning the period after the first trimester, the Court proceedings read

> the state . . . may, if it chooses, regulate and even prescribe abortion . . . for the preservation of life or health of the mother.

Non-treatment of newborns

Logically, the same arguments used to permit deliberate elimination of malformed foetuses identified by prenatal diagnosis also apply to the deliberate elimination of infants having the same abnormality but who for various reasons are identified at or after the time of birth. Selective abortion, infanticide, homicide, and even voluntary euthanasia are a spectrum representing the consensus view of society rather than distinct independent entities. The view that the first is acceptable whilst the others are deeply abhorrent is illogical, although widely held by members of the medical profession and the general public (Motulsky 1974). These stark choices, however, are not usually those presented. The position is rather that of legally authorizing death of abnormal newborns, non-treatment of particular subgroups, or various forms of active euthanasia (Burt 1975, Robertson 1975, 1975*a*). Two studies serve to highlight this current dilemma.

Duff and Campbell (1973) describe the care of 229 infants who died in the special-care nursery of the Yale–New Haven Hospital during the period from January 1970 to June 1975. They suffered from a variety of conditions including respiratory distress, extreme prematurity, and congenital anomalies including spina bifida. Some 43 (19 per cent) of these deaths were due to 'discontinuance or withdrawal of treatment' over the study period. Although this policy was decided after careful consideration between parents and physicians and is viewed by Duff and Campbell as a 'group decision', Robertson (1975) is of the opinion that both parents and physicians are violating a number of criminal laws in virtually every US state. He states:

present criminal sanctions should be enforced more fully or legislation permitting non-treatment should be enacted.

In England, Zachary (1977) has documented a similar, but perhaps more subtle medical regime specifically relating to spina bifida infants. So-called 'no treatment' methods include administering large doses of hypnotics such as chloral hydrate at eight times the recommended dose and giving morphine without the parents' knowledge. Withholding of food also is mentioned. This active euthanasia would appear to go far beyond Lorber's (1971, 1972) original policy of conservative and non-surgical management and undoubtedly brings death more quickly to certain infants. Lorber (1974*a*), describing the aims of selective non-treatment as the early painless death of the infant, emphasizes that nothing must be done to prolong life. He writes

This means no antibiotic therapy for infections, no 'intensive care', no oxygen or tube feeding and infants should be fed on demand, no more. . . . If they [spina bifida infants] do survive for about six months and appear likely to survive indefinitely, such infants must be taken back into the 'fold' and all their problems treated as if they had been treated from birth.

Attempts to draw up criteria authorizing the withholding of treatment are fraught with problems. Despite this, evaluation of a legal policy and identification of a non-treatment group of spina bifida infants is required. Lorber and others in the United Kingdom and Duff and Campbell in the United States presumably wish parents and physicians to have the final discretion to decide whether a severely handicapped infant with spina bifida should be treated or not treated. Reasons for this view vary. Non-treatment is put forward as being in the best interests of the child owing to a painful future life of physical and mental handicap. The child or newborn infant is totally helpless and cannot express any personal view in this situation, an important distinction when compared with voluntary euthanasia in adults. A fate which may seem worse than death to an individual who has experienced normal health, for example sudden blindness or sudden deafness, may be quite tolerable to another who has known no other existence due to congenital blindness or deafness. Other reasons for identifying a group of spina bifida infants not to be treated include the burden which their survival imposes on the immediate family and on society. The argument that the only feasible solution is non-treatment is incorrect because better public and other support for these families could relieve part of the burden. Finite limitations to the financial resources of state health and social services are another reason advanced in support. Despite justifications for these interpretations of non-treatment many members of society are in strong disagreement and even the medical profession itself is unsure of the accuracy of selected clinical signs and symptoms as predictors of the future quality of life of spina bifida infants. A sample of such infants, who according to the criteria of Lorber (1971) would have been selected for non-treatment, were found to fare quite well when treated by Ames and Schut (1972) in the United States.

Are there then, processes other than this informal physician–parents group-decision method for selecting spina bifida infants for non-treatment or conservative management? Robertson (1975) addressing the problem of anomalous newborns irrespective of aetiology, has well summarized the situation by stating

> Despite the substantial costs flowing from identification of a class of infants who are selected for non-treatment, many persons might still reasonably conclude that the costs of treating all defective newborns are not worth the benefits of treatment and therefore should not be required. While they will differ as to which situations justify non-treatment, and perhaps limit the practice to a few extreme cases, they accept in principle a policy of selection for non-treatment. The important question then for society and legal policy is the circumstances and process by which non-treatment decisions are to be made . . . Otherwise we risk creating a non-treatment policy, the total costs of which are greater than those of treatment when the original justification for non-treatment was that it was the less costly method of resolving a tragic dilemma.

Robertson goes on to identify three types of costs dependent on this acceptance of a non-treatment group and puts forward suggestions for improving the present legal position. Infants from whom treatment cannot be reasonably withheld but who fall into the non-treatment subgroup will occur because all spina bifida infants do not comprise clearly distinct treatment and non-treatment groups. Furthermore, this policy may change attitudes towards and lessen respect for handicapped persons resulting, over a period of time, in society regarding spina bifida individuals as using an unduly large amount of limited health resources. Thirdly, the mechanism involved in making these non-treatment decisions may be a bureaucratic nightmare. Nonetheless, if a less open selection procedure rather than a formal decision process is favoured, major problems arise due to the arbitrariness and furtive nature with which such a policy may be implemented and this system may be open to abuse.

Of Robertson's suggested alternative policies, the first would alter the law to relieve parents and physicians of the possible risk of criminal prosecution for non-treatment as for example in cases where the views of Lorber, Duff and Campbell, and others are followed. Their decisions then would become independent of the law but as a safeguard the physician could seek legal authority if his judgement and that of the parents differed with respect to whether their particular offspring should or should not be treated. This approach places great responsibility on the physician and parents and leads to a policy of active euthanasia. In the United Kingdom it is possible to contract out of liability for negligence and Clive (1978) considers that a doctor could get the parents to absolve him from all liability for injury however caused. This aspect of the law may be changed if the Avoidance of Liability (England and Wales) Bill (1976), which also will extend to Scotland, is passed because this prohibits contracting out of liability for death or personal injury resulting from negligence. The Society for the Protection of the Unborn Child in the United Kingdom reported to a Chief Constable the deaths of three newborn infants with neural-tube defects in a Nottingham hospital as possible instances of unlawful killing (*Lancet* 1978). A report of the Department of Health prepared by a standing medical advisory committee on guidance about the care of children born with these defects has been available since 1973 and an ethical working party (*Lancet* 1975*a*) also has published its views. Physicians however, already appear to be taking to themselves too much responsibility in the decisions to be made under these conditions. Secondly, non-treatment could be limited to certain classes of malformed infants identified by clinical signs and symptoms closely associated with an unacceptable biosocial prognosis. This would greatly reduce the element of arbitrariness and subjective bias but in the process would seriously diminish the respect for life generally recognized by all civilized communities. An Orwellian scenario might not be too distant. Robertson's third decision-making model envisages an impartial body such as a court of review committee taking over the non-treatment decision. The latter could only take place if the views of this committee, parents, and physicians were in agreement. The accompanying bureaucracy might make any such system unworkable in practice and would be extremely costly. The fourth alternative

> is the present system of formal illegality, and through prosecutional decisions not to prosecute, informal delegation to parents and physicians of discretion to make these decisions.

As with the first alternative, bias and subjectivity mainly on the part of the physician might occur leading to unnecessary deaths. By comparison with the first alternative, this risk should be less because physicians might be more cautious in agreeing with a parental choice of non-treatment due to the knowledge that they may be prosecuted. Robertson concludes that the choice among these four alternatives

> will depend on whether society finds the danger of the unstructured discretion of parents and physicians to be greater than the dangers of direct governmental involvement in the taking of life to benefit others.

Ethics

These observations on selective abortion, infanticide, treatment or non-treatment of spina bifida infants, together with a brief examination of some legal aspects have so far not questioned the bases for these actions which stem from ethical, moral, and religious beliefs. These, however, have changed throughout history. Some groups such as the Roman Catholic Church take an absolutist position that abortion is morally indefensible under any circumstances. Thus the introduction of maternal serum AFP screening and a selective abortion programme at present is impossible in the Republic of Ireland despite the high prevalence of anencephalus and spina bifida in that country. Lejeune (1970) also considers abortion unacceptable for biological and not strictly religious reasons. Much of what we have discussed from the legal point of view could very well be argued on moral and ethical grounds. Weighing the rights of the foetus against the rights of society requires great judgement and yet society desires to minimize the amount of ill health in the community. Whether the influence of medicine on demography has been beneficial or a mixed blessing is open to debate (Illich 1975).

Taking of life by capital punishment for the general good of the community is now deemed unacceptable in most Western democratic countries mainly on moral and ethical grounds. In this debate much emphasis is placed on the likelihood of condemning an innocent man to death even though the victim's life has been forfeited. Thus, what is the motive for deliberately eliminating a malformed foetus, especially if there is a risk of unintentionally terminating the life of a normal foetus *in utero*?

In many ways all these observations converge in the concept of eugenics, an applied science which seeks to maintain or improve the genetic potentialities of the human species. Although Galton first used the term eugenics, Darwin pesented an interpretation several years earlier in *The descent of man and selection in relation to sex* published in 1871. He wrote:

> With savages, the weak in body or mind are soon eliminated; and those that survive commonly exhibit a vigorous state of health. We civilized men, on the other hand, do our utmost to check the process of elimination; we build asylums for the imbecile, the maimed, and the sick; we institute poor-laws; and our medical men exert their utmost skill to save the life of everyone to the last moment. There is reason to believe that vaccination has preserved thousands, who from a weak constitution would formerly have succumbed to smallpox. Thus the weak members of civilized society propagate their kind. No one who has attended to the breeding of domestic animals will doubt that this must be highly injurious to the race of man. It is surprising how soon want of care, or care wrongly directed leads to the degeneration of a domesticated race; but excepting in the case of man himself, hardly anyone is so ignorant as to allow his worst animals to breed . . .
>
> We must therefore bear the undoubtedly bad effects of the weak surviving and propagating their kind; but there appears to be at least one check in steady action, namely, that the weaker and inferior members of society do not marry so freely as the sound; and this check might be indefinitely increased by the weak in body or mind refraining from marriage, though this is more to be hoped for than expected.

Effects on the prevalence of genetic disease in man of intrauterine diagnosis and selective abortion have been explored by Fraser (1972, 1972*a*, 1973), Harris (1974), and others. Certain mathematical models may be of value for examining effects with respect to traits governed by Mendelian inheritance. Motulsky, Fraser, and Felsenstein (1971) estimate a policy of selective abortion of subsequent pregnancies following the birth of an affected infant having an autosomal recessive disease would reduce the number of subsequent cases by a minimum of 12.5 per cent and a maximum of 34 per cent. In relation to X-linked recessive conditions, selective abortion would be much less successful because a large proportion, as high as 50 per cent in some instances, of these diseases are due to new mutations. The application of genetics to man has made very little impact on the frequencies of any allelic or chromosomal variants according to Edwards (1974) and to use this argument to justify termination of pregnancies with neural-tube defects is invalid. The common complex birth defects such as spina bifida would have small reductions in proportion to the low recurrence risks in sibs. As anencephalus and spina bifida do not segregate along Mendelian lines, the effects of any long-term change in the population distribution of possible genetic factors that may play a part in determining the occurrence of these defects are totally unknown.

We are, therefore, in practice dealing with short-term effects and particularly the number of liveborn infants with spina bifida allowed to remain alive relative to the finite resources of society and the attitudes of parents and physicians. The object of diagnosis in medicine has been to treat the patient more effectively, and where this is impossible to reduce the patient's suffering. However, the aim of a maternal serum AFP screening programme is exactly the opposite because if a diagnosis is made that the foetus is abnormal the treatment is to do away with the patient by terminating the pregnancy.

Once the absolutist position is rejected the situation becomes a confused collection of value judgments. We have pointed out that normal foetuses have already been aborted on the erroneous assumption that they had neural-tube defects and selective treatment of affected newborns also raises problems when spina bifida infants originally categorized in a non-treatment group do not die but continue to cling to life. What is to be done in the situation when one member of a multiple pregnancy is diagnosed as having a neural-tube defect and the other foetuses are apparently normal? Just because medical research discovers that a certain procedure is possible is no reason to accept that such a policy should be implemented (*British Medical Journal* 1973). Regarding birth defects, even compulsory sterilization after the birth of an affected child would reduce prevalence rates at birth by trivial amounts (Edwards 1969*a*) although widespread use of abortion would alter malformation prevalence rates at birth within a short time. It is clear, therefore, that acceptance of any secondary preventive measures with respect to anencephalus and spina bifida depends not only on evaluating the medical evidence but also on legal and ethical considerations which in most societies will be the determining factors.

XIII

Aetiology and prevention

31

Aetiology, primary prevention, and directions for further research

IN summarizing our current understanding of the aetiology of anencephalus and spina bifida, we must present more questions than answers. We cannot yet identify the causative agent or the mechanism of production of these defects, or even present a tenable unifying hypothesis. We can only recapitulate some of the major features which characterize these defects, and suggest certain further lines of inquiry.

Are anencephalus and spina bifida likely to have the same cause? Most of the evidence is consistent with a common aetiology. The embryology of the two conditions is similar and around 10 to 30 per cent of cases of anencephalus have associated spina bifida lesions. Teratological experiments demonstrate that in general the same agents may produce either defect and it seems possible that the time of application is the critical factor, a slightly later exposure resulting in spina bifida rather than anencephalus. The strongest human evidence for a common aetiology is the linked genetic pattern with the sibling risks of either defect being comparable in affected families. The main epidemiological features are common to the two conditions. Prevalence rates at birth are similar at least in Caucasian populations as are the major long-term secular trends and the associations with social class, ethnic origin, maternal age, and parity. Nevertheless, further assessment demonstrates certain dissimilarities between the two conditions. In human family pedigrees, although the risk to siblings of either defect is much greater than the risk in the general population, siblings show a weak tendency to preferentially exhibit the same defect as the propositus. In the British Isles, seasonal trends for each defect show excesses of affected births in winter but the peak date of conception for spina bifida is some two months later than that for anencephalus. Secular trends in the prevalence of the two defects are not identical, especially with regard to short-term increases over one or two years; for example, there were short-term increases in Canada in the prevalence of anencephalus in the early 1950s and in spina bifida in the 1960s neither trend being seen with respect to the other defect at the same time. Two differences in their epidemiology are very striking. Firstly, the sex distribution is different, with about 30 per cent of anencephalics being male, compared to a male proportion of spina bifida of 40 per cent. Secondly, oriental populations have prevalence rates of anencephalus similar to those of Caucasian populations living in the western areas of North America, Australia, and other regions where the rate is around 1 per 1000 births, whereas spina bifida prevalence rates in oriental populations are around 0.2

per 1000 births. This is much lower than the spina bifida rates in any Caucasian communities and points to some essential difference in aetiology. Whether this means that the two defects result from different aetiological factors, which happen to be somewhat similar in their occurrence, whether they have the same primary aetiological mechanism which is modified by other agents including genetic factors related to race and to the sex of the affected foetus, or whether the two defects have a common set of aetiological factors, plus subsidiary sets of factors which are specific to one defect, remains to be resolved. At the moment, it seems reasonable to extrapolate the more extensive data available on anencephalus in human populations to supplement the much more restricted information relating directly to spina bifida.

The relative importance of genetic and environmental factors is a major question. The most striking features of neural-tube defects in human populations are the large differences in prevalence rates between populations of similar genetic and racial stock and the large variations in prevalence rates over relatively short periods of time. Associations with social class and with maternal reproductive history complement these major features in demonstrating that the predominant aetiological component most probably is a set of environmental factors which shows variation by time, place, and person. The siblings of affected cases have high risks but no Mendelian inheritance pattern is seen. The observation of familial aggregation alone provides little support for a genetic mechanism as this is also to be expected in any environmentally determined congenital disease. Some years ago, it was suggested that environmental factors might totally account for the defects without any genetic contribution (Yen and MacMahon 1968). Since then the higher concordance rate in monozygotic than in dizygotic twin pairs has become apparent and this provides the strongest evidence for a genetic component. The multifactorial model involving environmental agents interacting with a polygenic predisposition, as suggested by Fraser (1959), and Carter (1970), thus seems the most reasonable model despite its unattractiveness due to the lack of parsimony and the resultant inability to indicate a discrete testable hypothesis. The current world data suggest a concordance rate of around 3 per cent for dizygotic twin pairs and as high as 11 per cent for monozygotic twin pairs. These rates are compatible with a multifactorial model as are other features such as the higher recurrence risk after two affected siblings and the variation in the sibling risk with the prevalence rate in the population. The data do not fit all the theoretical requirements of such a model as there is no higher sibling risk after a male propositus and sibling risks for anencephalic and for spina bifida propositi are similar. A separate feature suggesting a genetic aetiology is the stability of prevalence rates in certain ethnic groups, notably blacks and Jews, who have low rates even when they reside in areas where Caucasians have high rates. The difference between Caucasian and oriental populations with regard to the relative frequencies of anencephalus and of spina bifida noted above also may be explicable in terms of a genetic influence.

The most practical application of knowledge of the occurrence patterns of neural-tube defects is the use of recurrence risks reported by various studies in counselling situations. We would emphasize, however, that these recurrence risks are empiric estimates and are not related to any specific aetiological model. Two recent North American family studies are of great interest as they demonstrate in areas with a low population prevalence that the recurrence risks are closer to 2 per cent than the frequently used figure of 5 per cent which is based on British studies and on one earlier North American study from the relatively high prevalence area of New England. This estimate of a 2 per cent recurrence risk probably applies to most Caucasian populations having prevalence rates at birth of anencephalus and spina bifida combined of 2 per 1000 births or less, which include the white populations of the western area of North America, Australia, and South Africa. Neither the 5 per cent nor the 2 per cent figures may be applicable to non-Caucasians such as blacks, Jews, or orientals. Moreover, the recurrence rate in high prevalence areas such as Ireland may well be greater than 5 per cent.

While the multifactorial model is acceptable as an explanation of causation, it is evident that the main factors determining prevalence originate in the environment. Caucasian populations show a prevalence rate of anencephalus and spina bifida combined of over 8 per 1000 births in Ireland, but rates as low as 1.5 per 1000 births are seen in other areas including British Columbia, where three-quarters of the population are of British stock. In areas with rates higher than about 1.5 , including the whole of the British Isles, it is likely that environmental factors are contributing to the excess and even in British Columbia they probably have a major influence. The potential then exists that these factors can be identified and modified. There are a large number of hypotheses relating to various environmental factors, all of which are supported by some of the data but none fully explain the epidemiological features observed. Several of these hypotheses require further studies.

We suspect a dietary mechanism may play a major role. The social-class association, long-term secular trends, seasonal variation, and some of the geographical variation may be explicable on a dietary basis. It seems evident from the very few and rather poorly designed studies conducted so far that mothers of infants with these defects have an unbalanced diet with a probable excess of carbohydrate and low-quality foodstuffs. One of the more viable specific hypotheses is that of folic acid deficiency although certain epidemiological features of neural-tube defects clearly are not explained by this mechanism. The potato-blight hypothesis suffered from premature promulgation with insufficient evidence but in fact was a reasonable and testable hypothesis consistent with at least some of the major features of neural-tube defects in human populations, notably the high rate in Ireland. We would point out that a positive association between the prevalence rates of anencephalus and spina bifida and the production and consumption of potatoes in different areas is present, albeit with many inconsistencies, even though there is no association in time between the occurrence of neural-tube defects and potato-blight outbreaks. The high-potato diet therefore may be a clue to a more specific dietary component. Our current studies in Canada suggest water hardness is unlikely to play a direct causal role although it is possible that hard and soft water supplies may be an indicator of an important difference with regard to other aspects of diet.

The possible relationship of these defects to infectious organisms is worthy of attention. The rapidity with which prevalence rates change over time, the seasonal variation, the social class, and the geographic associations may be explicable by an infectious aetiology. The available evidence in humans is sufficient to exclude rubella, toxoplasmosis, and cytomegaloviruses as likely causative agents and although the evidence on influenza is predominantly negative, it must still be regarded as unproven. In animals central nervous system malformations are seen in sheep after infection with blue-tongue virus, and Parvo, H–1 and RV viruses can produce such defects in small laboratory mammals (Sever, J. L. 1975). The effects of less common viral infections in humans, and the possibility of a latent virus infection require further study. Two types of investigation would be particularly useful. In areas in which screening programmes are operative it would be valuable to obtain serum samples and conduct multiple viral antibody tests when maternal blood is taken for estimation of serum alpha-foetoprotein concentrations. Initially, sera from mothers suspected of carrying an infant with a neural-tube defect could be compared with sera from comparison mothers, and sequential determinations could be performed when a specific infectious agent was suspected. Secondly, material from spontaneous abortuses or from induced abortions as well as from stillborn and liveborn affected infants, could be examined in detail for the presence of viruses in the tissues and the placentae.

Suggestions that a dietary or infectious aetiology may involve exposure not during the affected pregnancy, but a late effect of either nutritional deprivation of the mother during early childhood or infection of the mother during that time or at puberty, deserve serious consideration. These hypotheses are very difficult to test but it is intriguing that at least some epidemiological evidence is in their favour. The hypotheses put forward by Janerich (1974) which postulate differences in gonadotrophin levels between mothers of infants with anencephalus and spina bifida and mothers of normal infants, and which possibly involve ovarian damage during childhood by infectious or other agents, could be tested by hormonal studies during and after affected pregnancies. A primary hormonal mechanism reflecting pathological processes starting well before the first pregnancy could have its major impact on the first pregnancy and perhaps a somewhat lesser impact on subsequent pregnancies providing an explanation for the maximum rate of these defects being observed in first births. This primiparity effect is difficult to explain on the basis of most other hypotheses.

More complex hypotheses involving tissue interactions between foetuses in a twin pregnancy or between the affected pregnancy and cellular remnants of an earlier pregnancy also are intriguing and can explain some of the epidemiological features of anencephalus and spina bifida. The complex genetic models suggested by Knox (1970, 1974) are particularly interesting as they provide an explanation for the female predominance of these defects. This is one of the important epidemiological observations which is ignored by several other aetiological hypotheses. The postulate that a spina bifida lesion may represent the site of an absorbed second twin can be tested by detailed anatomical, histological and chromosomal examination of affected infants. Hypotheses relating to reactions between a conception and cellular rest material from an earlier pregnancy or spontaneous abortion have been supported by one small follow-up study of women who have had a spontaneous abortion, but require evaluation by further studies and laboratory investigations. The major counter evidence to such hypotheses is the increased risk of these defects in first births which appears to be a strong association in Canada and in several other communities. In Canada we have noted several epidemiological features of anencephalus and spina bifida are different in first births than in other births and this raises the question of whether the aetiology of the defects may differ in these two situations. This possibility should be further examined both by comparing the epidemiological features of neural-tube defects occurring in first and subsequent pregnancies in other communities, and by comparing the anatomical characteristics of such affected infants related to birth rank. If two distinct aetiological mechanisms are operating, one might expect to see some differences in the distribution of subtypes of these defects defined by anatomical structure and by the frequencies of other defects accompanying the major malformation.

The extent to which the prevalence at birth of anencephalus and spina bifida is influenced by differential early foetal loss rates is not at all clear. It is intriguing that the early foetal loss rate of affected infants appears to be higher in Japan than in the United Kingdom in contrast to the prevalence rate at birth which is lower in Japan. Mothers in geographical areas of South Wales which show high neural-tube defect prevalence rates at birth have lower rates of early foetal loss in other pregnancies than do mothers in areas of South Wales with lower neural-tube defects prevalence rates at birth. The available information on spontaneous abortions with neural-tube defects shows these cases have an approximately equal sex distribution unlike those surviving beyond 28 weeks of gestation. Although differences in early foetal loss rates may influence prevalence rates at birth, the observations made so far do not permit a general statement as to which characteristics of the prevalence rates at birth reflect different early foetal loss rates and which reflect different rates of true incidence.

We have considerable information about the occurrence of anencephalus and of spina bifida and yet little is definitely known concerning aetiology. Why does this situation exist? Does this demonstrate that the methods of studying aetiology, and particularly the epidemiological method, are of little value? We believe that the lack of strong aetiological hypotheses in part reflects the limitations of the scientific methodologies used but to a much greater degree illustrates that they have been inadequately applied. Despite the fairly large number of epidemiological studies surveyed in this book, few are as rigorous in terms of design, scope and analysis as the epidemiological studies which have demonstrated specific aetiological mechanisms in other conditions such as chronic lung disease, heart disease, and cancer. It is only fair to point out, however, that funding for investigations of these major non-communicable diseases of adult life has been many times greater than for research relating to birth defects, and of the funding allocated to the latter, most is devoted to laboratory work rather than to studies of the affected infants and their families. There are particular difficulties in studying the aetiology of congenital abnormalities in human populations. The greatest is the impossibility of directly measuring incidence rates. We are attempting to examine features of a disease process which cannot be observed directly but is seen after the seven-month time interval between the probable initiation of the defect and the time of observation. Thus outlines are blurred and features which if observed directly when the malformation occurred might be recognizable but instead remain a mystery. In such circumstances an animal model is valuable. However, evidence from teratological experiments is difficult to interpret because of species differences and also because many experiments are designed without relevance to the human situation and little attempt is made to employ agents and dosages similar to those to which populations are exposed.

If we judge the epidemiological studies of neural-tube defects completed to date by the standards now accepted for studies of major adult chronic diseases, we must conclude that few studies are of the quality necessary to elucidate a complex problem. The great majority of the epidemiological studies we have reviewed are of the descriptive type where the investigator is limited to examining associations of the prevalence rate of these defects with factors such as social class, area of residence, time, maternal age, and parity. These factors cannot provide a direct biological explanation for the occurrence of the malformations but are merely indicators of exposure to the underlying process responsible for causation. Obviously, future investigations must go beyond these simple indices if they are to identify direct aetiological mechanisms. Few of the studies we have reviewed adopted a particularly good interview format. Most have used very simple interviews or else relied on routine medical records or on vital statistical information. The most useful study which could be mounted at present is a case–control design in which a detailed history, preferably conducted at home and carried out by a trained interviewer, would assess not only events during pregnancy but events earlier in life and gain detailed information about dietary patterns, occupational histories, exposures to drugs, infections, and chemicals, and data on other diseases existing in the family. The interview data could be complemented by haematological, chemical, and immunological tests and perhaps by studies of mutagens in foetal and maternal fluids and tissues. The major difficulty with a retrospective approach is again the seven months or so minimum waiting period between the time when data are collected and the probable time of exposure to the aetiological agent. This could be reduced greatly if the study were linked to an alpha-foetoprotein screening programme when mothers with affected pregnancies are ascertained at around 16 to 20 weeks of gestation.

Despite the attractiveness of a cohort design in which detailed information on current exposure can be gained early in pregnancy and in which laboratory investigations for nutritional deficiencies or exposure to infections can be made, such a study probably would not be very useful in the case of neural-tube defects. Despite being the most common fatal congenital anomaly, neural-tube defects are still relatively rare outcomes of pregnancy and therefore cohort studies need to be extremely large if adequate numbers of affected pregnancies are to be included. Obviously, a prospective design in which several pregnancy outcomes are assessed and several aetiological factors investigated is more attractive and feasible. In the past, experience with such surveys in the United Kingdom, Canada, and the United States has not been very encouraging in terms of gaining information on specific birth defects although valuable information relating to issues such as prematurity has been produced. In these large, expensive multicentre studies there have been considerable difficulties in ensuring a high and consistent standard of data recording, and data editing and analysis has been quite slow. The particular value of a prospective design in the future is that all pregnancy outcomes, including therapeutic and spontaneous abortions, should be ascertained in the population under investigation and where possible detailed anatomical examination of abortuses should be made together with necropsy examination of stillbirths and perinatal deaths. A large epidemiological project of this nature would be time consuming, expensive, and may not command sufficient priority at present.

More attention should be given to ensuring that birth-defect registries and routine vital statistics are put to greater use. Vital statistical systems and congenital malformation registries are expensive to maintain and yet their return to date in terms of furthering understanding of the causes of disease has been fairly small. One reason for this is that although much attention and financial support is given to the setting up and operation of the registry, often very little attention is given to ensuring that the data are adequately evaluated and analysed and that persons with good training in epidemiology and genetics and with a capacity for original work are supported by the registry and encouraged to use the data to the full. All too often registries become bureaucratic organizations content to produce routine reports only. The same applies to most systems of vital statistics. These were originally set up as practical public health measures to warn the community of impending epidemics and to demonstrate inequalities in terms of mortality and morbidity. The production and reporting of vital statistics in the nineteenth century was not a sterile administrative exercise, but a powerful tool which led to many social and medical reforms. Not only the reports of such leading figures as Edwin Chadwick and William Farr, but even routine vital statistical reports produced by Registrars General or by Medical Officers of Health are often documents of considerable interest; they rarely present statistics alone but often include commentaries calling for specific direction of medical and social resources. In comparison, vital statistical reports from Britain, Canada, and the United States at the present time often are devoid of any interpretation or reference to the implications they hold for the health of the community. This may be largely due to the demise of the medical statistician as someone employed both to supervise the collection of such statistics and to interpret them. Vital statistics are a powerful tool for studying the aetiology not only of neural-tube defects but of most serious diseases in our society and should return to being flexible and dynamic modes of investigation rather than unchangeable administrative procedures.

Our ability to detect a specific aetiological mechanism of a human disease is greatest under two circumstances: where a large proportion of the disease entity is caused by a certain exposure, and where a specific exposure produces the disease in a relatively high proportion of those individuals exposed. An example of the first is phocomelia produced by thalidomide, and of the second is asbestos leading to lung cancer and mesothelioma. The efficiency of the epidemiological method is greater if the aetiological factor is an event not frequently experienced by a large proportion of the population. It follows that if the total incidence of disease is not produced by one characteristic factor but comprises the end results of several aetiological agents it will be difficult to detect such mechanisms. This may well be one reason for the failure of studies to delineate a single aetiological mechanism for anencephalus and spina bifida. It seems likely that not one but several aetiological factors are involved. It may even be that these defects result from a necessary combination of a finite number of factors, each of which in itself may be neither an unusual exposure nor a pathogenic agent. Thus it may be that only a mother with a certain genetic background, who is exposed simultaneously to a relatively common chemical or infectious agent and a diet deficient in some essential constituent, produces an infant with a neural-tube defect. Obviously such mechanisms are much more difficult to elucidate than the simple direct action of one powerful teratogen. A similar argument applies if what is now regarded as one homogeneous entity, anencephalus and spina bifida, is in fact a mixture of a number of different disease entities, each with its own aetiological mechanism. If this were so the epidemiological features of each specific condition, which might be quite clear and consistent individually, become blurred when combined into one group. In view of these points it is disappointing that very few adequate series of affected infants are available in which detailed anatomical and histological examination of each infant has been made. The small number of detailed anatomical observations are equally disappointing in that little or no attention is given to comparing anatomical features in a total series of infants representing all affected births in one community and time period. It would be valuable in future studies to distinguish defects which may be part of a specific syndrome, to study the frequency of occurrence of other defects in association with the primary anomaly and to classify cases on anatomical grounds using systems such as that suggested by Nishimura and Okamoto (1976).

Further research

As mentioned, we consider the most useful further investigation of the aetiology of anencephalus and spina bifida would be a well-designed case–control study. Further family surveys in different geographical areas would be valuable as the number completed so far is small and more are required to evaluate different genetic models and to provide empiric risk estimates for local populations. A family study in Ireland would be particularly useful to see if the recurrence risk is higher than elsewhere. Certain laboratory investigations which could be made using relatively small numbers of subjects might be valuable. These include viral antibody tests, a search for infectious agents in spontaneous abortuses, comparison of blood groups and tissue between mothers of affected infants and mothers of normal infants and between mothers and their affected infants, and studies of disease history prior to the affected pregnancy searching particularly for chronic diseases of an infectious or autoimmune origin. As with most other diseases, investigations of certain population groups who demonstrate characteristic features could provide very useful information. These include women who experienced adverse conditions *in utero* or during early childhood, or who had a severe illness around the time of puberty. Such groups might be defined as particular cohorts of migrants or persons who have lived through major social upheaval or war conditions. Certain ethnic or religious groups with uncommon dietary customs, religious practices, or patterns of contraceptive use and sexual behaviour are worthy of study. Communities having a large proportion of very high parity mothers, or pregnancies at early maternal ages as occur in South America, Africa, and Asia may provide valuable contrasts with industrial Western societies. Women who are members of groups whose use of medical and other drugs can be adequately ascertained, for example, subscribers to prepaid group insurance plans in North America or possibly women in employment groups such as the Armed Forces, may be worthy of study to further evaluate risks associated with drug use during pregnancy. Further studies of women exposed to anaesthetic agents and to occupational chemical exposures are indicated.

Additional work could be conducted using vital statistics or existing birth-defect registries, especially if there are opportunities for record linkage. These include surveys of the prevalence at birth of anencephalus in areas of the world for which such information is unknown; an estimate of this frequency can be obtained from mortality data and even mortality rates from spina bifida are of some value. Associations of these defects with the occupations of either parent have not been sufficiently studied; congenital defect registries which do not collect such data should consider including information on parental occupation. Vital statistical systems, especially if mortality data are linked to other information, may clarify how risks are modified by ethnic origin and migration. Unfortunately some very good opportunities for this type of study are lost by administrative decisions. For example, the Canadian birth certificates include information on both ethnic origin and birthplace and if both these items were available they would allow a distinction to be made between recent migrants and first generation migrants which would be very valuable. However, in the 1950s the information on place of birth of the parent, while recorded, was not coded and entered into the computerized record and in recent years vital-statistic authorities have not collected information on ethnic origin. Record linkage systems, as in British Columbia, have great potential because important and accurate studies may be conducted at minimum expense once the system is set up. For example, how do malformation rates attributed to other defects in siblings, parents, and children of propositi affected with anencephalus and spina bifida compare with rates in relatives of propositi with other conditions? What are the causes of death of parents of the infants with anencephalus and spina bifida, and do these give any clue to an association with any chronic diseases? Are the siblings of propositi with anencephalus and spina bifida atypical in terms of birth weight, gestation time, sex distribution, or the frequency of multiple births?

We have outlined hypotheses which suggest an increased rate of multiple births in sibships including infants with anencephalus and spina bifida and hypotheses related to a general inadequate diet, smoking and maternal nutritional deprivation early in life might be expected to be shown by differences in the birth-weight distribution of other members of neural-tube defect sibships. Linked registry data also would allow a study of the survival patterns of infants with spina bifida, as no good data are available which include all cases of spina bifida occurring in a defined population. Registries which include spontaneous or induced abortuses are particularly valuable, although there are many difficulties in assuring adequate and representative sampling of abortuses in a defined maternal population and in making detailed anatomical and chromosomal examination of each specimen. Abortus registry data from areas with contrasting prevalence rates at birth would be particularly valuable in elucidating the natural history of neural tube defects, and abortus monitoring systems may be particularly useful in identifying new embryotoxic exposures in the population (Oakley 1975).

In keeping with the title of this work, we have discussed mainly epidemiological approaches to the aetiology of neural-tube defects. In fact, the majority of important aetiological relationships are first suggested by alert clinicians and the epidemiological role is to test and confirm or refute these suggestions. Experimental work with animals has so far produced few findings relevant to the aetiology of the condition in humans, but is particularly valuable in screening drugs and chemicals for toxic effects. Much progress may result from further exploration of the cellular mechanism which produces these defects; for example, Luduenna and Wessells (1973) have proposed that neurulation is due to cell contraction controlled by a microfilamentous system containing actin, which may be blocked by chemicals which bind to actin such as cytochalasin; Linville and Shepard (1972) demonstrated that cytochalasin B could produce neural-tube defects in the chick embryo, which was of particular interest at that time as similar compounds are present in blighted potatoes. The causative model may also involve a necessary role for chance; thus if, as is likely, more than one event must occur at a cellular level to produce a neural-tube defect, the effect of multiple factors will depend on whether they affect the same cells and on their precise timing. Therefore even if we could measure the polygenic predisposition of the individual and quantitate the environmental factors we would still be unable to predict precisely the outcome of each pregnancy.

The high-risk mother

We can summarize some of our work in a brief sketch of the mother who is at a higher risk than her contemporaries of bearing a child affected with anencephalus and spina bifida. The most important factor is a prior history of a stillbirth or liveborn child affected with anencephalus or spina bifida, or the occurrence of spina bifida in the mother herself or in the father; any one of these attributes confers a risk of approximately 5 per cent in British populations and approximately 2 per cent in North American populations and in other low prevalence areas. Detailed figures for more complex family histories are given by Bonatti-Pellié and Smith (1974). We can delineate other factors which are associated with the occurrence of anencephalus and spina bifida but we emphasize that all these, while of interest from the aetiological point of view, are of little help in predicting the outcome of pregnancy for an individual woman. Women with a prior history of a spontaneous abortion, a stillbirth or a child death from causes other than neural-tube defects appear to be at higher risk. If any of these events has occurred more than once, the risk is higher again. Births to mothers who have not previously borne a normal liveborn child have higher rates of these defects and the rate decreases with the number of previous livebirths born to that particular mother. It follows that women with a history of a number of sponanteous abortions and no liveborn children are at particularly high risk. We have discussed the associations with area of residence and ethnic origin. Within North America and the British Isles, women whose ethnic origin is Celtic (Irish, Scottish, Welsh) have higher risks than those who come from England. Furthermore, English mothers have higher risks than mothers from most other European countries and Jews, blacks and orientals have low rates of these defects. Mothers of Sikh origin and possibly those from the Arab countries of the Middle East may have relatively high risks. In general it appears that these ethnic associations pertain to women born in their country of origin, and to their daughters born in the migrant's new area of residence; the ethnic factor has then very little influence in further generations. We have no information yet on whether migration from a high- to a low-risk country or vice versa in infancy or at puberty has different consequences compared with migration shortly before the affected pregnancy. The defects are more common in births to mothers in poor economic circumstances, and possibly independently of this factor, to mothers of short stature. It is possible that the social-class gradient may reflect not so much current social class as social class during childhood. Women with a history of dizygotic twinning, or who have had closely spaced pregnancies, may be at increased risk compared to the general population. In the British Isles and Canada, births conceived in the spring have a slightly higher prevalence rate than those conceived at other times of the year. Women who have a generally poor diet with the possibility of nutritional deficiences or excesses, those exposed to certain drugs including anaesthetic agents and those who smoke may be at increased risk, although all these associations have yet to be confirmed. We emphasize, however, that the main value of these associations is in elucidating aetiology rather than for medical counselling. With the exception of the prior occurrence of an affected infant, correlations with these factors are not high enough to give a useful predictive value when applied to individuals. In the Canadian 14-city study the multivariate model incorporating eleven predictive factors, while demonstrating several associations which may be aetiologically important, had a low discriminatory power in separating affected and unaffected infants.

32

Antenatal diagnosis and induced abortion

THE demonstration that measurement of the concentration of alpha-foetoprotein (AFP) in amniotic fluid or in maternal serum may indicate the presence of a foetus with a neural-tube defect has for the first time, along with two other recent developments, provided society with an opportunity of lowering the prevalence at birth of anencephalus and spina bifida thereby reducing the number of children handicapped by spina bifida and their substantial needs in terms of special care and education. The two other developments, without which AFP test would be merely an intriguing procedure, are a change of view in most Western democracies concerning the ethics of induced abortion and the resultant changes in legislation. Antenatal diagnosis and selective abortion must therefore be discussed with the realization that technical, ethical, and legal considerations are unavoidably interrelated. At the present time no authority, and certainly not the present authors, may claim to possess the judgement of Solomon required to pronounce on this issue. We are fully aware of our limitations and will not attempt to present any overall conclusion but simply highlight what appear to be the more important considerations concerning this subject.

Measurement of AFP concentration in amniotic fluid samples is a diagnostic rather than a screening test. Since first described by Brock and Sutcliffe (1972) it has been shown to be a very accurate test for anencephalus and open spina bifida. Most cases of anencephalus have AFP concentrations which are well outside the normal range; a small proportion of open spina bifida lesions may have concentrations which are low enough to give difficulty in diagnosis and closed lesions will tend to have normal concentrations. Amniocentesis should be preceded by ultrasonography and possible contamination by maternal urine or by foetal blood must be excluded. As well as AFP determination, the diagnosis of neural-tube defects may be assisted by studies of the total and proportional macrophage counts, the proportion of viable cells which rapidly adhere to glass or plastic surfaces, and studies of the morphology of adherent cells. Amniotic fluid AFP determination cannot be regarded as a screening test, except where the anmiocentesis has been performed for another indication such as advanced maternal age. It is most used of course in women with a history of a prior affected child. The proportion of positive results expected in this situation is quite small, being around 5 per cent in Great Britain, but lower in North America; Milunsky (1978) had a positive result in 1.6 per cent of a large series of amniotic fluid assays done because of a previous child being affected; this accords with the low recurrence rate reported by recent North American family studies. The probability of a positive result from an amniocentesis performed because of a previous affected birth is in fact considerably lower than that of an amniocentesis performed on the basis of an elevated serum AFP level. Thus in women with a previously affected child, the value of serum AFP determinations and ultrasound examinations conducted in order to avoid unnecessary amniocenteses requires further assessment.

Even if all women who had had a previously affected child received an amniocentesis, and if this were totally successful at identifying affected infants, the reduction in the prevalence at birth of neural-tube defects in the general population would only be some 5 per cent in Great Britain and even less in North America. Thus it is the use of AFP estimation on maternal serum samples which is the major issue at present. Potential benefits in terms of a reduction in the prevalence at birth of neural-tube defects are quite high. Correspondingly, the legal and ethical problems together with the technical aspects involved in total population screening are considerably more complex than those involved in offering a diagnostic test to women who already have an affected child. We must not only consider the performance of the test as such, but also the efficiency of the entire screening programme.

The best information currently available on maternal serum AFP screening comes from the retrospective multicentre British study (United Kingdom Collaborative Study Group 1977) and the prospective studies performed in Scotland. The retrospective study included a very large number of pregnancies and provides information on the accuracy of the test. It showed that the percentage of defects correctly diagnosed (the sensitivity of the test) for anencephalus increased sharply up to 15 to 16 weeks of gestation and thereafter increased much more slowly up to 21 weeks, while the sensitivity for open spina bifida was maximal at 17 to 18 weeks (Brock 1978*a*). At 16 to 18 weeks of gestation, which gave the optimum sensitivity consistent with an early enough diagnosis to give time for an induced abortion before 20 weeks of gestation, the sensitivity was 88 per cent for anencephalus and 79 per cent for open spina bifida, using a cut-off point of 2.5 times the median AFP level in unaffected pregnancies. Most cases of anencephalus have markedly elevated serum AFP levels which produce few difficulties of interpretation. In this study, 76 per cent of the cases of spina bifida were classified as having open lesions. The detection rate for the remainder was around 38 per cent and within this group there were probably some entirely closed lesions which are not accompanied by any appreciable elevation of AFP, and certain other lesions which are associated with some elevation in the AFP level. This distinction between open and closed spina bifida lesions is of great importance and a source of considerable difficulty. Although the distinction has been made critical by the screening procedures, we have little information about the relative frequencies of open and closed lesions in different populations. The specificity of the screening test, that is the proportion of true negative pregnancies which are correctly classified, depends directly on the cut-off point selected. A higher cut-off point will give greater specificity as fewer unaffected pregnancies will have AFP levels above the cut-off point, but correspondingly more affected pregnancies will have levels below the limit used and so the sensitivity of the test will fall. Most cases of anencephalus have such high levels of AFP that raising the cut-off point from, for example, the 95th to the 99th percentile of normal, produces little change in the sensitivity but for open spina bifida an appreciable decrease will occur. The Collaborative Study Group advised the use of a cut-off point of 2.5 times the median level for the laboratory concerned and estimated that at a prevalence rate at birth of 4 per 1000 births for anencephalus and spina bifida combined (a figure typical of much of the United Kingdom), about 10 per cent of pregnancies with an elevated serum AFP level would have a neural-tube defect.

These test sensitivities give the upper limit of the detection rate of a screening programme. To avoid performing amniocentesis on the large number of unaffected pregnancies with elevated serum AFP levels, a repeat serum sample and ultrasound examination should be performed. Some affected pregnancies which show an initial elevated serum AFP level may be misdiagnosed as normal after the additional tests, thus reducing the detection rate. Failure to interpret correctly the AFP results, for example by errors in estimating gestation time, communication failures, laboratory errors, and failure of the patient to attend for further tests will also reduce the effectiveness of the programme. Thus in the large prospective study from Glasgow (Ferguson-Smith *et al*. 1978) 48 per cent of the cases of spina bifida screened had an initially raised serum AFP level but only 29 per cent were finally diagnosed as affected. On the credit side, the great majority of unaffected pregnancies which had an initially raised serum AFP level were correctly diagnosed by further AFP estimation and by ultrasound so that amniocentesis was performed on only 20 per cent of the pregnancies with a false positive initial serum AFP level and no unaffected infants were aborted in error. In the Edinburgh prospective study (Brock *et al*. 1978), a lower initial cut-off point and perhaps somewhat less rigorous follow-up was used, and all of the 50 per cent of cases of spina bifida which showed an initially high serum AFP level were correctly diagnosed; however 35 per cent of pregnancies with false positive serum AFP levels were submitted to amniocentesis and one unaffected infant was aborted. The most encouraging aspect of these prospective studies is the demonstration that the risk of mistakenly aborting an unaffected foetus is very small if the programme includes repetition of the serum AFP estimation after an initial high level together with carefully performed ultrasound examinations. The risk of deliberately aborting an unaffected child is probably less than the risk of accidentally inducing a spontaneous abortion after amniocentesis, which appears to be around 1 to 2 per cent (Medical Research Council of the United Kingdom Working Party on Amniocentesis 1978). However, the price of this careful follow-up of initially positive AFP levels is to make a final false negative diagnosis on a number of affected pregnancies whose initial serum AFP level was high.

Let us now consider the question of the advisability of instituting routine maternal serum AFP screening for all expectant mothers in a community and the associated ethical and legal issues. If the deliberate termination of an affected pregnancy is regarded as beneficial by society and the accidental termination of an unaffected pregnancy is viewed as an error of moderate consequence, then acceptance of population AFP screening depends on the balance between benefits and costs. These may be expressed in financial terms or alternatively in terms of the numbers of births affected. Using the latter index we can estimate the number of normal infants aborted as the major deficit and a further deficit is the number of normal women who are exposed unnecessarily to the screening test, ultrasonography, amniocentesis, and other investigations. What to count as a benefit is more difficult. If we include every neural-tube defect diagnosed antenatally and aborted as a benefit, the results appear favourable largely due to the very high detection rate for anencephalus. We would argue, however, that this is illogical. The great majority of anencephalic infants are stillborn and the rest die within hours of birth at a median time of around 36 weeks of gestation. Antenatal diagnosis merely replaces a stillbirth or neonatal death with a late induced abortion, reducing the average duration of pregnancy by some 16 weeks. We could argue that this is a substantial benefit to the mother, but we could also argue that the benefits are as yet undocumented, at most very minor and that there may be some negative effects even in these women. Similarly, a high proportion (some 15 to 30 per cent) of cases of spina bifida are stillborn. A much smaller percentage (5 per cent to 10 per cent) of infants with spina bifida have no, or a very minimal, handicap and the deliberate abortion of this latter group is really little different from the accidental abortion of an unaffected child. Thus if a risk benefit argument is to be used, we would argue strongly that the benefit side of the equation must be based on that proportion of spina bifida births which would survive but be moderately or severely handicapped. If we use the detection rates shown by the Scottish prospective studies, we would therefore expect only a 30 to 50 per cent reduction in the prevalence at birth of spina bifida. The minimally handicapped cases of spina bifida will be those with closed lesions which have the lowest detection rate, whereas the effect of the higher detection rate for large open spina bifida lesions is diminished as a high proportion of these infants would be stillborn anyway. These detection rates apply to that subgroup of the total population of pregnant mothers who have an initial serum AFP estimation performed at the appropriate gestation time. A further major limitation of population screening is that a fairly high proportion of women do not present early enough for this to be carried out; this proportion is around 15 to 30 per cent in most centres and is highest in the lowest socio-economic groups who have the greatest risk of an affected pregnancy. It is evident from the prospective studies that failure to diagnose an affected infant is as often due to administrative difficulties as to technological failure. There are difficulties in communication of test results to the physician, in ensuring that women return for subsequent examinations, and in correctly interpreting serum AFP levels in terms of gestation time. These difficulties cannot be ignored. In fact it is most likely that errors will be minimal in the prospective studies already carried out which are relatively small and have been performed by highly motivated research orientated groups based on a small number of teaching hospitals. A national programme in the United Kingdom most likely would run into more administrative difficulties in proportion to the large number of laboratories and hospitals involved. The difficulties are likely to be even greater in a less centralized medical-care system as in the United States or Canada. It is more difficult in such societies to ensure a constant standard of care and adherence to prescribed guidelines, and particularly in the United States it may be impossible to restrict AFP determinations to a small number of laboratories. For similar reasons, the excellent results of the Scottish prospective studies in terms of correctly diagnosing unaffected pregnancies without resort to amniocentesis would probably not be replicated by a routine programme. The low complication rates of amniocentesis when conducted in specialized centres may well be unobtainable if a large screening programme is instituted which results in greatly increased demands on facilities and staff. The final factor which will limit the effectiveness of any screening programme is the size of the group of mothers who will not accept abortion, and this must be taken into account.

It is important that predictions of the effects of a national or regional screening programme for neural-tube defects should be based on the most valid available data, and not give an over-optimistic forecast as has been presented by several investigators. North American statements have at times directly applied the results of the British experience to their situations; this is invalid. The proportion of mothers with elevated serum AFP levels who have infants with neural-tube defects is approximately proportional to the prevalence rate in the community and so in most areas of North America the cost benefit balance will be less favourable than in Great Britain. It should be clear that because of the differences in prevalence rates, in medical care organization and the relative lack of experience with serum AFP estimations, pilot prospective surveys analagous to the Scottish studies should be conducted in areas of North America where population screening is to be considered before any large programme is instituted. Similar arguments apply to attempts to estimate the cost–benefit aspects of a screening programme in financial terms. The overwhelming importance of the surviving but handicapped spina bifida cases is very evident in any costing. The pronouncement of grossly underestimated costs must be avoided; the figure of one million pounds annually for a national screening programme in the United Kingdom as used by Hampson in his parliamentary campaign is such a figure, as it ignores the costs of the necessary increase in facilities for ultrasonography and amniocentesis. A more realistic estimate may be at least twice this sum plus capital outlay. The relative cost in North America would be considerably higher reflecting the higher cost of medical services generally. Epstein (1978) estimates that a screening programme for the state of California, with 300 000 livebirths per year, would cost about 4.5 million dollars annually, or $44 000 for each infant with spina bifida identified. Even if such costs are regarded as acceptable, the mere provision of the money will not immediately allow such a service to be instituted. Whereas the initial serum AFP estimation is a simple matter, the provision of ultrasonography and amniocentesis requires more skilled personnel and appropriate facilities than are currently available in either the United Kingdom or in most areas of North America. For example, in British Columbia amniocentesis for the detection of Down's syndrome can only be offered to mothers aged over 38 years, although medical opinion is that it should be available to mothers aged 35 years or over. Currently about 1 in 5 mothers aged over 38 years requests amniocentesis but even so all facilities are fully utilized.

Having alluded to some of the technical aspects, let us consider again the ethical and legal implications of prenatal diagnosis. Each geneticist, physician, and mother must make a personal decision concerning the ethics of prenatal diagnosis and selective abortion. For this reason we deplore any attempt by professional groups or learned committees to set standards in this area. To regard, for example, antenatal diagnosis and abortion as 'prevention' is at the least a misnomer. The objective of antenatal diagnosis is the deliberate killing of a malformed infant, and whether we find this idea acceptable or not, it should not be disguised by inappropriate terminology. We can identify three ethical positions. Firstly, to those who regard abortion as unacceptable, attempts at antenatal diagnosis of untreatable defects are nonsensical and the issue is closed. Secondly, at the other extreme if there is total acceptance of abortion, there would be support for a liberal screening programme which allows a high sensitivity by accepting a large number of abortions of unaffected infants. Such a situation exists in Japan where under the Eugenic Protection Law 1948 (Carle 1948), induced abortion has been used as a major means of birth control. One million terminations annually were performed in the 1950s and concomitantly with the decline in the birth rate, the prevalence at birth of certain abnormalities such as Down's syndrome has been reduced by about 30 per cent. The third position is the consensus held in Great Britain and North America at present that selective abortion is permissible but abortion of unaffected infants is undesirable. The risk–benefit comparisons we have just described have been based on this premise. However, the majority who hold this position must be cognizant of the minority who find abortion unacceptable. The proportion of women in this category will reduce the effectiveness of screening and for this reason antenatal screening presents no solution to the problem of neural-tube defects in one country in which they are very common, namely the Republic of Ireland. Efforts must be made to avoid putting such mothers in difficult positions. The screening test should not be carried out without the informed consent of the mother. We are concerned that in the United States some authorities suggest a legal mandate should be placed on obstetricians or hospitals to ensure that all pregnant mothers obtain an AFP test. A similar consideration applies to the recognition of the freedom of conscience of family doctors, obstetricians, and genetic counsellors who must not be forced into contributing to a course of action which they regard as ethically wrong. This is especially applicable in the United States where medical practice is mainly influenced by legal considerations. It is clear that failure to advise a patient who has had a previously affected infant of her risk of having a further affected child constitutes malpractice. The American situation is such that if serum AFP estimation were available at all, there is considerable legal pressure to make it available to every woman, and failure to do so might result in legal action. For similar reasons, it may be essential that a full chromosome analysis is made on all amniotic fluids sampled, even if there is no indication of a chromosomal defect. This greatly increases the cost of any programme. These legal constraints may mean that it will be difficult to introduce pilot programmes of AFP screening on a selective basis, and once introduced there may be great pressure on every obstetrician and every hospital to provide other diagnostic services, which would almost certainly lead to increased error rates and suboptimal results.

In summary, the development of methods which may detect anencephalus and some cases of spina bifida *in utero* represents a major scientific advance. However, it by no means presages the disappearance of neural-tube defects as a major health problem. We believe that the United Kingdom Collaborative Study and the prospective trials carried out in Scotland represent excellent sources of information. Occasionally these data have been wrongly interpreted and forecasts of the risks and benefits of a national screening programme have overestimated any reduction in the amount of care for affected infants which might result. Also, they have underestimated the costs and the risks of screening. The British findings cannot be applied directly to North American populations and small-scale prospective trials are essential if screening programmes are to be considered in Canada and the United States. We are concerned by the uncritical acceptance of a medical procedure which, in contradistinction to the traditional Hippocratic philosophy of medicine, has as its objective the termination rather than the preservation of life. While this policy may relieve part of the burden on the parents and society, obviously it does not benefit the foetus. Although the deliberate elimination of malformed infants might be acceptable to some members of society, we should remain aware of the precise nature of any intervention and take into account the sincere views of those who do not agree with this procedure. Furthermore, we must continue to search for adequate primary preventive measures which will provide a much more satisfactory solution. The infants, children, and adults with neural-tube defects must never be regarded as anything less than full human beings and worthy of the highest standards of medical care.

APPENDIX 1

Worldwide prevalence rates of anencephalus

TABLE A1.1 *Selected surveys of the prevalence of anencephalus per 1000 births in various countries*

Area	Rate per 1000	Births (number)	Study period	Sources of ascertainment	Reference
British Isles					
Birmingham	2.31	158 307	1940–7	H, M	Record and McKeown 1949
Birmingham	2.41	190 236	1950–9	R	Leck, Record *et al*. 1968
Camden	1.20	17 102	1964–7	M, B	Jepson 1969
Exeter	3.00	8117	1954–60	M, B	Ward and Irvine 1961
Leicester	2.31	46 312	1953–62	M, B	Moss 1964
Liverpool	3.15	13 964	1923–32	H	Malpas 1937
Liverpool	3.14	91 176	1960–4	R	Smithells 1968
London	1.56	52 593	1938–53	H	Penrose 1957
London	1.41	409 466	1965–8	H, M, B	Carter and Evans 1973
Northamptonshire	1.03	62 224	1944–57	M, B	Pleydell 1960
Oxford	1.36	35 960	1962–6	R	Hobbs 1969
Oxford	1.49	118 675	1965–72	R	Fedrick 1976
Reading	2.20	12 951	1958–63	M, B	Griffin and Sorrie 1964
Southampton	1.95	14 907	1958–62	H, M	Williamson 1965
Scotland	2.59	1 945 813	1939–58	M	Record 1961
Scotland	2.79	1 162 939	1961–72	M	Fedrick 1976*a*
Aberdeen	1.60	37 585	1938–55	H, B	Anderson *et al*. 1958

TABLE A1.1 *continued*

Area	Rate per 1000	Births (number)	Study period	Sources of ascertainment	Reference
British Isles (continued)					
Dundee	3.30	33 596	1950–9	H, M, B	Walker and Smith 1961
Dundee	3.33	40 573	1956–66	M	Elwood, J. H. and MacKenzie 1971
Edinburgh	2.83	92 007	1956–66	M	Elwood, J. H. and MacKenzie 1971
Glasgow	3.20	250 526	1956–66	M	Elwood, J. H. and MacKenzie 1971
Glasgow	2.80	104 431	1964–8	H, M, B	Wilson 1971
South Wales	3.55	102 786	1956–62	H, M, B	Laurence *et al*. 1967
South Wales	3.09	90 921	1964–6	R	Richards and Lowe 1971
Northern Ireland	3.07	157 725	1969–73	R	Elwood, J. H. 1976
Belfast	3.95	147 825	1950–66	R	Elwood, J. H. 1970
Belfast	4.20	41 351	1964–8	R	Elwood, J. H. and Nevin 1973
Cork	2.05	37 135	1962–6	M, B	Spellman 1969
Dublin	3.79	246 356	1936–65	H	Leck and Rogers 1967
Dublin	4.69	62 495	1936–45 1960–5	H	Leck and Rogers 1967
Dublin	5.93	23 085	1953–5	H	Coffey and Jessop 1957
Dublin	4.23	328 109	1953–73	H	Coffey 1974
Co. Galway	3.90	5367	1958–60	H, B	Cahalane *et al*. 1965
Rest of Europe					
Czechoslovakia	0.50	500 000	1956–62	B	Kučera 1965
Denmark: Copenhagen	1.01	167 940	1911–49	H	Buchi 1950

TABLE A1.1 *continued*

Area	Rate per 1000	Births (number)	Study period	Sources of ascertainment	Reference
Rest of Europe (continued)					
Finland: Helsinki	0.29	17 084	1935–44	H	Hiilesmaa 1945
Finland: Viipuri	2.98	11 425	1935–44	H	Hiilesmaa 1945
Finland:	0.32	621 026	1965–73	R	Granroth *et al*. 1977
France (76 cities)	0.54	746 276	1945–55	H	Frézal *et al*. 1964
France: Paris	0.45	144 611	1945–55	H	Frézal and Lamy 1956
France: Lyon	0.12	59 406	1945–55	H	Frézal and Lamy 1956
Germany: Munich	0.83	141 706	1929–41	H	Hegnauer 1951
Germany: Berlin, Hamburg	1.26	882 634	1930–63	H	Lenz 1965
West Germany	1.42	271 821	1950–6	R	Tünte 1965
Greece: Athens	0.60	34 978	1951–5	H	Louros and Kyriakis 1956
Holland	1.03	1 148 097	1950–4	M	Van Den Bosch 1956
Hungary: Budapest	1.10	692 670	1963–7	H, M, B	Czeizel and Révész 1970
Iceland: Reykjavik	0.47	10 655	1949–55	H	Steffensen 1956
Italy: Naples	4.00	8994	1943–51	H	Candido 1953
Italy: Parma	1.45	8228	1938–47	H	Spoto 1947
Italy: Turin	0.13	7991	1949–55	H	Dellepiane 1956
Spain: Barcelona	0.78	12 969	—	H	Dexeus Tria de Bes 1950
Spain: Madrid	0.81	19 714	1961–4	H	Stevenson *et al*. 1966

TABLE A1.1 *continued*

Area	Rate per 1000	Births (number)	Study period	Sources of ascertainment	Reference
Rest of Europe (continued)					
Sweden: Lund	0.56	48 179	1923–45	H	Böök and Rayner 1950
Sweden: Malmo	0.71	56 633	1917–49	H	Böök and Rayner 1950
Sweden	0.37	159 500	1964–6	R	Källén and Winberg 1968
Switzerland: Geneva	0.80	27 732	1936–55	H	Wertheimer 1957
Switzerland: Zurich	0.54	49 539	1921–44	H	Ehrat 1948
Yugoslavia: Ljubljana, Zagreb	0.59	8416	1961–4	H	Stevenson *et al*. 1966
North America					
CANADA					
Total	0.97	1 855 638		M	
British Columbia	0.65	169 722		M	
Alberta	0.57	156 331		M	
Saskatchewan	0.56	94 217		M	
Manitoba	0.82	91 436	1965–9	M	Elwood, J. M. 1974
Ontario	1.00	665 058		M	
Quebec	1.19	530 054		M	
New Brunswick	1.33	63 394		M	
Nova Scotia	1.05	74 391		M	
Prince Edward Island	1.54	11 035		M	

TABLE A1.1 *continued*

Area	Rate per 1000	Births (number)	Study period	Sources of ascertainment	Reference
North America (continued)					
British Columbia					
Total	0.67	228 391	1952–60	R	Miller 1964
Total	0.64	243 149	1964–70	R	Trimble and Baird 1978
Manitoba	1.20	94 167	1964–8	R	Choi *et al*. 1972
Nova Scotia: Halifax	1.49	49 704	1946–55	H, M	Alter 1963
Quebec					
Total	1.45	656 000		H, M	
French	1.43	564 000		H, M	
British	1.77	57 000	1961–5	H, M	Horowitz and McDonald 1969
Jewish	0.33	6000		H, M	
Other	1.38	29 000		H, M	
UNITED STATES					
Alabama	0.83	444 325	1961–6	M	Cassady 1969
Boston, Mass.					
Total	0.98	311 437		H	
Protestant	0.90	92 200		H	
Catholics	1.19	161 344	1930–65	H	Naggan and MacMahon 1967
Jews	0.40	45 000		H	
Other	0.69	7247		H	

TABLE A1.1 *continued*

Area	Rate per 1000	Births (number)	Study period	Sources of ascertainment	Reference
North America (continued)					
Charleston, S.C.	0.53	55 156	1946–55	H, M	Alter 1962
Chicago, I11.	0.71	19 615	1950–9	H	Wacker 1963
Fall River, Mass.	2.80	5264	1948–54	H	Hurwitz 1955
Iowa	0.58	58 686	1963	H, M, B	Hay 1971
Los Angeles, Calif.	0.49	97 381	1948–58	H	Smilkstein 1962
New York State (excluding New York City)	0.79	3 144 056	1945–62	M, B	Janerich 1973
New York State	0.61	1 580 499	1963–71	M, B	Janerich 1973
Providence, R.I.	1.57	222 538	1885–1965	H	MacMahon and Yen 1971
Rochester, N.Y.	1.39	129 600	1918–38	M	Biggar *et al*. 1976
Rhode Island	1.93	168 654	1936–52	H	MacMahon, Pugh, and Ingalls 1953
Rochester, Minn.	0.90	26 500	1935–67	H	Kurtzke, Goldberg, and Kutland 1973
Rochester, Minn.	0.57	8716	1944–50	H	Harris and Steinberg 1954
Rochester, Minn.	0.90	30 314	1935–71	M, H	Haynes *et al*. 1974
Virginia	0.98	23 381	1961–9	H	Solowy and Shepard 1971
Wilmington, Delaware	0.87	12 529	1954–5	H	Monahan 1956
Hawaii					
White	0.62	40 221	1948–58	H, M, B	Morton, Chung, and Mi 1967
Japanese	0.56	45 103	1948–58	H, M, B	Morton, Chung, and Mi 1967
Atlanta, Ga.					
White	1.06	18 870	1967–8	H, B	Center for Disease Control 1969
Black	0.14	7138	1967–8	H, B	Center for Disease Control 1969

TABLE A1.1 *continued*

Area	Rate per 1000	Births (number)	Study period	Sources of ascertainment	Reference
North America (continued)					
United States (12 hospitals)					
White	1.40	16 385	1961–6	H	Chung and Myrianthopoulos 1968
Black	0.41	16 959	1961–6	H	Chung and Myrianthopoulos 1968
American Indians	0.32	24 000	1965–6	B	Adams and Niswander 1968
Asia and Australia					
India: Bombay	1.15	23 568	1960–3	H	Master-Notani *et al*. 1968
India: Calcutta	0.36	19 191	1961–4	H	Stevenson *et al*. 1966
Singapore					
Total	0.77	88 069		H	
Chinese (all)	0.62	72 660		H	
Chinese (Hakka)	—	7490		H	
Indians (Sikhs)	6.50	1230	1953–6	H	
Indians (others)	0.69	12 990		H	Searle 1959
Malays	1.22	2458		H	
Eurasians	1.45	690		H	
Europeans	2.15	930		H	
Singapore	0.97	8267	1953	H	Searle 1956
Malaysia (Kuala Lumpur)	1.13	15 937	1961–4	H	Stevenson *et al*. 1966
Philippines (Manila)	0.15	29 664	1961–4	H	Stevenson *et al*. 1966

TABLE A1.1 *continued*

Area	Rate per 1000	Births (number)	Study period	Sources of ascertainment	Reference
Asia and Australia (continued)					
Taiwan	1.17	25 814	1965–8	H	Emanuel *et al*. 1972
Taiwan	1.15	14 834	1955–62	H	Wei and Chen 1965
Hong Kong	0.56	32 176	1951–3	H	Penrose 1957
Japan (all)	0.43	6 229 762	1969–71	M	Imaizumi 1974
Japan (Nagasaki and Hiroshima)	0.63	63 796	1948–54	M, H	Neel 1958
Australia					
Melbourne	0.72	225 250	1942–62	H	Stoller and Collman 1965
Melbourne	0.76	69 760	1949–58	H	Betheras 1962
Sydney	0.74	90 864	1942–64	H	Jones 1967
Victoria	0.48	700 909	1954–61	M	Green 1964
Victoria	0.72	753 097	1954–65	B	Collman and Stoller 1968
Middle East and Africa					
Egypt (Alexandria)	3.75	9598	1961–4	H	Stevenson *et al*. 1966
Iran	1.58	14 520	1966–70	H	Damyanov and Dutz 1971
Israel	0.87	531 985	1959–60	H, M	Naggan 1971
Israel	0.68	90 793	1959–60	H, M	Halevi 1967
Lebanon	2.00	7940	1956–62	H	Mufarrij and Kilejian 1963
Uganda (Kampala): Coloured	0.36	5498	1953–5	H	Simpkiss and Lowe 1961
South Africa					
Johannesburg					
Coloured	0.19	32 186	1951–5	H	Kahn 1956
White	0.77	7779	1952–3	H	Kahn 1956

TABLE A1.1 *continued*

Area	Rate per 1000	Births (number)	Study period	Sources of ascertainment	Reference
Middle East and Africa (continued)					
Pretoria					
Coloured	0.23	4404	1953–5	H	Kahn 1956
White	0.95	8413	1953–5	H	Kahn 1956
Cape Town					
Coloured	0.80	3695	Not stated	H	Horner and Lanzkowsky 1966
White	0.70	2807	Not stated	H	Horner and Lanzkowsky 1966
South Africa	0.80	74 000	1961–4	H	Stevenson *et al*. 1966
South America					
Mexico City	0.80	38 783		H	
Panama	0.57	15 852		H	
Brazil (Sao Paulo)	0.62	14 421	1961–4	H	Stevenson *et al*. 1966
Chile (Santiago)	0.30	23 720		H	
Columbia					
Bogota	0.11	18 812		H	
Medellin	0.29	20 459		H	
Chile	0.20	3 446 000	1960–71	M	Cruz-Coke 1972
West Indies (Jamaica)	0.41	29 363	1956–67	H	Thorburn *et al*. 1969

H Hospital records; M Mortality data; B Birth certificates; R Registry Data. — Not recorded.
Most rates are calculated per 1000 (live and still) births but some are per 1000 livebirths.

APPENDIX 2

Analysis of seasonal variation

STEPHEN D. WALTER
Assistant Professor of Public Health (Biometry)
Yale University School of Medicine
New Haven, Connecticut, USA

TIME is the third component in the often-quoted trio of 'person, place, and time' which characterizes epidemiologic phenomena (MacMahon and Pugh 1970). This position may, however, only reflect alphabetic convention rather than practical significance, because there exist many examples in a variety of areas where temporal variation has been the primary instrument in uncovering an aetiologic mechanism.

Various kinds of temporal variation can arise, either singly or in combination. First, one may consider the long-term or secular changes which have taken place in disease incidence; the method of cohort analysis is frequently used here. Second, the time interval between one disease-related event and another may be used to characterize the disorder; for example, the time between vaccination and onset of symptoms, or the time between exposure to contaminated food and illness. Third, point outbreaks (or epidemics) of disease display isolated peaks in incidence which one may attempt to relate to a corresponding change in the environment. Finally, a disease may vary cyclically, with a given pattern of increase and decrease in incidence being repeated several or many times.

Seasonal changes fall into the larger category of cyclic fluctuation, having the particular characteristic that the incidence pattern repeats once per year. They are perhaps the most common kinds of cyclic patterns encountered by epidemiologists because so many human disorders are related to factors (for example viruses, climate, nutrition, activity patterns) which are themselves fundamentally related to the seasons. In particular, seasonality in congenital abnormalities may reflect cyclic changes in risk to the mother or her foetus either near the time of conception or later in the pregnancy.

To infer the existence of a seasonally related hazard for a particular defect from epidemiologic information, the data analyst is ultimately concerned with the rate for the defect rather than with the absolute number of cases which may be affected by other extraneous influences. For instance, when examining a series of abnormal births, one may wish to take into account the total number of births which occurred in the same period; this is because the total fertility rate is itself seasonal, but this seasonal trend is not of direct interest in this context. Similarly, when researching the possibility of a seasonal factor acting early in pregnancy, one may wish to make some adjustment for possibly different foetal survival rates by season.

We shall review below some of the common methods for analysing seasonal trends, with the emphasis on current statistical practice among epidemiologists. There will also, however, be some reference to more sophisticated statistical methodology which would be appropriate in this context. The technical aspects will not be discussed in detail, and the reader is advised to consult the original references provided if he wishes to explore further the various advantages of each method and the necessary calculations for their application. Because the statistical techniques have relevance, and indeed have sometimes been developed, in areas of epidemiology other than that of congenital abnormalities, references to other diseases and disorders will occur.

Early development

One of the first suggestions that congenital abnormalities might be seasonally distributed was by McKeown and Record (1951) who identified a winter excess of anencephalic stillbirths during the period 1939–47 in Birmingham, England. The peak was initially demonstrated graphically, but its statistical significance was established by using the t test to compare the number of births in the first and last quarters of the year versus the second and third quarters; at the time this simple method of pairwise comparisons of time periods by the t test (or an equivalent χ^2 test) was the only one in common usage. Despite the subsequent development of other methods of analysis, results have continued to be reported in this way, or indeed by simply using the 'eyeball' test (Cridland 1961; Laurence *et al.* 1968; McDonald 1971; Revill and Barker 1972). Some authors have extended this approach slightly by using a χ^2 test on case frequencies in several time periods for example, four quarters or twelve months (Slater *et al.* 1964; Hayes 1961; Lee 1962) or by using the pairwise method with all possible sets of six-month divisions of the year (January to June versus July to December, February to July versus August to January, and so on; Vianna and Polan 1976).

While valid in principle, these methods are inadequate in certain respects. First, the nominal p value resulting from a pairwise comparison of two six-month periods is only appropriate if the choice of periods has been determined *a priori*. This is so in some instances where a previously suggested seasonal pattern is to be validated in new data; for example, Guthkelch (1962) attempted to reproduce the winter excess of anencephalus reported by McKeown and Record (1951). In other studies, however, the comparison actually made is clearly suggested by the data themselves, leading to an overoptimistic estimate of statistical significance. Second, when several or all possible comparisons are made, using the same data, the conclusions are statistically dependent; ideally the resulting p values should be adjusted to take this into account, but this is not always done. Similar considerations apply when several different abnormalities are being analysed simultaneously; for example, if a large number of significance tests are being performed, then a certain fraction of them would be expected by chance alone to indicate significance even if no seasonal effect existed. Finally, a t test or χ^2 test on data grouped by time period (six months, three months, one month) will not have very great power to detect the seasonal patterns which might actually be anticipated, if indeed such patterns exist. For example, the usual χ^2 for differences between monthly frequencies has 11 degrees of freedom (d.f.); a given set of 12 frequencies would lead to the same value of χ^2 regardless of their ordering (this is neglecting, for the moment, differences in the 'expected' monthly frequencies due to the variable month length); it is clear, therefore, that this test will not have as great a chance of detecting an excess of cases occurring during, say, four to six winter months as would a test which is designed specifically to exploit this ordering in the structure of monthly fluctuation. In the following section, we will describe some parametric tests which have this objective.

Parametric tests

In many diseases with a known seasonal behaviour the incidence may sometimes change abruptly as a result of temporary environmental effects; for example, the rate of respiratory disorders may increase during an exceptionally cold spell of weather. Nevertheless, the general pattern is one of a gradual fluctuation from month to month, the pattern being essentially repeated each year. For diseases where seasonality has not been clearly established, it may be reasonable to suppose that the seasonal effect, if real, also acts smoothly over relatively long periods of time. At the expense, then, of assuming a particular kind of seasonality to be operative, one can devise statistical tests which are specific for this kind of variation, and which may evaluate the significance of its associated parameters—hence parametric tests. In a subsequent section, we will also consider tests which do not make any such assumption, and which are therefore non-parametric.

One simple and convenient parametric form of variation which has been used is the sinusoidal or simple harmonic pattern. Here the incidence is assumed to have one symmetric peak per year and a similar symmetric trough six months later. Edwards (1961) proposed a test procedure for variation of this kind, based on a geometric argument; the computations are quite simple, and the test has enjoyed widespread use by epidemiologists (Wehrung and Hay 1970; Roberts, Lowe, and Lloyd 1972; Rothman and Fyler 1974). The method requires that the data from one or several years be grouped by calendar month, and consists of arranging the 12 resulting frequencies as a set of weights on the rim of a circle representing the year. The months are assumed to be of equal length, and the test compares the observed centre of gravity of the data with its observed position, the origin of the circle, under a null hypothesis of no seasonality. The vector between the origin and observed centre of gravity points to the estimated month of peak incidence or prevalence at birth (the 'phase' of the sinusoidal curve), and the distance between these two points provides an estimate of the amplitude of the oscillation, defined as the proportional difference between the average and peak rates. The phase and amplitude are the two parameters which completely specify a particular sinusoidal curve from among this general class of curves. If the null hypothesis is true (no seasonality), the distance squared between the origin and centre of gravity follows approximately a distribution with 2 d.f., and this fact leads to an appropriate test statistic. If a significant variation is found, one may then calculate the expected monthly frequencies on the basis of the estimated parameters of the curve; these may be compared with the observed frequencies by a goodness-of-fit χ^2 test statistic with 9 d.f. to see if the sinusoidal characterization of the monthly variation is indeed adequate, or if some more complex form is required. It should be pointed out that Edwards's test is, strictly speaking, only valid in large samples; the properties of this test in small sample situations will be discussed later.

A number of variants of Edwards's test have been published to deal with departures from its idealized assumptions which occur frequently in epidemiologic practice. Hare and Price (1968) developed a test which would compare the seasonal trend in two related series of frequencies for the 'numerator' and 'denominator' of a rate, regarding this statistically as a two-sample problem; an obvious application in this context is if one wished to evaluate the seasonality of a particular congenital abnormality (the numerator) while allowing for the total number of births (the denominator). Walter and Elwood, J. M. (1975) also addressed this problem by weighting the frequencies of one series according to the frequencies in the other; they also allowed for the data to be grouped into any number of time intervals, of unequal length in general; thus this method could be applied to quarterly, monthly, weekly, or any other kind of grouped data. Cave and Freedman (1975) reformulated Edwards's approach to test for a sinusoidal oscillation with a peak every six months (instead of annually); the approach is not completely general for all disorders suspected of having a bimodal behaviour, because the two maxima are required to be of the same size. A more common kind of epidemiologic hypothesis is one where there is a dominant and a secondary peak during the year; this type of behaviour would probably be detected by Cave and Freedman's test, but theirs would not be the most powerful approach to use in this case. It may be noted that if the two peaks are in fact equal, then Edwards's test will have a very small probability of rejecting the null hypothesis because the expected centre of gravity of the system would be the origin of the circle.

Some non-geometric approaches to the sinusoidal model are available. Johnson (1971) discusses this in a nonlinear model framework for the special case of four observations per cycle (quarterly data in this context). Roger (1977) also uses this method, calculating maximum likelihood estimates of the general simple harmonic curve, with data arbitrarily grouped and possibly weighted according to the frequencies in another series of data. St Leger (1976) also considered this model in a similar fashion. Glasser (1970) in investigating absenteeism used a sinusoidal function for the probability of a spell of absence to be initiated for an individual, and combined this with a gamma distribution for the average probability of absence in different individuals.

Given these two main choices of method (geometric and maximum likelihood) available for the basic sinusoidal model, the question naturally arises as to which is to be preferred. Unfortunately the answer to this has not been fully investigated at this time, but certain general indications are possible. Useful here are the simulation results of St Leger who compared the two tests by repeatedly generating in the computer sets of artificial data which were distributed sinusoidally with a known amplitude; by this means it was possible to compare the empirical properties of each test with their theoretical equivalents. Of particular interest was the behaviour of the tests when small samples were involved. The maximum-likelihood test produces a statistic which is distributed as χ^2 with 2 d.f. in large samples. The simulations showed, however, that this statistic approximated to a χ^2 distribution much more closely in small samples than did Edwards's test statistic. The latter in fact tended to produce significance much too often if the null hypothesis were true and the usual percentage points of the χ^2 distribution were used as critical values. Both tests appeared to have enough power to detect an amplitude of 20 per cent with at least 200 observations in the year, but amplitudes of 30 per cent and 50 per cent were necessary to have reasonable power of detection with samples of 50 and 20 respectively. Although maximum likelihood estimates of the amplitude parameter are unbiased in large samples, this is not the case in small samples where (as shown by the simulations) overestimates are obtained, particularly when the amplitude is itself small. It turns out, however, that Edwards's test also gives upwardly biased estimates of amplitude, and in fact the bias is generally greater than that for maximum likelihood estimates. In certain cases, Edwards's method may even give inadmissible amplitude estimates greater than unity. The main counteradvantage of Edwards's method appears to be that of computational simplicity; the maximum-likelihood estimates must be found iteratively using a special computer algorithm, but even this may not be a great problem with the ready access of most investigators to computing facilities. Roger also carried out some simulation experiments to compare the maximum-likelihood and geometric methods and reaches a similar conclusion to St Leger that maximum likelihood is to be preferred if the probability values arising from the test statistics are to be taken literally.

A desirable characteristic of any significance test is that it has as much power (or probability) as possible to reject the null hypothesis if it is not true, that is, to have a good chance of detecting a given size of effect with as small a sample as possible. It is clear that the geometric and maximum likelihood approaches have greater power than the usual χ^2 test for any variation between monthly frequencies (James 1976*a*); this is less important when few observations per cycle are made (for example, with quarterly data), but analyses which take an ordered structure of variation into account should be more powerful even in this case. Both approaches lead to a χ^2 statistic with 2 d.f., regardless of the number of observations per cycle and so from this point of view one should subdivide the data into as many segments as possible without creating excessively small frequencies in each. The power of Edwards's test was evaluated for the annual sinusoidal alternative model by Walter (1977*a*) using sample sizes from 50 to 100 000; the method used can be adapted to evaluate the power against any other parametric alternative. Roger (1977) remarks that the square-root transformation used in the geometric tests may not be optimal; nevertheless there is an asymptotic equivalence between tests using transformed and untransformed data (Smith 1961). A discrepancy between the maximum-likelihood and geometric test statistics may arise if either the denominator (if any) or the sector lengths are highly variable but in most applications this will not be important (Roger 1977, 1977*a*). Thus with large samples the choice between the parametric tests will usually make little difference to the substantive conclusions. With small samples the parametric tests suffer from deficiences as described above, in that their apparent test significance levels may not be valid and their parameter estimates may be biased. The basic reason for this is that the parametric tests assume that the grouped frequencies (for example, by month) are approximately normally distributed; this is only true, however, if the average frequencies are quite large. To avoid such difficulties there have been some attempts to construct tests which do not make this assumption, or alternatively do not assume a particular parametric form for the variation by season. These will now be briefly discussed.

Non-parametric tests

The most notable test in this category is that of Hewitt, Milner, Cisima, and Pakula (1971), who incidentally were also motivated in this work by the clear indication from simulation experiments that Edwards's test gave results which were overly significant in small samples. The test procedure is first to assign a rank to the case frequency or rate of each month, with rank 12 being given to the month with the most cases, 11 to the month with the next highest number, and so on down to rank 1. Two kinds of hypothesis may then be tested. In the first, a predetermined six-month segment of the year (for example, March to August) is postulated to have a higher case rate than the other six-month segment (September to February); the sum of ranks for these six months is calculated, and then compared against an empirical distribution which was established by computer sampling by Hewitt *et al*. (1971). It turns out that any rank sum greater than 49 is significant at the 0.05 level, and any sum greater than 52 is significant at the 0.01 level. Thus if the months March to August had ranks 8, 11, 7, 9, 5, and 12, the rank sum is 52 which has $0.01 < p < 0.05$. The second kind of hypothesis which may be tested is where the six-month interval with elevated rate is not specified *a priori*, but where one is interested in testing for seasonality with a peak in any six-month period. Here one computes rank sums for all possible six-month periods, and then uses the maximum as the test statistic which is again compared to a table of empirical probabilities given by Hewitt and colleagues. In this case the maximum rank sum must be 55 or greater to be significant at the 5 per cent level, but not even the value 57 (which is the highest rank sum obtainable, equal to 12 + 11 + 10 + 9 + 8 + 7) is significant at the 1 per cent level.

In using this test one is restricted to monthly data because no comparable tables for other data groupings are available. Also one must avoid ties between months when assigning ranks, although ties are quite unlikely if one adjusts the case frequencies by the number of days in the month or by an appropriate denominator. Ties are of course more likely in small samples. The advantage of this test is that it does not assume any particular kind of seasonal fluctuation to be operative, and can be used with very small samples without fear of violating distributional assumptions. Nothing is known about the power of this test when applied to the usual kinds of seasonal variation. A somewhat similar test is due to David and Newell (1965), and is based on the maximum difference in the numbers of cases in all possible pairs of six-month divisions of the year. This test also is not directed to detecting a particular kind of seasonal variation, but does nevertheless assume the monthly case frequencies to be approximately normally distributed. In this sense the test is a compromise between the parametric tests and that of Hewitt *et al*. Tables given by the authors must be consulted to evaluate the significance of a particular data set.

Other methods

The techniques discussed above have been developed largely in the context of epidemiologic applications, and have arisen almost independently of the methodology available for time-series data in general. Good overviews of statistical time-series analysis are given by Box and Jenkins (1970), Anderson (1971), and Kendall (1973). Although this methodology is quite extensive, relatively little emphasis is placed on the analysis of frequency data in particular, and this may be one contributing factor to the rather limited use which has been made of these methods by epidemiologists. Another reason may be that the computations are generally more complex than those for the previously described tests; none the less a little investment in this more refined technology can yield the potential for a much more thorough and detailed analysis. Again, not wishing to be drawn into a description of the technicalities, we will content ourselves here with a brief description of the salient practical aspects.

One of the main analytic devices in time-series analysis is the use of Fourier analysis. Here the data in a time series are approximated by a set of trigonometric functions with various 'wavelengths'. Thus, for example, one might choose to model the incidence at birth of a congenital abnormality by a combination of an annual cycle and a semi-annual cycle. These two seasonal trends could be in phase, in which case there would be a dominant and a secondary peak during the year, or out of phase in which case there would be three separate peaks. By various combinations of these cycles, appropriately weighted, it is possible to approximate the behaviour of most time series which arise in practice. Pocock (1974) applied this method to the analysis of sickness data for a five-year period, and was able to attribute about half the variation of absences to seasonal effects. His model originally involved a large number of harmonics, but became simplified when non-significant terms were excluded from consideration. Pocock (1972) has also used a variant of this approach to relate sickness to climate; included in the model here were harmonics to represent the seasonal effects as before, and also terms corresponding to weather variables, the occurrence of holidays, and sickness levels in the previous few weeks. A stepwise method of selecting significant terms into the model was used, similar to that adopted in other regression calculations. Rogot, Fabsitz, and Feinleib (1976) have used a similar methodology using daily data on mortality from various causes.

One assumption required by all the methods discussed so far is that the time series is 'stationary' meaning that it is not experiencing any long-term or secular trend. If the series is in fact influenced by both seasonal and secular effects, analysis is more difficult. One approach is to 'remove' the trend by applying a moving average, and then to examine the seasonal behaviour of the 'detrended' series. It is not always possible to remove the trend in this way without affecting the seasonal component which may be somewhat obscured or exaggerated in the adjusted series; whichever occurs depends on the extent of the moving average compared to the period of oscillation, and on the nature of its weights (for example, Kendall and Stuart 1976, Chapter 46). A moving average may even induce spurious cyclicisms in a stationary series (known as the Slutsky–Yule effect); in general terms, it may tend to mask long-period cycles and augment short-period cycles. In certain cases it is possible to correct the adjusted series to take account of trend fitting, but in most problems the distortion of the seasonal components will only be recognized in a rather general way. Similar problems arise if one wishes to examine the trend after adjusting for seasonality; for example, it may be difficult to differentiate between a trend and a slow oscillation, of which perhaps only part has been observed. On the other hand it is undesirable to forego making any such adjustment. An analysis of the seasonal components alone in a series which in fact contains only a monotonic secular increase would reveal a spurious seasonal pattern with the response values rising steadily through the year. Conversely a test for trend alone on a short series which in fact behaves in a stationary simple harmonic fashion with a peak in March to April would indicate a spurious downward trend through the year. In less extreme situations, the effect of one component can mask or augment the effect of the other if not taken into account. One solution to this dilemma might be to make two analyses, for trend adjusting for seasonality, and vice versa, but one then has to make simultaneous inferences from statistically dependent analyses.

A somewhat different approach to seasonality which falls into the general category of regression analysis is where the frequency of the disorder under study is related to variables which are in turn seasonally variable. An example would be to regress the rate of a congenital abnormality on the mean local temperature by month (for example, Elwood, J. H. and MacKenzie 1971). One advantage of this method is that it may be possible to choose regressor variables which have a central role in the postulated causal origin of the disorder. At the same time, one is not restricted to any particular form of seasonal fluctuation in the outcome. On the other hand, it is necessary (as with other regression work) to evaluate whether the model adequately summarizes the data, or whether additional predictor variables are needed.

Pooling of data

It is a somewhat common practice with frequency data to pool over years before analysing for seasonality. By this means the data are reduced to 12 monthly frequencies and methods such as Edwards's test may be used. This is done particularly often with sparse data, such as the monthly numbers of cases of a rare disease, but it is not unusual even when the unpooled data would be amenable to analysis. A danger here is that a secular trend may induce a spurious seasonal pattern in the pooled data; for example, if the rate of a particular disease is progressively increasing, then more cases will occur in December than in January each year, and this will remain true in the pooled data even if no seasonal effect exists. A more subtle instance of this occurs in the analysis of deaths in the elderly (Roger 1977*a*); because the death rate by month of age increases quite rapidly after 80 years, an apparent increase in the probability of death following a birthday may be induced.

One counteradvantage of pooling frequency data is that the resulting aggregated frequencies will be 'smoother' from month to month, and in particular may behave more like normally distributed variables; an assumption required in many of the techniques described here. In practice one has to weigh this against the lost potential to examine the trend in detail, or indeed to answer more detailed questions such as whether the seasonal effect has changed over the years of the series. With respect to the latter, tests are available via Fourier analysis to determine if a cyclic effect has changed its phase (time of peak) or strength (amplitude).

Computation

The data manipulations required for some of the simpler techniques described here can be carried out by hand or with a pocket calculator, as long as the data are already in aggregated form, for example in monthly frequencies. Even this becomes tedious if more than a few applications are desired, and at this point resort to the computer is recommended. Many of the easier methods such as those of Edwards and Hewitt *et al*. may be quickly programmed, with the option of reading the data in on a case-by-case basis. In using the computer one also has the option of doing additional calculations, such as evaluating the goodness-of-fit of an 'expected' seasonal curve, which might be omitted using hand calculation.

Some of the common computer programme suites contain certain routines which can be adapted for applications in seasonality analysis. In particular, the subprogramme REGRESSION of SPSS (Nie, Hull, Jenkins, Steinbrenner, and Bent 1975), the procedure of NLIN of SAS, (Barr, Goodnight, Sall, and Helwig 1976) and programmes P3R and PAR of BMD (Dixon 1977) can be used for non-linear regression analysis; this permits the specification of a few harmonic functions to predict the level of an outcome variable such as a case frequency. Also, the more familiar linear regression programmes can be used to regress a case frequency on appropriate seasonally affected predictor variables. The procedure SPECTRA of SAS is particularly useful to carry out a complete Fourier analysis of a time series, allowing the possibility of an arbitrary pattern of seasonal variation whose components may be tested for statistical significance.

APPENDIX 3

The Canadian fourteen-city study

SOME of the information on the epidemiology of anencephalus in this book is from a study in which we compared certain characteristics of all fatal cases of anencephalus ('cases') with those of a random sample of livebirths ('controls') in Canada. Some methodological issues of this study are now described.

The Canadian 14-city study is based on the information available on stillbirth certificates and on birth certificates. The study is therefore restricted in scope, especially as the information requested on these statutory certificates is included for reasons which are diverse, but which do not include any conscious attempt to clarify the aetiology of birth defects. A survey in which a specially designed questionnaire would be completed by mothers of infants with anencephalus or spina bifida and by comparison mothers would be preferable to the current design, but would be much more costly. Moreover, it would have to be carried out over many years to amass sufficient subjects, and a special notification system would be required as most provincial authorities in Canada will not permit individuals to be identified from vital statistical records for research purposes. The 14-city study included a large number of cases of anencephalus and a large comparison group without such difficulties. The investigation was made possible by the generous co-operation and resources of Statistics Canada, where all vital registrations from 1950 onwards are stored on computer tape. We considered using information on all or a random sample of anencephalic births or deaths from anencephalus in Canada. However, as our major purpose was to consider the geographical variation in mortality rates in terms of other factors, we selected all fatal cases of anencephalus occurring to mothers resident in a small number of major cities, chosen to provide a large geographical range. We hoped this would avoid most of the problems of comparability of diagnosis and certification, as infants born in major urban centres are more likely to be exposed to consistent standards of medical care than those born in small towns or in rural areas. The largest cities in each of eight provinces were selected. Unfortunately, the largest cities of all, the conurbations of Toronto and Montreal, could not be used as there had been several major boundary changes with the creation of new administrative areas, making it impossible to gather comparable information over a long period of time. The cities chosen were Vancouver (British Columbia), Edmonton and Calgary (Alberta), Regina and Saskatoon (Saskatchewan), Winnipeg (Manitoba), Hamilton, Kitchener, London, Windsor, and Ottawa (Ontario), Quebec (Quebec), St John (New Brunswick), and Halifax (Nova Scotia) (Fig. 9.1).

The case series consisted of all stillbirths or infant deaths certified as being due to anencephalus or monstrosity, occurring between 1950 and 1969, to mothers resident in any of these cities. There were 1391 cases thus defined. Most of these infants (73 per cent) were stillborn, while the remainder were liveborn and presented as infant deaths. The records of all stillbirths coded under the *International Classification of Diseases* codes Y.38.0 (7th revision, 1950 to 1968) or P.69 (8th revision, 1969) were extracted from the main Statistics Canada tape and transferred to a new tape after removal of the name, parents' names, and addresses to satisfy confidentiality requirements. Infant deaths recorded under codes 750 (7th revision) or 740 (8th revision) were extracted from the main mortality tapes. From these, the names and addresses were noted and a manual search of microfilmed birth certificates was performed by Statistics Canada staff to obtain the matching birth certificates. As the deaths occurred within a few days of birth and the records are grouped in chronological order by place of occurrence, this linkage operation was completed successfully for all records. Data from the birth certificates, excluding identifying information, and with the addition of the length of survival in days, were merged with the stillbirth data. To provide a control group, the records of all livebirths in the 14 cities in the years 1952, 1957, 1962, and 1967 were transferred, minus identifying information, to a new tape. From this data base of 238 720 records a sample of 5000 was chosen using random numbers, giving a ratio of controls to cases of approximately 4:1.

Information available

In Canada, the registration of births and deaths is under the jurisdiction of the provincial governments, and the format and wording of statutory certificates differ from province to province. Birth certificates and stillbirth certificates are completed by the parents and physician respectively and are sent to the Registrar of Births, Deaths, and Marriages in each province. Since 1921, the certificates from each province, except Newfoundland and the northern territories, have been forwarded to the Dominion Bureau of Statistics, now Statistics Canada, and there the data are coded, using as far as possible the same coding system and format for the whole country. All birth and death information since 1950 is currently stored on computer tape. The data recorded are as follows:

(1) Place of birth and residence of mother, each recorded by province, area (county or census tract), and municipality. Case and control births were selected on the basis of the place of residence of the mother rather than the place of birth, as many births occurring in urban areas are to mothers resident elsewhere who are delivered in an urban hospital. The 'area' coded refers to large divisions, and in general no unit smaller than a municipality is coded. This unfortunately prevents the use of local area of residence, which would be a useful indicator of socio-economic status.
(2) Place of birth—home, hospital, or other.
(3) Attendant at birth—physician, midwife, nurse, or other.
(4) Sex of the infant.
(5) Plurality of birth—single, twin, triplet, etc.
(6) Legitimacy—legitimate or illegitimate.
(7) Month of birth (from date of birth).
(8) Year of birth (from date of birth).
(9) Age of mother.
(10) Number of previous children born alive to the mother.
(11) Number of previous children stillborn to the mother.
(12) Number of previous children born alive to the mother and since deceased.
(13) Total number of children previously born to the mother.
(14) Ethnic origin of the mother. The question is expressed as 'to which national or ethnic group do you belong?' and is further defined in a footnote as referring to descent through the paternal grandfather. Several provinces in more recent years include a separate question on citizenship.
(15) Age of the father.
(16) Ethnic origin of the father.
(17) Occupation of the father; recorded only in a few provinces and only prior to 1955.
(18) Birth weight of the infant.
(19) Gestation in completed weeks.

For each subject information on nineteen factors was given by birth or stillbirth certificates. Eight of these factors were omitted from the main analysis. Length of gestation and birth weight are influenced by the presence of anencephalus and are not involved in the causal pathway producing this defect and so were not included in the model. The sex of the infant similarly is best not regarded as a cause and is thus omitted; however, modifications of the associations with other factors by the sex of the infant were considered. Paternal age and occupation were omitted because they were unknown for a considerable proportion of subjects. There was no problem of missing data for any other factor except maternal ethnic origin, where the unknown category was retained as such. As the associations with maternal and paternal ethnic origin were similar, and for 55 per cent of subjects maternal and paternal ethnic origins were identical, paternal ethnic origin was excluded. 'Total previous births' also was excluded as it is derived from previous livebirth and previous stillbirth history. Only five subjects did not have a physician present at the birth, so the variable attendant present at birth was excluded.

In each of the three methods of analysis, we examined eleven factors: city of residence, year of birth, month of birth, maternal age, previous livebirths, previous stillbirths, previous child deaths, maternal ethnic origin, plurality of birth, legitimacy, and place of birth. Each of these factors was represented by a number of binary variables, the number being one less than the number of categories of the factor. Thus city of residence, a factor with 14 categories, was represented by 13 binary variables. The use of binary variables avoids the problems of ordering the categories of a factor and assuming a specific relationship of risk over the ordered categories. In the present data several factors do not have categories which have a clearly logical order (for example, city of residence, ethnic origin) and in several of those that do a non-linear association with risk seemed likely (such as livebirths). The eleven factors were represented by 47 binary variables.

Methodological considerations in the study design

There are several advantages in basing the study on a small number of selected cities. One of the objectives of the study is to determine if the geographical variation in mortality rates persists after removal of the effects of parity, ethnic origin, and other variables. A small number of geographical locations allows each to be studied individually. If a random sample of all anencephalic deaths had been chosen, it would have been necessary to assume a specific type of relationship between anencephalus risk and a geographic parameter such as longitude, or to group the observations into larger units such as provinces. The study of geographical location in terms of a manageable number of binary variables makes no assumption as to the form of the relationship between mortality rate and location. Moreover, with a less restricted sample, difficulties would have arisen as coding of place of residence is complex and has changed frequently over the 20-year study period and often no detailed information is available for residents of rural areas or unincorporated small communities.

The urban population studied is not representative of the Canadian maternal population, although the mortality rate of anencephalus shows no consistent urban–rural difference. It seems likely that compared to the total Canadian population, the urban population has narrower maternal age and parity ranges, higher illegitimacy rates, and a different ethnic structure with over-representation of some groups, for example Jewish and Italian, and under-representation of others such as Dutch and Scandinavian. However, such differences are likely to be similar for the case and for the control groups and so will not bias the results. Bias could result if urbanization varied by social class, for example if the urban concentration of women in a certain ethnic group were more marked in the lower social classes, that group's rate of anencephalus would be overestimated. Such differential effects as do occur are probably of minor importance.

We selected a sample of livebirths, rather than of all non-anencephalic live and stillbirths, as a control group as we wished to compare the characteristics of mothers of infants with anencephalus to those of mothers of healthy children. A better control group would be livebirths from which infants with abnormalities were excluded, but this would produce only a very slight improvement in validity. The study was not designed to test one specific hypothesis but to estimate the associations of anencephalus risk with each of the factors on which data were available. If one factor had been the sole object of inquiry, we could have controlled confounding by matching the control series to the anencephalus cases on as many as possible of the other factors. However, this would mean we could not have assessed the association of anencephalus risk with the factors on which matching had been performed, and would have greatly reduced the scope of the study. We obtained the livebirth sample by taking random samples from the records of all livebirths delivered to mothers resident in the 14 cities for each of the four years 1952, 1957, 1962, and 1967. Systematic sampling was used as a first stage because the original tapes are arranged by year of birth. The non-randomness thus produced is probably of little consequence.

The possibility of bias in the recording of information must be considered. For several factors, the percentage of records with missing information was higher for the anencephalus cases than for controls, notably paternal age (unknown for 8 per cent of cases and 6.8 per cent of controls) and length of gestation (31 per cent of cases and 11 per cent of controls). The excess missing data may reflect less careful recording for stillbirths than for livebirths. Many anencephalic foetuses are macerated or accompanied by hydramnios making the estimation of length of gestation more difficult. There was no problem of missing data for other factors. However, it is conceivable that certain information, for example that on previous stillbirths or infant deaths, might be more carefully recorded for the mothers of abnormal infants; if so this could produce an overestimate of a positive association with the risk of anencephalus.

The need for a multivariate method of analysis

The aim of this study was to estimate the association of each of several factors (maternal age, parity, race, city of birth, etc.) with the outcome of the pregnancy. The outcome is a binary variable—anencephalic or not anencephalic. Some of the other factors are continuous, such as age, or have a meaningful order, as does parity. Others are discrete and cannot be logically ordered, such as race and city of residence. A simple method of analysis is to use multiple cross-tabulations. To estimate the association of anencephalus with one factor while controlling for another, a 2-by-n table, where n is the number of categories of the factor under study, is prepared within each category of the factor to be controlled. Thus to control for city of birth, fourteen 2-by-n tables are needed. The association can then be assessed by a summary risk ratio such as that of Mantel and Haenszel (1959), or a direct standardization technique may be used, as the control series is a random sample of the total livebirths with a known sampling fraction. Thus, in each cell of the tables, a mortality rate (deaths from anencephalus per 1000 livebirths) can be calculated, and these rates can then be standardized. The limitation of cross-tabulation is that to control all factors requires a very large number of tables. To control for a single confounding factor with three categories requires three tables; for I factors each with k_i categories we require $\prod_{i=1}^{I} k_i$ tables. For example, to control simultaneously for maternal age, race, city and quinquennium of birth requires $5 \times 10 \times 14 \times 4 = 2800$ tables. Clearly even with large number of subjects this method quickly becomes impracticable.

The use of multivariate mathematical models offers a solution to the problem of dealing with many variables, but raises other issues. In this study, as in many other epidemiological situations, one of the chief limitations is that the outcome variable (anencephalus or not) is binary, and few of the factors under examinations have normal distributions. We chose to use a relatively new technique as our main method of analysis, that of stratification by a multivariate confounder score, and also to use two other approaches—binary multiple regression and a multiple logistic function. All of these methods are mathematically fairly straightforward, and the statistical reader may find much of our discussion rather simplistic. An alternative to our choice of analyses would be methods based on contingency tables as reviewed by Bishop, Feinberg, and Holland (1975).

Stratification by a multivariate confounder score

This method has been developed recently by Miettinen (1976) and was first applied to a case–control study of myocardial infarction designed to estimate the effect of one risk factor, coffee drinking, while controlling simultaneously for seven other factors (Jick, Miettinen, Neff, Shapiro, Heinonen, and Slone 1973). It has also been used in the analysis of case–control studies of trigeminal neuralgia (Rothman and Monson 1973) and endometrial cancer (Elwood, J. M., Cole, Rothman, and Kaplan 1977). An outline of the method will now be given but further details are described by Miettinen (1976).

One of the methods most frequently used to control confounding in epidemiological analysis is stratification, as discussed in Section 5. Miettinen has extended this approach to allow stratification on a multivariate function rather than on only one variable; thus the approach used is derived principally from epidemiological reasoning, in contrast to other multivariate models which are primarily derived from mathematical distribution theory. Let us consider the estimation of the association between anencephalus or control status and legitimacy, a binary 'exposure' variable, and suppose we wish to control this association for the effects of maternal parity, expressed in five categories (0, 1, 2, 3, 4+). Five 2-by-2 tables are compiled, giving disease status (case or control) by legitimacy for each category of parity. A method such as that of Mantel and Haenszel (1959) then is applied to calculate a risk-ratio estimate based on the data in all five 2-by-2 tables. This estimates the association between disease status and legitimacy controlled for the confounding effect of parity. The rationale behind this approach is that the risk of a subject being in the anencephalic rather than in the control group is associated with parity and also the probability of illegitimacy is independently related to parity. Any factor which is independently associated with the exposure factor being assessed and with case status is a confounding factor (Miettinen 1970) and may be controlled by this stratification analysis. This method is limited by the large number of strata required to deal with the confounding effects of several variables. However, it is possible to gain efficiency by combining strata, without introducing confounding. A sufficient criterion which will allow combination of strata is if the risks of anencephalus in two or more strata of the confounding variable are the same in subjects not exposed to the factor being assessed, the strata may be combined. For example, if the risks of anencephalus, indicated by the case–control ratio, for parity groups 2, 3, and 4+ are identical there is no confounding effect of parity over these strata, and so to estimate the association of anencephalus risk with legitimacy only three strata (parity 0, 1, 2+) are required, allowing greater efficiency. Let us now extend this approach. Rather than just looking at parity, we use all the information available to group cases and controls into a small number of strata based on each subject's risk of anencephalus, as conferred by all factors except legitimacy. We prepare, within each stratum of the risk function, a 2-by-2 table sharing the distribution of cases and controls by legitimacy, and then estimate the association between anencephalus status and legitimacy controlled for the joint confounding effects of the other study factors. To define the strata, we rank the cases and controls in order of their anencephalus risk conferred by all study factors except the one under investigation. We refer to this risk estimate as the 'risk score' and to the function used as a multivariate risk or confounder score.

The confounder score

One method of assessing the risk for each subject from data in a case–control study is a linear discriminant function separating cases and controls. For each subject, information on outcome (anencephalus or control) and on each factor studied is included. The factors analysed may be entered as continuous or as discrete variables. An additive model is used and interaction terms may be included. The linear discriminant function as developed by Fisher (1936) employs a simple least-squares approach to estimate the coefficients giving the greatest separation of the case and control populations. This method assumes multivariate normality of the independent variables, and equal variance–covariance matrices in the two populations. If these assumptions are fulfilled the estimates of the discriminant coefficients are maximum likelihood estimates (Cornfield 1967). Even when these conditions are not met, as is the case if dichotomous variables are used, the function may perform adequately, as assessed empirically (Truett, Cornfield, Kannel 1967) and by formal evaluation (Gilbert 1968, 1969). Under some circumstances, a more precise risk score may be produced by other models such as a quadratic discriminant function or a log–linear risk-function (Miettinen 1976). However, as the discriminant function is used solely to achieve a ranking of risk scores, only major errors in the assessment of the risk score which would place a subject in the wrong stratum are of consequence, and therefore it is unlikely that more complex models would provide a useful increase in precision. For the same reason, the method should be more robust than those where estimation of the effect of a factor is based on the value of the discriminant coefficient for that factor. As the risk score should reflect the risk among the subjects conditional on 'non-exposure' with respect to the factor being assessed, the linear discriminant function could be applied only to unexposed subjects; however, if the function is computed by including the exposure variable, the risk conditional on non-exposure may be assessed for all subjects by setting the exposure variable to 'non-exposure'. Non-exposure is defined as a reference category of the factor being studied, for example for parity 'non-exposure' may be defined as nulliparous. When the discriminant function is fitted using all predictor variables, the coefficients of many of these may be small and not statistically significant. This lack of significance of a factor in contributing to the risk score does not mean that it cannot be a confounding factor and so reduction of the model without introducing confounding is possible only if the discriminant coefficient of the exposure variable remains unchanged after any reduction. Generally, there is little advantage in model reduction in a study with several controls per case (Miettinen 1976).

Thus the risk score for each subject is calculated from the linear discriminant function in which the variables representing the factor under investigation are set to a referent 'non-exposure' level. We would expect there to be cases having a risk score greater than that of the highest control, and controls with a lower risk score than that of the lowest case, assuming a higher value of the dependent variable indicates the case group. These extreme subjects are excluded as there are no comparison subjects with similar risk scores. Within the common range of scores, the strata are then defined. The number of strata and the divisions between them are arbitrary. Five strata are usually sufficient as any improvement in the control of confounding produced by using a greater number is usually small (Cochran 1968). Where there are fewer cases than controls, the analysis may be made more efficient by placing a similar number of cases in each stratum, for example by using a quintile division of the ranked risk-score for the cases. Having defined the strata, the distribution of each variable except the one being assessed is examined within each stratum. If stratification is to succeed in controlling confounding, each major confounding factor should be present in a similar proportion of cases and controls within each stratum. If there are large differences between cases and controls within a stratum, confounding may still exist and that stratum should be further divided. If two strata are very similar, no confounding will be introduced by combining them into one new stratum, and some gain in efficiency may result. After ranking and stratification of scores, cross-tabulations of case–control status by the factor under assessment are made for each stratum of risk score. The remainder of the analysis is based on these cross-tabulations.

Application to the 14-city study

This method was applied to the study of 1391 deaths from anencephalus and 5000 comparison livebirths. The risk score was estimated from a linear function of eleven factors: city of residence, year of birth, month of birth, maternal age, numbers of previous livebirths, stillbirths, and child deaths, ethnic origin, plurality of birth, legitimacy status, and place of birth. These eleven factors were represented by 47 binary variables. The risk score based on all factors was computed by a linear discriminant function. The distributions of cases and controls by values of this discriminant score are shown in Table A3.1 and in Fig. A3.1. As the dependent variable was defined as one for the cases and zero for the controls, the risk scores for the cases were higher than those for the controls. Inspection of the distributions of cases and controls by several of the risk factors, in simplified form, within five strata of the discriminant score allows an appraisal of the stratification as a means of controlling confounding (Table A3.2). For example, a history of a previous stillbirth is recorded for 9.0 per cent of the cases and 2.3 per cent of the controls, and thus the estimation of the association of anencephalus occurrence with another factor based on the whole sample may be confounded by stillbirth history. However, within each stratum of risk a similar proportion of the cases and of the controls have a history of a previous stillbirth; thus if the association of risk with another factor is estimated within each of the strata of risk score and then a summary estimate of association is computed over the five strata, confounding by stillbirth history as well as by other factors will be controlled.

The calculations for one risk factor—maternal residence in Halifax—will be described in more detail. For the factor city of residence, Vancouver was chosen as the reference category and thus the 14 cities were represented in the linear discriminant function by 13 binary variables, residence in Vancouver being represented by all of these variables being zero. To estimate the effects of city of residence, the risk score with residence set at Vancouver was used; the risk score was thus calculated from the discriminant function ignoring the contribution of the 13 variables representing places of residence other than Vancouver. The subjects were then divided into five strata by this risk score. A cross-tabulation of case–control status by city of residence within strata of risk score was generated. Various analyses were applied to these cross-tabulations using the 'Relrisk' programme developed by Dr K. J. Rothman at the Harvard School of Public Health. The numbers of cases and of controls in the 'exposure' city of Halifax and the reference city of Vancouver in each of the five risk strata are shown in Table A3.3. The odds ratio (Cornfield 1951) calculated from the total number of cases and controls is $(57 \times 621)/(170 \times 119)$ or 1.75; this estimates the unadjusted risk ratio. The stratum-specific risk ratios range from 0.81 to 2.24. We used the method of Zelen (1971) to test for homogeneity of risk ratio over the strata; here it yields a non-significant result. This test has since been criticized (Mantel, Brown, and Byar 1977) and an alternative test proposed (Halperin, Ware, Byar, Mantel, Brown, Koziol, Gail, and Green 1977). Three estimates of the unconfounded risk ratio are shown, those given by the methods of Mantel and Haenszel (1959), the iterative maximum likelihood procedure of Gart (1970), and the standardized mortality ratio of Miettinen (1972, 1972*a*). The 95 per cent confidence limits of Gart's estimate are shown and limits for the Mantel–Haenszel estimate may be calculated assuming a log–normal distribution of risk ratio. Where Z is the square root of the chi-square statistic, these are given by

$$\text{limits} = \exp\{\ln \hat{RR}(1 \pm 1.96/Z)\}$$

TABLE A3.1 *Distributions of discriminant scores, based on all variables for cases and controls, Canadian 14-city study*

Range of score	Number of cases	Number of controls
−2.118 to −1.897	0	7
−1.897 to −0.425	278	1936
−0.425 to 0.076	278	1448
0.076 to 0.570	278	865
0.570 to 1.260	277	483
1.260 to 4.972	277	261
4.972 to 5.271	3	0

Categories of risk score are based on quintile divisions of the number of cases within the common range of scores. A higher score implies a higher rate of anencephalus.
See also Figure A3.1.

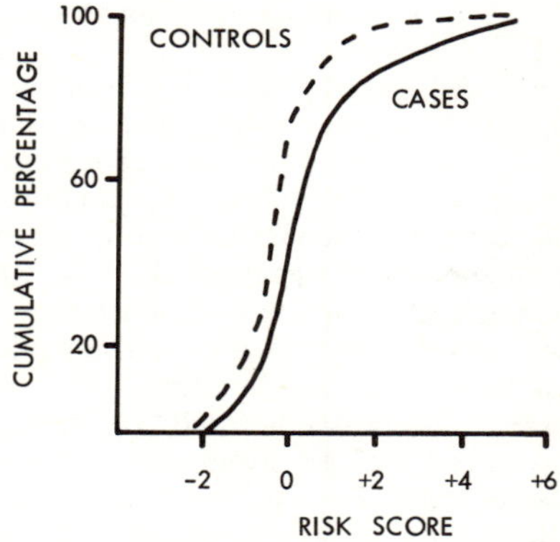

FIG. A3.1. Distributions of linear discriminant function risk scores relating to 1391 cases of anencephalus (stillbirths and infant deaths) and a random sample of 5000 livebirth controls calculated by including all study variables (city of residence, year and month of birth, legitimacy, maternal age, parity, number of previous stillbirths, number of previous livebirths, ethoric group, plurality of birth, and place of delivery—Canadian 14-city study.

TABLE A3.2 *Percentage distribution of cases and controls exposed to selected risk factors by stratum of risk score computed using all factors, Canadian 14-city study*

		Stratum of risk score											
		1		2		3		4		5		Total	
Factor	Category	Cases	Controls	Cases	Controls	Cases	Controls	Cases	Controls	Cases	Controls	Cases	Controls
Place of birth	Vancouver	19.8	17.5	12.6	13.5	4.0	5.7	2.5	3.5	4.0	6.5	8.6	12.5
	Winnipeg	2.9	3.7	11.2	10.6	15.1	15.1	15.1	13.5	9.4	8.4	10.7	8.9
	Windsor	5.8	5.1	3.2	3.6	5.0	4.9	6.1	6.0	4.0	5.7	4.8	4.7
	Quebec	2.5	2.5	8.3	7.2	11.2	14.8	11.2	8.3	16.6	13.4	10.0	7.1
	Halifax	2.2	1.7	5.4	3.6	6.8	6.7	2.5	2.3	3.6	6.5	4.1	3.4
Year	1950–4	5.0	6.2	18.7	17.9	34.5	39.8	59.0	58.5	51.6	42.4	33.9	22.3
Parity	0	16.2	12.1	50.7	53.2	65.1	60.2	64.0	54.4	20.2	24.0	43.3	37.1
Previous stillbirths	1	0	0	0	0	0	0.1	1.4	3.8	43.3	35.9	9.0	2.3
Infant deaths	1	0	0.1	1.4	0.3	2.5	2.3	15.8	19.2	41.5	45.0	12.2	4.7
Ethnic group	Canadian/ unknown	32.0	25.2	20.1	22.1	7.6	7.8	4.0	6.5	7.9	10.3	14.3	18.7
	Irish	4.3	5.0	10.1	8.8	11.9	11.4	13.3	14.0	15.2	14.1	11.0	8.5
	French	6.1	6.7	13.7	13.2	20.9	24.1	21.2	19.0	30.3	24.4	18.4	13.7
	Russian	5.0	8.8	4.3	2.4	2.2	1.9	0.4	1.9	1.1	2.3	2.6	4.7

Stratum 5 represents the stratum of highest risk.

which here yields limits of 1.10 and 2.27, similar to those obtained by Gart's method. The standardized mortality ratio is a better estimate of association when the risk ratio is not uniform over the strata. However, non-uniformity implies an interaction between the factor under study and one or more of the other factors contributing to the risk score, and so a summary measure in this situation is difficult to interpret. The confounding risk ratio (Miettinen 1972) provides an estimate of the amount of confounding which has been removed by the stratification. This is the ratio of the crude risk ratio to the standardized mortality ratio, and is 1 when there is no confounding.

TABLE A3.3 *Estimation of the risk of anencephalus in births to mothers resident in Halifax compared to births to those resident in Vancouver*

Stratum of risk score	Halifax Cases	Halifax Controls	Vancouver Cases	Vancouver Controls	Stratum-specific risk ratio
1 (low risk)	4	29	26	153	0.81
2	15	42	28	176	2.24
3	15	51	29	185	1.88
4	12	29	20	75	1.55
5 (high risk)	11	19	16	32	1.16
Total	57	170	119	621	

Crude risk ratio	= 1.75	
Heterogeneity chi-square (4 d.f.)	= 3.48	
Maximum likelihood estimate	= 1.59	95% two-sided confidence limits = 1.10, 2.29
Mantel–Haenszel estimate	= 1.58	
Standardized mortality ratio	= 1.55	
Confounding risk ratio	= 1.13	
Mantel–Haenszel normal deviate	= 2.47	p value (one tail) = 0.007

Effect modification

The term 'effect modification' is used to describe a situation in which the association of anencephalus risk with one factor is modified by the presence of another factor. The method of stratification by a multivariate risk score allows the study of joint effects of two or more factors. To study two factors simultaneously, the discriminant score is computed setting both factors to 'non-exposure' or reference categories, and stratification is carried out in the usual way. For each stratum, tables of the distributions of cases and controls by the two factors under consideration are generated. Rather than using summary estimates of risk ratio, a simpler presentation is possible by computing category-specific mortality rates using direct standardization over the strata of the multivariate score. The standard population used was the total number of controls in each stratum. These rates and their standard errors are derived as follows (Elwood, J. M., Raman, and Mousseau 1978).

Let there be A anencephalics and B livebirths in the total population under study who are in the relevant three-factor-specific category (the three factors being the two under study and the risk score). As the case group includes all cases of anencephalus in the population, and as the control group is a random sample of all livebirths with a known sampling fraction f, the numbers of cases and controls in the category are A and b respectively, where $E(b) = f \cdot B$.

The mortality rate in the category r_i is thus Af/b. If a number of these category-specific rates are standardized over i strata of risk score, each with a standard population n_i, the direct standardized rate is equal to

$$\frac{\sum_{i=1}^{I} r_i n_i}{\sum_{i=1}^{I} n_i}.$$

The sampling error of the category-specific mortality rate is determined by the variance of $1/b$, as A has no sampling variation. Considering b as a binomial random variable, being taken from a population B with sampling fraction f, then

$$\text{variance } (b) = B \cdot f \cdot (1-f).$$

The variance of $1/b$ can be approximated by the first term of a Taylor series as

$$\left[-\frac{1}{E(b)^2}\right]^2 \cdot \text{var}(b)$$

$$= \frac{1}{B^4 \cdot f^4}\{B \cdot f(1-f)\}$$

$$= \frac{(1-f)}{b^3},$$

and the variance of $A \cdot f/b$ is thus

$$(A \cdot f)^2 \cdot \text{var}(1/b) = \left[\frac{A \cdot f}{b}\right]^2 \cdot \frac{1-f}{b}.$$

In the current data $f = b/B = 5000/1\,193\,600 = 0.004189$, so $(1-f)$ can be approximated to 1, hence the variance of the category-specific rate r_i is given by $\text{var}(r_i) = r_i^2/b$.
The variance of the direct standardized rate is given (Armitage 1971) by

$$\frac{\sum_{i=1}^{I} \{n_i^2 \cdot \text{var}(r_i)\}}{(\sum n_i)^2}.$$

The standard error of the standardized rate is of value in showing the stability of an individual rate. It is not of great value in the assessment of the existence and nature of an interactive effect as this depends on the presence of regular trends or patterns in the mortality rates in the several cells of a two-way table rather than on the significance of differences between a particular pair or group of rates.

This study has several examples of effect modification, which are discussed in the relevant chapters. The differences in the associations of risk with several factors between first and later births are perhaps the most interesting. The combination of the multivariate confounder score technique and the use of a known sampling fraction of controls makes the comprehension and illustration of effect modification straightforward in our study. This contrasts with the difficulties inherent in understanding the meaning of an interaction term in some other multivariate models, even though the statistical significance of such a term may easily be demonstrated. For example, the distributions of cases and controls, and the derived anencephalus mortality rates, by year, season, and number of previous livebirths are shown in Table A3.4. Several effects are apparent. In all season–parity categories except one the rates are lower in the later years. In all year–parity categories except one, the rates are higher in winter. In all year–season categories, the lowest rates are at parities 1–3 with higher (in one instance equal) rates at parity 0 or at parity 4 or more. However, these results are uncontrolled for other factors such as maternal age, ethnic origin, or place of residence. The standardized rates in which other factors have been controlled demonstrate effect modification (Table A3.5). Both the winter

TABLE A3.4 *Canadian 14-city study: numbers of cases and controls and crude mortality rates from anencephalus per 1000 births, by year and season of birth and number of previous livebirths born to the mother*

			Number of previous livebirths		
Year	Season		0	1–3	4+
1950–9	Summer	Cases	165	187	31
		Controls	449	682	113
		Rate	1.54	1.15	1.15
	Winter	Cases	190	175	37
		Controls	397	610	120
		Rate	2.00	1.20	1.29
1960–9	Summer	Cases	115	130	41
		Controls	548	663	143
		Rate	0.88	0.82	1.20
	Winter	Cases	131	143	40
		Controls	457	648	164
		Rate	1.20	0.92	1.02

TABLE A3.5 *Standardized mortality rates from anencephalus per 1000 livebirths by year and season of birth and number of previous livebirths*

		Number of previous livebirths		
Year	Season	0	1–3	4+
1950–9	Summer	1.54 (0.12)	1.06 (0.05)	0.66 (0.07)
	Winter	2.70 (0.61)	1.06 (0.06)	0.59 (0.05)
1960–9	Summer	1.24 (0.12)	1.10 (0.08)	0.85 (0.07)
	Winter	1.96 (0.31)	1.15 (0.08)	0.90 (0.08)

Rates are standardized over 5 strata of risk score with year, month, and parity set to referent levels. Standard population taken as total number of controls in each stratum. Risk-score controls for city of residence, history of stillbirths or infant deaths, maternal age, ethnic origin, legitimacy, and kind of birth and place of delivery. Standard errors are given in parentheses.

excess and the decrease in prevalence over time are now seen to be restricted to first births (parity 0). In the other parity categories, there is no seasonal variation and the anencephalus rates show a small increase over time. The U-type association of risk with parity is replaced by a simple negative association.

Binary multiple regression

We applied two other multivariate models to the same data as analysed by Miettinen's method in order to allow empiric comparisons of our results. A multivariate model specifically incorporating binary variables has been described by Feldstein (1965, 1966). The method has been used for estimating the independent associations of several factors with pregnancy outcomes (Feldstein and Butler 1965), infant mortality (Elwood, J. H., MacKenzie, and Cran 1971), perinatal and post-perinatal mortality (Elwood, J. H., MacKenzie, and Cran 1974*a*, 1974*b*).

The binary multiple regression model is the same as that of a least squares regression technique using continuous variables and may be represented as:

$$\mathbf{Y} = \mathbf{X}\boldsymbol{\beta} + \mathbf{U},$$

where $\mathbf{Y}$ is the vector of observations of the dependent variable, $\mathbf{X}$ the matrix of observations on the independent variables, $\boldsymbol{\beta}$ the vector of regression coefficients, and $\mathbf{U}$ the vector of stochastic errors. A least-squares technique is used to derive the vector of estimated regression coefficients $\mathbf{b}$. Of the assumptions required for optimal estimation, those of independence of observations and additivity of terms are not affected by the binary nature of the variables. However, the assumptions of normality of the distributions of variables, and constancy of the error variance, are not fulfilled. Thus the least-squares estimates of the regression coefficients will be unbiased, but the statistical significance of the regression coefficients cannot be tested in the usual way. Feldstein (1966) has shown that the variance of the error term is not constant but is given by

$$\begin{aligned}\mathrm{var}(u_i) = E(u_i)^2 &= (-\mathbf{X}_i'\boldsymbol{\beta})^2(1-\mathbf{X}_i'\boldsymbol{\beta}) + (1-\mathbf{X}_i'\boldsymbol{\beta})^2(\mathbf{X}_i'\boldsymbol{\beta}) \\ &= (\mathbf{X}_i'\boldsymbol{\beta})(1-\mathbf{X}_i'\boldsymbol{\beta}).\end{aligned}$$

This heteroscedasticity results in non-optimal but unbiased estimates of β; a generalized least-squares method will give greater efficiency (Johnston 1963), but in large data sets the small improvement is not worth the large amount of extra calculations required (Feldstein 1966; Elwood, J. H. *et al.* 1971).

The estimated regression coefficients are derived from

$$\mathbf{b} = (\mathbf{X}'\mathbf{X})^{-1}\mathbf{X}'\mathbf{Y}.$$

The matrix $(\mathbf{X}'\mathbf{X})$ and the vector $\mathbf{X}'\mathbf{Y}$ take simple forms and may be derived from simple cross-tabulations. $\mathbf{X}'\mathbf{X}$ is a $(k+1)$ by $(k+1)$ matrix, where k is the number of regressor variables, and an element $x_{i,j}$ is the number of subjects for which both variables i and j are equal to 1. $\mathbf{X}'\mathbf{Y}$ has elements x_i, where x_i is the number of 'cases'—in this case anencephalics—where x_i is equal to 1.

As a single factor (e.g. age) with $t+1$ subcategories is represented by a number t of binary variables, the regression coefficients cannot be interpreted as they stand. Feldstein defined adjusted deviations which represent the deviation from the overall rate in the study population for subjects in each category of the factor.

For the category i of a factor with $t+1$ subcategories, the estimated deviation d_i is given by

$$d_i = b_i - \frac{1}{N}\sum_{j=1}^{t} b_j n_j,$$

where b_i is the estimated regression coefficient for subclass i, n_j is the number of subjects in subclass j, and N is the total number of subjects. The estimated proportional deviation is $d_i/\bar{y}$, where $\bar{y}$ is the overall rate in the study group. For the default subgroup of the factor, represented by all variables being zero, the deviation is estimated by

$$d_{t+1} = \frac{1}{N}\sum_{j=1}^{t} b_j n_j,$$

i.e., b_{t+1} is taken as zero (Elwood, J. H. 1969).

The standard errors of these adjusted deviations can be derived from the error variance matrix

$$\mathbf{V} = \text{var}(\mathbf{b}) = S^2(\mathbf{X'X})^{-1},$$

where

$$\mathbf{S}^2 = (\mathbf{y'y} - \mathbf{b'X'y})/(N - k - 1).$$

For the factor under consideration the relevant submatrix of $\mathbf{V}$ is $\mathbf{V}_1$ and

$$\mathbf{W}'_i = \left[-\frac{n_1}{N}, -\frac{n_2}{N}, \ldots, \left(1 - \frac{n_i}{N}\right), \ldots, -\frac{n_r}{N}\right]$$

and

$$\text{var}(d_i) = \mathbf{W}'_i(\mathbf{V}_1)\mathbf{W}_i,$$

thus giving the variance of the adjusted deviation d_i. As these deviations are not normally distributed, a precise test of significance cannot be performed; however, the ratio of the deviation to its standard error may be used as an asymptotic test. To provide an approximate significance test for the association between risk and one category of a factor under study, we have compared the risk difference between that category and the reference category

$$\bar{y}(d_i - d_r)$$

to its standard error

$$\bar{y} \cdot \sqrt{(\text{var } d_r + \text{var } d_i - 2 \text{ covar } d_r d_i)}$$

making a further approximation by ignoring the covariance term.

Results expressing the risk in one category of a risk factor in terms of the overall risk in all subjects can be converted into risk ratio estimates by taking one category as the referent: the anencephalus mortality rate in this category is $\bar{y}(1 + d_r)$ where d_r is the proportional deviation and $\bar{y}$ the mortality rate in the study population, while the relative risk in any other category i is given by

$$\begin{aligned}\text{relative risk} &= \bar{y}(1 + d_i)/\bar{y}(1 + d_r) \\ &= (1 + d_i)/(1 + d_r).\end{aligned}$$

The multiple logistic model

Ideally, in constructing a mathematical model to relate the risk of disease (given by the prevalence rate at birth in our context) to a number of putative risk factors, the form of the model should be decided on the grounds of a precise biological hypothesis specifying the relationship between risk factors and outcome. In practice however, there is rarely sufficient information available to justify the use of one specific model, and the type of model used is thus decided on arbitrary grounds. Moreover, is most real situations, the predictions of different models will be sufficiently similar and the amount of data sufficiently limited that several models will adequately fit the data and even a post hoc decision as to the best model may not be possible.

The multiple logistic model, developed by Cornfield (1962), Cox (1970), and others, relates a linear combination of putative risk factors x_i to the logit of disease risk p and takes the form

$$\ln\left(\frac{p_j}{1-p_j}\right)=\alpha+\beta_1 x_{1j}+\cdots+\beta_n x_{nj},$$

where p_j is the probability of disease in the jth individual, x_{ij} is the value of the ith risk factor for that individual, and α and the β_i are the parameters of the model. This function has been used extensively in epidemiological work, both for prediction of outcome in individuals and in case–control studies where the aim is to identify risk factors and estimate their associations with outcome. The model has certain attractive properties. The logit transformation ensures that the maximum range of the dependent variable $\ln\left(\frac{p}{1-p}\right)$, $-\infty$ to $+\infty$, transforms to values of p limited by 0 and 1; thus non-admissible values of p cannot be generated. If a dichotomous risk factor is represented by a binary variable x_i with values 0 or 1, the odds ratio associated with that variable is given simply by the exponential of the coefficient, exp (b_i).

Two somewhat different approaches have led to computational methods which may be used to estimate the coefficient β_i of the logistic function. One invokes the relationship between the multiple logistic function and the linear discriminant function. As mentioned, the discriminant function computes for each subject a discriminant score y_j from a linear combination of predictor variables, using estimated coefficients b_i chosen to maximize the separation of two populations: the model is thus

$$y_j=b_1x_{1j}+b_2x_{2j}\cdots+b_kx_{kj}.$$

The discriminant score is related to the risk of disease. An expression which will estimate the risk in one subject was derived by Cornfield (1962) using Bayesian reasoning. The probability of a subject in population 1 having a set of x values (x_1 $\ldots .x_k$) is f_1 (**t**) and the probability of a subject in population 0 having that set is f_0 (**t**) where (**t**) represents the vector (x_1 .... x_k). If the prior probability of being in population 1 is p, then the probability p_j of a subject j being in population 1 given the vector (x_{1j}. . . . x_{kj}) is

$$\begin{aligned}p_j&=p\cdot f_1(\mathbf{t})/\{p\cdot f_1(\mathbf{t})+(1-p)\cdot f_0(\mathbf{t})\}\\&=1/\{1+R(\mathbf{t})(1-p)/p\},\end{aligned}$$

where $R(\mathbf{t}) = f_0(\mathbf{t})/f_1(\mathbf{t})$, i.e. the likelihood ratio associated with (**t**). The risk of disease in the jth subject is given by

$$p_j=1/\left\{1+\exp\left(-\alpha'-\sum_{i=1}^{k}\beta_i x_{ij}\right)\right\}$$

or equivalently

$$\ln\left(\frac{p_j}{1-p_j}\right)=\alpha'+\sum_{i=1}^{k}\beta_i x_{ij}.$$

This derivation shows that the multiple logistic function is a reasonable model, and it may be easily seen that the coefficients $\boldsymbol{\beta}_i$ are given by the coefficients of the discriminant function, which can be estimated by non-iterative procedures. However, this derivation assumes that in the diseased and non-diseased populations the variables $(x_1 \ldots . x_k)$ are multivariate normal, with the same variances and covariances, but with different means. Such distributional criteria are unlikely to be met in practice—for example, important risk factors may be binary. The consequences of departures from normality were examined by Truett *et al.* (1967). Using 12 years of data from the Framingham study they compared the observed numbers of subjects in deciles of risk for coronary heart disease with the numbers expected by applying the multiple logistic model using seven predictor variables, of which five were continuous (e.g. age, systolic blood pressure), one discrete (cigarettes smoked per day, in four groups), and one binary (electrocardiogram normal or abnormal). Agreement between observed and expected numbers was good, and it was shown that for the purposes of prediction, a sufficient criterion is that the linear combination of predictor variables $y = a + \sum_{i=1}^{k} b_i x_i$ be univariate normal. Approximate normality is likely even with a number of dichotomous variables, given a large number of subjects, as shown by the central limit theorem (Munroe 1951). However, for interpretation of an individual discriminant coefficient, the assumption of normality of the associated independent variable is still important.

Other approaches to the multiple logistic function avoid distributional assumption. Walker and Duncan (1967) demonstrated that if we assume the multiple logistic model is applicable, an iterative technique provides maximum likelihood estimates of α and $\boldsymbol{\beta}_j$ without any assumption of normality of the x variables. Halperin, Blackwelder, and Verter (1971) showed that these estimates are asymptotically unbiased for a dichotomous predictor variable. The discriminant function estimates will be asymptotically biased. With multiple variables, the discriminant function estimates of those coefficients which are zero will not converge to zero if two or more of the other independent variables have non-zero coefficients. Halperin and colleagues compared empirically results obtained by the discriminant function method of Truett *et al.* (1967) and by the method of Walker and Duncan (1967) applied to the same data. They found that where the assumptions of multivariate normality and equal variance-covariance matrices were not met, regression coefficients estimated by the two methods often were substantially different, both for discrete and continuous variables, but the ratios of the estimated coefficients to their standard errors had less variation. The absolute values of the coefficients estimated by the discriminant function model tended to be higher than those estimated by maximum likelihood. Halperin and colleagues concluded that the discriminant function approach gave results similar to those from maximum likelihood in terms of identifying statistically significant risk factors, but that the estimates of the magnitude of the coefficients could be misleading. Clearly, in a situation having several discrete or binary predictor variables, as in our study, the Walker–Duncan method is preferable. However, it is an iterative procedure involving considerably more complex computations and we were unable to use it because of financial and time constraints.

The logistic model assumes that the logit of disease risk is related to a linear combination of predictor variables. This implies a multiplicative model in terms of relative risks; the relative risk in the presence of two factors is equal to the product of the relative risks for each factor separately. The different sets of parameters $\boldsymbol{\beta}$ are linearly related to one another for the discriminant function, binary regression and logistic regression models in populations where the joint distributions of the covariates are multivariate normal. In finite sets of data the estimated *b*s will not be identical as fitting algorithms are different which will lead to non-linear variation in the estimates. If it is desired to confer an additive structure on the covariates of the model then a regression model may be used where the dependent variable is not an indicator zero–one variable but is a function which is directly proportional to the rate. Such an additive regression model was used in our pilot study of drinking water composition, the dependent variable being the mortality rate from anencephalus in each city studied (Section 19).

Comparisons of the results given by three methods of analysis

The point estimates of risk ratio for each category of each factor examined are shown in Table A3.6 as produced by each of the three methods of analysis (stratification by a multivariate risk score, binary multiple regression, and a multiple logistic model). For most factors, the estimates of risk ratio produced by each method are similar. Where there is a disparity, usually the estimates given by binary regression are more conservative (nearer to the null value of one) than are those given by the two other methods. The differences are considerable where the risk ratios are substantially different from one, for example for stillbirth or infant death history. Here the highest estimates are given by the logistic model, where a discriminant function was used to estimate the coefficients.

We also compared the significance levels given by the three methods, using the results of the Mantel–Haenszel (1959) or Mantel (1963) tests in conjunction with stratification by a multivariate risk score, and the asymptotic tests for the binary regression and multiple logistic models. The three methods of analysis show very little difference in terms of the factors showing significant associations with anencephalus (Table A3.6). Of the 45 variables examined, there is disagreement between the methods in terms of significance as the 5 per cent level in only four, and in a further six variables the level of significance reported (expressed as $p<0.05$, 0.01, or 0.001) varies between the three methods. None of the three methods of analysis appears consistently to give different results than the others. Thus in this study, each of the three methods indicate the same factors as having significant associations with anencephalus risk, although the estimates of risk ratio produced vary between the methods in instances where the risk ratio is considerably different from one.

The three multivariate models applied to the case–control study were chosen because each allows the consideration of binary independent variables. The binary regression model has been extensively investigated, both from theoretical and applied aspects (Feldstein 1966; Feldstein and Butler 1965; Elwood, J. H., MacKenzie, and Cran 1971, 1974). It can be shown that the point estimates of the regression coefficients are unbiased, although they are not of optimal efficiency owing to the heteroscedasticity of the independent variables (Feldstein 1966; Elwood, J. H. *et al.* 1971). The estimated regression coefficients may be used to calculate the deviation between the risk associated with each category of a factor and the mean risk in the population. This type of result is reasonably simple to present and understand but the extension used in this work to produce category-specific risks relative to the risk in one reference category may be regarded as somewhat clearer, especially if the factor has a few categories with greatly different numbers of subjects.

In fitting a multiple logistic model, the use of the linear discriminant function to obtain estimates of the coefficients assumes normality of the independent variables. When this condition is violated, as here, the results are biased even in the large sample case. In the data used by Halperin *et al.* (1971), the risk-ratio estimates derived by the discriminant function were larger in absolute value than those obtained by the Walker–Duncan iterative procedure which does not assume multivariate normality. In our study the risk-ratio estimates based on a discriminant

TABLE A3.6 *Canadian 14-city study: point estimates of the crude risk ratios of the associations with anencephalus of each factor studied, the risk ratios obtained after control of confounding effects of all other factors by three methods and approximate significance levels*

		Point estimates of risk ratio				Approximate tests of significance		
Factor	Category	Crude	SMVRS†	Binary‡	Logistic§	SMVRS†	Binary‡	Logistic§
City	Vancouver (R)	1.0	1.0	1.0	1.0			
	Edmonton	1.18	1.17	1.15	1.19	—	—	—
	Calgary	0.98	0.97	0.99	0.98	—	—	—
	Regina	0.78	0.77	0.87	0.86	—	—	—
	Saskatoon	0.98	1.02	1.17	1.14	—	—	—
	Winnipeg	1.76	1.74	1.56	1.96	***	***	***
	Hamilton	1.73	1.86	1.74	2.37	***	***	***
	Kitchener	1.53	1.73	1.77	2.46	**	***	***
	London	1.44	1.57	1.61	2.04	**	***	***
	Windsor	1.49	1.54	1.58	1.97	**	***	***
	Ottawa	2.07	2.24	1.89	2.85	***	***	***
	Quebec	2.02	1.67	1.48	1.76	***	***	***
	St John	2.55	2.46	1.97	3.12	***	***	***
	Halifax	1.75	1.59	1.35	1.51	**	—	*
Year	1950–4 (R)	1.0	1.0	1.0	1.0			
	1955–9	0.60	0.64	0.71	0.56	}***M	***	***
	1960–4	0.57	0.80	0.82	0.70		***	***
	1965–9	0.52	0.67	0.76	0.61		***	***

TABLE A3.6 *continued*

Factor	Category	Point estimates of risk ratio				Approximate tests of significance		
		Crude	SMVRS†	Binary‡	Logistic§	SMVRS†	Binary‡	Logistic§
Month	January–March (R)	1.0	1.0	1.0	1.0			
	April–June	0.79	0.77	0.83	0.74	**	***	***
	July–September	0.85	0.83	0.91	0.80	*	**	*
	October–December	0.92	0.90	0.93	0.87	—	—	—
Legitimacy	Legitimate (R)	1.0	1.0	1.0	1.0			
	Illegitimate	1.04	1.04	0.99	0.99	—	—	—
Maternal age	≤19	1.19	1.18	1.10	1.18	—	—	—
	20–4 (R)	1.0	1.0	1.0	1.0			
	25–9	1.03	1.02	1.04	1.07	—	—	—
	30–4	0.89	0.88	0.98	0.97	—	—	—
	35+	1.16	1.19	1.15	1.26	—	*	*
Previous livebirths	0 (R)	1.0	1.0	1.0	1.0			
	1	0.75	0.64	0.76	0.61	***M (1–4+)	***	***
	2	0.72	0.60	0.70	0.55		***	***
	3	0.80	0.59	0.66	0.51		***	***
	4+	0.84	0.49	0.54	0.40		***	***
Stillbirths	0 (R)	1.0	1.0	1.0	1.0	***M (0–2+)		
	1	4.30	3.91	2.37	8.45		***	***
	2+	3.11	3.09	2.05	5.17		***	***
Infant deaths	0 (R)	1.0	1.0	1.0	1.0	***M (0–2+)		
	1	2.89	3.25	2.74	5.60		***	***
	2+	4.94	5.98	2.83	16.00		***	***

TABLE A3.6 *continued*

Factor	Category	Point estimates of risk ratio				Approximate tests of significance		
		Crude	SMVRS†	Binary‡	Logistic§	SMVRS†	Binary‡	Logistic§
Maternal ethnic origin	England and Wales (R)	1.0	1.0	1.0	1.0			
	Ireland	1.04	0.99	0.99	0.98	—	—	—
	Scotland	0.85	0.89	0.93	0.87	—	—	—
	France	1.08	0.95	0.94	0.90	—	—	—
	Germany	0.68	0.83	0.88	0.80	—	**	—
	Central Europe	0.62	0.64	0.72	0.59	**	***	**
	Scandinavia	0.63	0.81	0.86	0.76	—	—	—
	Mediterranean	0.79	0.89	0.89	0.82	—	—	—
	Russia	0.44	0.49	0.62	0.48	***	***	***
	Oriental	0.61	0.81	0.89	0.82	—	—	—
	Other	0.47	0.50	0.59	0.45	**	***	**
	Canada/unknown	0.61	0.61	0.57	0.44	***	***	***
Kind of birth	Single (R)	1.0	1.0	1.0	1.0			
	Multiple	0.96	1.07	1.07	1.13	—	—	—
Delivery	Hospital (R)	1.0	1.0	1.0	1.0			
	Home	1.97	1.2	1.19	1.37	—	**	—

* = $p<0.05$ or ratio of result:standard error >2
** = $p<0.01$ or ratio of result:standard error >2.6
*** = $p<0.001$ or ratio of result:standard error >3.3

† Stratification by a multivariate risk score: Mantel–Haenszel estimates or, where a Mantel test for linear trend is used, maximum-likelihood estimates. Significance values based on the Mantel–Haenszel χ^2 or on the Mantel normal deviate (marked M).

‡ Point estimates from a binary regression analysis including all study factors. 'Significance' levels are approximate, based on the ratio of the difference in deviations in the test and referent categories to the pooled standard error, for a reduced regression model.

§ Logistic model using the linear discriminant function. Risk-ratio estimate given as the exponential of the discriminant coefficient; 'significance levels' are based on the ratio of the coefficient to its standard error.

function were higher than those produced by the binary regression model, especially when the latter risk ratios were substantially different from unity. Significance testing of the estimates obtained by the discriminant function, as with binary multiple regression, is possible only in an approximate fashion by comparing the value of the discriminant coefficient to its standard error. The significance of a factor represented by a group of variables may be assessed in either method from discriminant functions or regressions performed with and without that factor.

Analysis based on stratification by a multivariate confounder score is a fairly new technique, and the conditions under which it is adequate have not been defined. The methods of obtaining risk-ratio estimates from stratified data have been shown to reduce efficiently confounding by the factor on which stratification is based (Mantel and Haenszel 1959; Cochran 1965, 1968; Mantel 1963). The validity of the analysis used here is conditional on the validity of the linear discriminant function in ranking subjects according to risk. The estimates of the discriminant coefficients are biased by the non-normality of the independent variables, but the resultant errors in the rank order of risk scores are unlikely to be of as much consequence as are errors in the risk-ratio estimates based directly on the value of the discriminant coefficients. In the present context the similarity of the results based on stratification by a multivariate risk score and on binary multiple regression suggests that the errors involved in the computation of the risk scores are not large. However, further work is needed to assess the robustness of the method under such conditions as the use of non-normal and heteroscedastic variables. The tests used to assess statistical significance do not take into account any error in the categorization of subjects into strata of risk, and some adjustment may be necessary in this regard. The method, however, has certain advantages. The discriminant function used need only be computed once, and further analysis is simple and flexible; the results may be expressed in terms of risk ratios or deviations from the mean rate, or as absolute measures of risk if, as in this case, the controls are a random sample from a population of known size. Statistical tests may be applied to either one category of a factor or to test for a trend in risk over all categories. Although such a statement is subjective, it could be claimed that the form of the final results is more easily understood by a non-statistical audience than are the results of other multivariate techniques. A further advantage is the ability of the method to study interactions. Methods such as binary multiple regression allow the detection of interactions by the inclusion in the regression model of suitable terms, and several other approaches to the detection of interactions in multidimensional contingency tables are known (for example Darroch 1962; Plackett 1969; Bishop 1969). However, in epidemiological work it is desirable not only to detect such interactions but to be able to describe their form, and inspection of estimated rates displayed in two- or three-dimensional tables is a useful technique. The stratification method allows calculation of such rates standardized for all factors except the two or three under study. Thus stratification by a multivariate risk score appears to have some advantages over other multivariate techniques but further examination is required.

References

ABELEV, G. I. (1971). Alpha-fetoprotein in ontogenesis and its association with malignant tumors. *Adv. Cancer Res.* **14**, 295–358.

—— ALPERT, E., HULL, E. W., MASSEYEFF, R., DE NECHAND, B., TATARINOV, Y., AND URIEL, J. (1970). Les proteines sériques foeto-spécifiques. Recommendations en vue d'une normalisation de la terminologie. *Bull. Org. mond. Santé* **43**, 311–12.

ÃBERG, A., MITELMAN, F., CANTZ, M., AND GEHLER, J. (1978). Cardiac puncture of fetus with Hurler's disease avoiding abortion of unaffected co-twin. (letter) *Lancet* **ii**, 990–1.

ABRAMOVICH, D. R. (1968). The volume of amniotic fluid in early pregnancy. *J. Obstet. Gynaec. Br. Commonw.* **75**, 728–31.

ABRAMOVICI, A., SHAKLAI, M., AND PINKHAS, J. (1978). Myeloschisis in a six weeks embryo of a leukaemic woman treated by Busulfan. *Teratology* **18**, 241–6.

ACHESON, E. D. (1967). *Medical record linkage.* Published for the Nuffield Provincial Hospitals Trust by the Oxford University Press, London.

ADAMS, M. S. AND NISWANDER, J. D. (1968). Health of the American Indian: congenital defects. *Eugen. Q.* **15**, 227–34.

ADELMAN, H. B. (1937). Experimental studies on the development of the eye. IV. The effects of the partial and complete excision of the prechordal substrate on the development of the eyes of *Ambylstoma punctatum. J. exp. Zool.* **75**, 199–238.

ADINOLFI, A., ADINOLFI, M., AND COHEN, S. (1971). Isolation and characterisation of human foetal-α-globulin (α_1F) from foetal and hepatoma sera. *Biochim. biophys. Acta* **251**, 197–207.

——, —— AND LESSOF, M. H. (1975). Alpha-feto-protein during development and in disease. *J. med. Genet.* **12**, 138–51.

AGAR, W. E., DRUMMOND F. H., AND TIEGS, O. W. (1935). A first report on a test of McDougall's Lamarkian Experiment on the training of rats. *J. exp. Biol.* **12**, 191–211.

AHLFELD, F. (1880–2). *Die Missbildungen des Menschen*. F. W. Grunow, Leipzig.

AHLGREN, M., KÄLLÉN, B., AND RANNEVIK, G. (1976). Outcome of pregnancy after clomiphene therapy. *Acta obstet. gynec. scand.* **55**, 371–5.

AKESSON, H. O., SMITH, G. F., AND THRYBOM, B. R. (1970). Twinning and associated stillbirth in Sweden 1871 to 1960. *Hereditas* **64**, 193–8.

ALADJEIN, S. (1976). Fetoscopy: an experimental approach. In *Intrauterine fetal visualization. A multidisciplinary approach*. Edited by M. M. Kaback and C. Valenti. Excerpta med. (Amst.), p. 157–61.

ALLAN, L. D., FERGUSON-SMITH, M. A., DONALD, I., SWEET, E. M., AND GIBSON, A. A. M. (1973). Amniotic-fluid alpha-fetoprotein in the antenatal diagnosis of spina bifida. *Lancet* **ii**, 522–5,

ALLEN, G. AND SCHACHTER, J. (1971). Ease of conception in mothers of twins. *Soc. Biol.* **18**, 18–27.

ALLUM, N. (1975). *Spina bifida. The treatment and care of spina bifida children.* George Allen and Unwin Ltd., London.

ALPERT, E. AND COSTON, R. L. (1975). Serum alpha-fetoprotein (AFP) in benign and malignant gastrointestinal diseases: evaluation of an immunoenzymatic assay. *Clin. chim. Acta* **58**, 77–83.

—— AND ZUCKERMAN, J. (1970). Absence of alpha-1-fetoprotein antigen or antibody in maternal sera. (letter). *Lancet* **ii**, 465.

—— HERSHBERG, R., SCHURR, P. H., AND ISSELBACHER, K. J. (1971). Alpha fetoprotein in human hepatoma: improved detection in serum and quantitative studies using a new sensitive technique. *Gastroenterology* **61**, 137–43.

ALSOP, F. M. (1919). The effect of abnormal temperatures upon the developing nervous system in the chick embryo. *Anat. Rec.* **15**, 307–31.

ALTER, B. P., MODELL, B., FAIRWEATHER, D., HOBBINS, J. C., MAHONEY, M. J., FRIGOLETTO, F. D., SHERMAN, A. S., AND NATHAN, D. G. (1976). Prenatal diagnosis of hemoglobinopathies. A review of fifteen cases. *New Engl. J. Med.* **295**, 1437–43.

—— (1962). Anencephalus, hydrocephalus and spina bifida epidemiology with special reference to a survey in Charleston, S.C. *Arch. Neurol.* **7**, 411–22.

—— (1963). Anencephalic births in a Northern and a Southern community. *Am. J. Dis. Child.* **106**, 536–44.

ALTHOUSE, R. AND KLINE, J. (1976). Neural-tube defects. (letter). *New Engl. J. Med.* **294**, 1462.

AMBROSINUS, B. (1642). *Ulysses Aldrovandus' Monstrorum Historia*. Bologna.

AMERICAN ACADEMY OF ORTHOPAEDIC SURGEONS (1972). Symposium on Myelomeningocele, Hartford, Connecticut, November, 1970. The C. V. Mosby Company, Saint Louis.

AMERICAN SOCIETY OF ANESTHESIOLOGISTS (1974). Occupational disease among operating room personnel a national study. *Anaesthesiology* **41**, 321–40.

AMES, M. D. AND SCHUT, L (1972). Results of treatment of 171 consecutive myelomeningoceles, 1963 to 1968. *Pediatrics* **50**, 466–70.

AMUSO, S. J. AND MANKIN, H. J. (1967). Hereditary spondylothesis and spina bifida. *J. Bone Jt Surg.* **49A**, 507–13.

ANCEL, P. (1955). Malformations determinées par des injections de substances chimiques localisee à la tête d'embryons de poule. *J. Embryol. exp. Morph.* **3**, 335–54.

ANDERSON, A. B. M., LAURENCE, K. M., AND TURNBULL, A. C. (1969). The relationship in anencephaly between the size of the adrenal cortex and the length of gestation. *J. Obstet. Gynaec. Br. Commonw.* **76**, 196–9.

ANDERSON, T. W. (1971). *The statistical analysis of time series*. James Wiley, New York.

ANDERSON, W. J. R., BAIRD, D., AND THOMPSON, A. M. (1958). Epidemiology of stillbirths and infant deaths due to congenital malformations. *Lancet* **i**, 1304–6.

ANDREWS, J. AND MCGARRY, J. M. (1972). A community study of smoking in pregnancy. *J. Obstet. Gynaec. Br. Commonw.* **79**, 1057–73.

ANTONOV, A. N. (1947). Children born during siege of Leningrad in 1942. *J. Pediat.* **30**, 250–9.

ARCHER, M. AND PATE, A. R. (1975). An analysis of 469 children with spina bifida treated in the Richmond Hospital between 1967–1973. *J. Irish med. Ass.* **68**, 293–9.

ARMITAGE, P. (1971). *Statistical methods in medical research*. Blackwell, Oxford.

ARNOLD, J. (1894) Myelocyste, transposition von Gewebskeimen und Sympodie. *Beit. path. Anat.* **16**, 1–27.

ARTHUR, A. B., BUSH, R. T., GUARD, F., AND WESTON, H. J. (1972). Spina bifida cystica: survey of 107 cases. *N.Z. med. J.* **70**, 272–7.

ASKROG, V. AND HARVALD, B. (1970). Teratogen effekt af inhalalionsanaestetika. *Nord. Med.* **83**, 498–500.

ASSEMANY, S. R., MUZZO, S., AND GARDNER, L. I. (1972). Syndrome of phocomelic diabetic embryopathy (caudal dysplasia). Am. J. Dis. Child. **123**, 489–91.

AVERY, M. E. (1975). Considerations on the definition of viability. *New Engl. J. Med.* **292**, 206.

AYLETT, M. J. (1973). Spina bifida in general practice. *Practitioner* **211**, 75–81.

—— (1974). Spina bifida and anencephaly: the search for a cause. *Update* **9**, 1177–9.

—— ROBERTS, C. J. AND LLOYD, S. (1974). Neural tube defects in a country town. *Br. J. prev. soc. Med.* **28**, 177–9.

BADGLEY, R. F. (1977). Chairman: *Report of the Committee on the operation of the Abortion Law*. The Queen's Printer, Ottawa.

BAILEY, N. T. J. (1975). *The mathematical theory of infectious diseases and its applications*. Charles Griffin, London.

BAIRD, D. (1973). Diet and congenital defects. (letter). *Br. med. J.* **1**, 291.

—— (1974). Epidemiology of congenital malformations of the central nervous system in (a) Aberdeen and (b) Scotland. *J. biosoc. Sci.* **6**, 113–37.

BALLANTYNE, J. W. (1894). The teratological records of Chaldea. *Teratologia* **1**, 127–42.

—— (1902). *Manual of antenatal pathology and hygiene. The foetus.* Wm. Green & Sons, Edinburgh.

—— (1904). *Manual of antenatal pathology and hygiene. The embryo.* Wm. Green & Sons, Edinburgh.

BANISTER, P. (1971). Evaluation of vital record usage for congenital anomaly surveillance. In *Monitoring, birth defects and environment: the problem of surveillance.* Proceedings of symposium, Albany, N.Y. 1970. Edited by Hook, E. B., Janerich, D. T., and Porter, I. H. Academic Press, New York, pp. 119–35.

Barden, G. A., Meyer, L. S., and Stelling, F. H. (1975). Myelodysplastics—fate of those followed for twenty years or more. *J. Bone Jt Surg.* **57A**, 643–7.

Barr, A. and Stevenson, A. C. (1961). Stillbirths and infant mortality in twins. *Ann. Hum. Genet. (Lond).* **25**, 131–40.

Barr, A. J., Goodnight, J. H., Sall, J. P., and Helwig, J. T. (1976). *A user's guide to S.A.S.* S.A.S. Institute.

Barrett, C. and Hakim, C. (1973). Anencephaly, ovulation stimulation, subfertility and illegitimacy. *Lancet* **ii**, 916–17.

Barry, A. P. (1958). Hydramnios. *Obstet. gynec.* **11**, 667–75.

Bayer, C. (1892). Zur Technik der Operation der Spina bifida und encephalocele. *Prag. med. Wchnschr.* **17**, 317, 332, 345.

—— (1897). Ueber die Endresultate der an der chirungischen Abtheilung des Kaiser Franz Joseph Kinder—Spitals in Prag seit dem Jahre 1882 operierten fälle von Spina bifida und Encephalocele. *Ztschr. f. Heilk. Berlin* **18**, 405–20.

Beckwith, J. B. (1966). The congenitally malformed VII. Exstrophy of the bladder and cloacal exstrophy. *Northw. Med.* **65**, 407–10.

Beckwith, J. R. (1975). Discussion on Geneticophobia and the implications of screening for the XYY genotype in newborn infants, Hook, E. B. In *Genetics and the Law*, edited by Milunsky, A. & Annas, G. J., Plenum Press, New York, p. 87.

—— and King, J. (1974). The XYY syndrome; a dangerous myth. *New Scientist* **64**, 474–6.

Beischer, N. A., Ratten, G. J., Fortune, D. W., and Macafee, C. A. J. (1973). Obstetric Complications when the Fetus has Potter's Syndrome. *Am. J. Obstet. Gynec.* **116**, 62–5.

Bélanger, L., Bélanger, M., Prive, L., Larochelle, J., Trembley, M., and Aubin, G. (1973). Tyrosinémie héréditaire et alpha-1-foetoprotéine. I. Interêt clinique de l'alpha-foetoproteine dans la tyrosinémie héréditaire. *Pathol. Biol. (Paris).* **21**, 449–55.

Bell, J. E. and Gosden, C. M. (1978). Central nervous system abnormalities—contrasting patterns in early and late pregnancy. *Clin. Genet.* **13**, 387–96.

Benirschke, K. and Kim, C. K. (1973). Multiple pregnancy (first of two parts). *New Engl. J. Med.* **288**, 1276–84.

Bennett, K. A. (1972). Lumbo-sacral malformations and spina bifida occulta in a group of proto-historic Modoc Indians. *Am. J. phys. Anthrop.* **36**, 435–40.

Bennett, M. J. (1978). Fetal loss after second-trimester amniocentesis in women with raised serum-alpha-fetoprotein. (letter). *Lancet* **ii**, 987.

—— Grudzinskas, J. G., Gordon, Y. B., and Turnbull, A. C. (1978). Circulating levels of alpha-fetoprotein and pregnancy specific β_1 glycoprotein in pregnancies without an embryo. *Br. J. Obstet. Gynaec.* **85**, 348–50.

Beolchini, P. E. and Bailo, U. (1965). Sulle 'sistenza di variazioni stagionali delta frequenza dell' anencefalia. *Minerva ginec.* **17**, 928–34.

Berg, K., Noer, G., Molne, K. and Bjøro, K. (1976). Maternal serum—Amniotic fluid protein interrelationship: relevance to diagnosis of disorders in the fetus. In *Prenatal Diagnosis* edited by Boué, A. Inserm, Paris, Vol. **61**, p. 245–52.

Bergstrand, C. G. and Czar, B. (1956). Demonstration of a new protein fraction in serum from the human fetus. *Scand. J. Clin. Lab. Invest.* **8**, 174.

Bernades, P., Smadja, M., Rueff, B., Bonnefond, A., Tursz, T., Martin, E., Bognel, C., Barge, J., and Uriel, J. (1971). Presence de l'alpha-foeto-proteine serique dans quatre cas de cancers digestifs primitifs autres que l'hepatoine. *Press Méd.* **79**, 1585–7.

Berner, H. W., Seisler, E. P., and Barlow, J. (1972). Fetal cardiac tamponade, a complication of amniocentesis. *Obstet. Gynec.* **40**, 599–604.

Betheras, F. R. (1962). Obstetrical aspects of foetal hydrocephalus and anencephalus. *Aust. N.Z. J. Obstet. Gynaec.* **2**, 31–7.

Biale, Y., Lewenthal, H., and Ben Aderet, N. (1975). Congenital malformations due to anticonvulsive drugs. *Obstet. Gynec.* **45**, 439–42.

Biggar, R. J., Mortimer, E. A. Jr., and Haughie, G. E. (1976). Descriptive epidemiology of neural tube defects, Rochester, New York, 1918–1938. *Am. J. Epidem.* **104**, 22–7.

—— Haughie, G. E., and Mortimer, E. A., Jr. (1976*a*). The relationship of supplemental iodine to neural tube defects in Rochester, New York, 1924–1932. *Am. J. Epidem.* **104**, 28–33.

Binney, C. (1968). Eugenic aspects of the English Criminal Law. *Eugen Rev.* **60**, 118–28.

Bishop, Y. M. M. (1969). Full contingency tables, logits and split contingency tables. *Biometrics* **25**, 383–400.

—— Feinberg, S. E., and Holland, P. W. (1975). *Discrete multivariate analysis: theory and practice.* The Massachusetts Institute of Technology Press, Cambridge, Massachusetts and London, England.

Blishen, B. (1967). A socio-economic index for occupations in Canada. *Can. Rev. Soc. & Anthrop.* 4–41.

Blyth, H. and Carter, C. O. (1969). A guide to genetic prognosis in paediatrics. *Develop Med. Child Neurol., Suppl.* **18**, 1–35.

Bobrow, M., Evans, C. J., Noble, J., and Patel, C. (1978). Cellular content of amniotic fluid. A predictor of central nervous system malformations. *J. med. Genet.* **15**, 97–100.

Bodman, J. (1959). Development of fetal protein. *Clin. chim. Acta* **4**, 103–9.

Bonaiti-Pellié, C. and Smith, C. (1974). Risk tables for genetic counselling in some common congenital malformations. *J. med. Genet.* **11**, 374–7.

Bond, E. B., Thompson, W., Elwood, J. H., and Cran, G. W. (1977). Evaluation of measurement of maternal plasma alpha-fetoprotein levels as a screening test for fetal neural tube defects. *Br. J. Obstet. Gynaec.* **84**, 574–7.

Bonnevie, K. (1936). Pseudencephalie als spontane recessive mutation bei der hausmaus. *Skr. Norske Vidensk.-Akad. Kl.* **1** (9), 1–39.

Böök, J. A. and Rayner, S. (1950). A clinical and genetical study of anencephaly. *Am. J. hum. Genet.* **2**, 61–84.

Boris, M., Blumberg, R., Feldman, D. B., and Sellers, T. F. (1963). Increased incidence of meningomyeloceles. *J. Am. med. Ass.* **184**, 768.

Boué, J. G., Boué, A., and Lazar, P. (1975). Retrospective and prospective epidemiological studies of 1500 karyotyped spontaneous human abortions. *Teratology* **12**, 11–26.

——, ——, —— and Gueguen, S. (1975). Outcome of pregnancies following a spontaeous abortion with chromosomal anomalies. *Am. J. Obstet. Gynec.* **116**, 806–12.

Bourreille, J., Metayer, P., Sauger, F., Matray, F., and Fondimare, A. (1970). Existence d'alpha-foeto-protéine au cours d'un cancer secondaire du foie d'origine gastricque. *Presse Méd.* **78**, 1277–8.

Box, G. E. P. and Jenkins, G. M. (1970). *Time series analysis forcasting and control.* Holden-Day Inc., San Francisco.

Bremer, J. L. (1906). Description of a 4 mm human embryo. *Am. J. Anat.* **5**, 459–80.

British Columbia Health Act (1971). Section 6. Regulations for the control of communicable diseases.

British Medical Journal (1973). New horizons in medical ethics. (Editorial) **2**, 680.

—— (1975). Risks of amniocentesis. (Editorial) **4**, 485–6.

—— (1977). Prevention of handicap. (Editorial) **4**, 1613.

—— (1978). Perspectives in spina bifida. (Editorial) **3**, (6142), 909–10.

Brock, D. J. H. (1974). The molecular nature of alpha-fetoprotein in anencephaly and spina bifida. *Clin. chim. Acta* **57**, 315–20.

—— (1975). Amniotic fluid alpha$_2$-macroglobulin and the antenatal diagnosis of spina bifida and anencephaly. *Clin. Genet.* **8**, 297–301.

—— (1975*a*). Antenatal misdiagnosis of neural-tube defects. (letter). *Lancet* **ii**, 495.

—— (1976). Prenatal diagnosis—chemical methods. *Br. med. Bull.* **32**, 16–20.

—— (1976*a*) The prenatal diagnosis of neural-tube defects. *Obstet. gynec. Surv.* **31**(1), 32–40.

—— (1976*b*). Mechanisms by which amniotic fluid alphafetoprotein may be raised in fetal abnormality. *Lancet* **ii**, 345–6.

—— (1978). Screening for neural-tube defects. In *Towards the prevention of fetal malformation*, edited by Scrimgeour, J. B. Edinburgh University Press, Edinburgh, p. 37–46.

—— (1978*a*). The use of maternal serum AFP screening for neural-tube defects. In *Prevention of neural-tube defects: the role of alpha-fetoprotein*. Edited by Crandall, B. F. and Brazier, M. A. Academic Press, New York, pp. 191–7.

—— and Olsson, J. E. (1976). Comparison of alphafetoprotein and β-trace protein in the antenatal diagnosis of anencephaly and spina bifida. *Clin. Genet.* **9**, 385–8.

—— and Scrimgeour, J. B. (1972). Early prenatal diagnosis of anencephaly. (letter). *Lancet* **ii**, 1252–3.

—— and Sutcliffe, R. G. (1972). Alpha-fetoprotein in the antenatal diagnosis of anencephaly and spina bifida. *Lancet* **ii**, 197–9.
—— —— (1973). Prenatal diagnosis of anencephaly. *Trans. Biochem. Soc.* **1**, 149–51.
——, Bolton, A. E., and Monaghan, J. M. (1973). Prenatal diagnosis of anencephaly through maternal serum-alphafetoprotein measurement. *Lancet* **ii**, 923–4.
——, Wald. N. J. and Cuckle, H. (1977). Organisation of maternal serum-α-fetoprotein screening for fetal neural-tube defects. (letter). *Lancet* **i**, 700.
——, Manson, J. C., Raeburn, J. A., Bolton, A. E., and McCrae, N. M. (1975). Serum alpha-fetoprotein in cystic fibrosis (letter). *Brit. med. J.* **2**, 392.
——, Barron, L., Jelen, P., Watt, M., and Scrimgeour, J. B. (1977). Maternal serum-alphafetoprotein measurements as an early indicator of low birth-weight. *lancet* **ii**, 267–8.
——, Scrimgeour, J. B., Steven, J., Barron, L., and Watt, M. (1978). Maternal plasma alpha-fetoprotein screening for fetal neural-tube defects. *Br. J. Obstet. Gynaec.* **85**, 575–81.
Brocklehurst, G., Editor (1976). *Spina bifida for the clinician.* Clinics in Developmental Medicine, No. 57. Heinemann, London.
Brody, S. and Carlström, G. (1965). Human chorionic gonadotrophin pattern in serum and its relation to the sex of the fetus. *J. clin. Endocr.* **25**, 792–7.
Brotherston, J. (1978). Implications of antenatal screening for the Health Service. In *Towards the prevention of fetal malformation.* Edited by Scrimgeour, J. B. Edinburgh University Press, Edinburgh, pp. 247–57.
Brothwell, D. R. and Powers, R. (1968). Congenital malformations of the skeleton in earlier man. In *The skeletal biology of earlier human populations.* Edited by Brothwell, D. R. Pergamon Press, Oxford, p. 173.
Brown, G. C. and Evans, T. N. (1967). Serologic evidence of Coxsackie virus etiology of congenital heart disease. *J. Am. med. Ass.* **199**, 183–7.
Brown-Séquard, M. (1859). De la transmission par hérédité chex les mammiféres, et particuliérement chez les cochons d'inde, d'une affection épileptiforme, produite chez les parents par des lésions traumatiques de la moelle épinière. *C.R. Soc. de biol. (Paris)* **11**, 194.
Bryan, E. M. and Kohler, H. G. (1974). The missing umbilical artery I. Prospective study based on a maternity unit. *Arch. Dis. Childh.* **49**, 844–52.
Bryant, E. M. and Hoehn, H. (1977). Adherent amniotic-fluid cells and neural-tube defects. (letter) *Lancet* **i**, 1203.
Büchi, E. C. (1950). Über das Verhältnis Zwischen Missbildungen und Gebäralter. *Bull. Schweiz. Ges. Anthrop. Ethn.* **26**, 11–12.
Buffé, D. (1973). Fetoproteins and children's tumours. In *Alphafetoprotein and hepatoma.* Edited by Hirai, H. and Miyagi, T. GANN Monograph on Cancer Research, University Press of Tokyo, **14**, p. 117–28.
Bulmer, M. G. (1958). The repeat frequency of twinning. *Ann. hum. Genet. (Lond.)* **23**, 31–5.
—— (1959). The effect of parental age, parity and duration of marriage on the twinning rate. *Ann. hum. Genet. (Lond.)* **23**, 454–8.
—— (1960). The twinning rate in Europe and Africa. *Ann. hum. Genet. (Lond.)* **24**, 121–5.
—— (1970). *The biology of twinning in man.* Clarendon Press, Oxford.
Bundey, S. (1974). Screening for spina bifida. (letter). *Lancet* **ii**, 1141.
Burns, J. M. (1973). Evidence that late fertilization is not a cause of Down's syndrome and spina bifida. In Motulsky, A. G., Ebling, F. J. G. (Eds) *Fourth International Conference on Birth Defects*, Abstract of Paper Excerpta Medica International Congress Series No. 297. Excerpta Medica, Amsterdam. Abstract No. 259.
Burt, R. A. (1975). Authorizing death for anomalous newborns. In *Genetics and the law.* Edited by Milunsky, A. and Annas, G. J. Plenum Press, New York, pp. 435–50.
Butler, N. R. and Alberman, E. D. (1969). *Perinatal problems. The Second Report of the 1958 British Perinatal Mortality Survey.* E. & S. Livingstone, Edinburgh.

Cahalane, S. F. and Jessop, W. J. E. (1970) Editors. *A study of perinatal mortality in Ireland 1958 to 1960.* Medical Research Council of Ireland, Dublin.
——, Kennedy, J. D., McNicholl, B., and O'Dwyer, E. (1965). Perinatal mortality survey for County Galway, 18 months, October 1958 through March 1960. *J. Irish med. Ass.* **57**, 135–41.

Callahan, G. B. and Mitchell, R. C. (1970). Conjoined twins—a geneological study. *Acta Genet. Med. Gemellol.* **19**, 213–16.

Campbell, D. M., Campbell, A. J., and MacGillvray, I. (1974). Maternal characteristics of women having twin pregnancies. *J. biosoc. Sci.* **6**, 463–70.

Campbell, S. (1974). The antenatal detection of fetal abnormality by ultrasonic diagnosis. In *Birth defects*. Proceedings of Fourth International Conference. Edited by Motulsky, A. G. and Lenz, W. Excerpta Medica, Amsterdam, pp. 240–7.

—— (1977). Early prenatal diagnosis of neural tube defects by ultrasound. *Clin. Obstet. Gynecol.* **20**, 351–9.

——, Grundy, M., and Singer, J. D. (1976). Early antenatal diagnosis of spina bifida in a twin fetus by ultrasonic examination and alpha-fetoprotein estimation. *Br. med. J.* **3**, 676.

——, Johnston, F. D., Holt, E. M., and May, P. (1972). Anencephaly: early ultrasonic diagnosis and active management. *Lancet* **ii**, 1226–7.

——, Wladimiroff, J. W., and Dewhurst, C. J. (1973). The antenatal measurement of fetal urine production. *J. Obstet. Gynaec. Br. Commonw.* **80**, 680–6.

——, Pryse-Davies, J., Coltart, T. M., Seller, M. J., and Singer, J. D. (1975). Ultrasound in the diagnosis of spina bifida. *Lancet* **i**, 1336.

Campbell, W. A. B. (1953). Influenza in early pregnancy: effects on the foetus. *Lancet* **i**, 173–4.

Candido, R. (1953). Rilievi sue casi dei anencefalia osservati nella clinica obstetrica—ginecologica di Napoli negli ultimi otto anni. *Arch. Obstet. Ginec. Napoli.* **58**, 238–44.

Cantuaria, A. A. and Jones, A. L. (1975). Immunoglobulin M in human amniotic fluid and its possible associations with neural-tube malformations. *Br. J. Obstet. Gynaec.* **82**, 262–4.

Carey, J. C., Greenbaum, B., and Hall, B. D. (1978). The OEIS complex (omphalocele, exstrophy, imperforate anus, spinal defects). *Birth Defects, original Articles Series* **14**, (6B), 253–63.

Carle, H. L. (1948). The new eugenic protection law in Japan. *Eugen. News* **33**, 21–3.

Carter, C. O. (1956). Changing patterns in the causes of death at the hospital for sick children. *Gt. Ormond St. J.*, **11**, 65–8.

—— (1965). The inheritance of common congenital malformations. In *Progress in medical genetics* edited by Steinberg, A. G. and Bearn, H. G. Vol. IV., 59–84, New York.

—— (1969). Genetics of common disorders. *Br. med. Bull.* **25**, 52–7.

—— (1970). Multifactorial inheritance revisited: In *Congenital Malformations: Proceedings of the Third Internatational Conference*. Edited by Fraser, F. C. anand McKusick, V. A. Excerpta med., (Amst.), 227–32

—— (1974). Clues to the aetiology of neural tube malformations. *Develop. med. Child Neurol., suppl.* **16**, 3–14.

—— (1977). Monogenic disorders. *J. med. Genet.* **14**, 316–20.

—— and Evans, K. (1973). Spina bifida and anencephalus in Greater London. *J. med. Genet.*, **10**, 209–34.

——, —— (1973*a*). Children of adult survivors with spina bifida cystica. *Lancet* **ii**, 924–6.

—— and Roberts, J. F. (1967). The risk of recurrence after 2 children with central nervous system malformations. *Lancet* **i**, 306–8.

—— David. P. A., and Laurence, K. M. (1968). A family study of major central nervous system malformations in South Wales *J. med. Genet.*, **5**, 81–106.

—— Laurence, K. M., and David, P. A. (1967). The genetics of the major central nervous system malformations, based on the South Wales socio-genetic investigation. *Develop. med. Child Neurol., suppl.* **13**, 30–34.

Case, R. A. M. (1956). Cohort analysis of mortality rates as an historical or narrative technique. *Br. J. prev. soc. Med.* **10**, 159–71.

Cassady,G. (1969). Anencephaly: a 6-year study of 367 cases. *Am. J. Obstet. Gynec.* **103**, 1154–9.

—— and Cailliteau, J. (1967). The amniotic fluid in anencephaly. *Am. J. Obstet. Gynec.* **97**, 395–9.

Cave, D. R. and Freedman, L. S. (1975). Seasonal variations in the clinical presentation of Crohn's disease and ulcerative colitis. *Int. J. Epidem.* **4**, 317–20.

Center for Disease Control (1969). Metropolitan Atlanta congenital defects program. Incidence of congenital defects, Oct. 1, 1967 to Sept. 30, 1968. Report No. 1.

Chance, P. F. and Smith, D. W. (1978). Hyperthermia and meningomyelocele and anencephaly (letter). *Lancet* **i**, 769–70.

Chandra, R. K., Madhavankutty, K., and Way, R. C. (1975). Serum α-fetoprotein levels in patients with cystic fibrosis and their parents and siblings. *Br. med. J.* **1**, 714–16.

Charles, E. (1951). Statistical utilisation of maternity and child welfare records. *Br. J. Soc. Med.* **5**, 41–61.

Chaube, S. and Murphy, M. L. (1966). The effects of hydrourea and related compounds on the rat fetus. *Cancer Res.* **26**, 1448–57.

Cheeseman, E. A. (1968). Medical record linkage in Northern Ireland—Reconnaissance and proposals with particular reference to problems of identification. In *Record linkage in medicine*, Acheson, E. D. editor, E. & S. Livingstone Ltd., Edinburgh, pp. 70–80.

Chemke, J., Czernobilsky, B., Mundel, G., and Barishak, Y. R. (1975). A familial syndrome of central nervous system and ocular malformations. *Clin. Genet.* **7**, 1–7.

—— Miskin, A., Rav–Acha, Z., Porath, A., Sagiv, M., and Katz, Z. (1977). Prenatal diagnosis of Meckel syndrome: alpha-fetoprotein and beta-trace protein in amniotic fluid. *Clin. Genet.* **11**, 285–9.

Cheng, D. W., Chang, L. F., and Bairnson, T. A. (1957). Gross observations on developing abnormal embryos induced by maternal vitamin E deficiency. *Anat. Rec.* **129**, 167–85.

Chiari, H. (1891). Über Veränderungen des Kleinhirns in Folge von Hydrocephalie des Grosshirns. *Dtsch. med. Wschr.* **27**, 1172–5.

—— (1896). Über Veränderungen des Kleinhirns, des pons und der medulla oblongata in folge von congenitaler hydrocephalie des Grosshirns. *Denkschr Akad Wiss. Wein* **63**, 71–116.

Choi, N. W. and Klaponski (1970). On neural tube defects: an epidemiological elicitation of etiological factors. (Abstract). *Neurology* **20**, 399–400.

—— —— Ateah, E., and Nelson, N. A. (1972). Some epidemiological aspects of central nervous system malformations in Manitoba. In *Drugs and fetal development* edited by Klingberg, M. A. Plenum Press, New York, pp. 511–25.

Christakos, A. C. and Simpson, J. L. (1969). Anencephaly in three siblings. *Obstet. Gynec.* **33**, 267–70.

Christie, A. D. (1977). See Donald, I. (1977), p 25.

Chung, C. S. and Myrianthopoulos, N. C. (1968). Racial and prenatal factors in major congenital malformations. *Am. J. hum. Genet.* **20**, 44–59.

—— , Ching, C. H. S., and Morton, N. E. (1974). A genetic study of cleft lip and palate in Hawaii. II. Complex segregation analysis and genetic risks. *Am. J. hum. Genet.* **26**, 177–88.

Clark, L. and Carlisle, C. H. (1975). Spina bifida with syringo-myelia and meningocoele in a short-tailed cat. *Aust. vet. J.* **51**, 392–4.

Clarke, C. A., McKendrick, O. M., and Sheppard, P. M. (1973). Spina bifida and potatoes. *Br. med. J.* **3**, 251–4.

——, Hobson, D., McKendrick, O. M., Rogers, S. C., and Sheppard, P. M. (1975). Spina bifida and anencephaly: miscarriage as possible cause. *Br. med. J.* **4**, 743–46.

Clarke, M. (1977). Feasibility of serum-α-fetoprotein screening for fetal neural-tube defects. (Letter) *Lancet* **i**, 1098–99.

Clarke, P. C., Gordon, Y. B., Kitau, M. J., Chard, T., and Letchworth, A. T. (1977). Screening for fetal neural tube defects by maternal plasma alpha-fetoprotein determination. *Br. J. Obstet. Gynaec.* **84**, 568–73.

Cleland, J. (1883). Contribution to the study of spina bifida, encephalocele and anencephalus. *J. Anat. Physiol.* **17**, 257–92.

Clive, E. M. (1978). Legal implications of antenatal screening. In *Towards the prevention of fetal malformation* edited by Scrimgeour, J. B. Edinburgh University Press, Edinburgh, pp. 227–39.

Cochran, W. G. (1965). The planning of observational studies of human populations. *J. roy. stat. soc., Series A* **128**, 234–66.

—— (1968). The effectiveness of adjustment by subclassification in removing bias in observational studies. *Biomet.* **24**, 295–313.

Coffey, V. P. (1970). Spina bifida in Ireland. *J. Irish med. Ass.* **63,** 343–8.

—— (1974). Twenty-one years study of anencephaly in Dublin. *J. Irish med. Ass.* **67**, 553–8.

——, and Jessop, W. J. E. (1957). A study of 137 cases of anencephaly. *Br. J. prev. soc. Med.* **11**, 174–80.

——, —— (1959). Maternal influenza and congenital deformities. *Lancet* **ii**, 935–8.
——, —— (1971). Associated factors in 737 cases of anencephalus. Paper presented at the XIII International Congress of Pediatrics, Vienna.
COHEN, E. N., BELLVILLE, J. W., AND BROWN, B. W. JR. (1971). Anesthesia, pregnancy and miscarriage: a study of operating room nurses and anesthetists. *Anesthesiology* **35**, 343–7.
COHLAN, S. Q. (1954). Congenital anomalies in the rat produced by excessive intake of vitamin A during pregnancy. *Pediatrics* **13**, 556–67.
COLE, P. AND MACMAHON, B. (1971). Attributable risk per cent in case-control studies. *Br. J. prev. soc. Med.* **25**, 242–244.
COLLMANN, R. D. AND STOLLER, A. (1962). Epidemiology of congenital anomalies of the central nervous system with special reference to patterns in the State of Victoria, Australia. *J. Ment. def. Res.* **6**, 22–37.
——, —— (1968). The occurrence of anencephalus in the State of Victoria, Australia. *J. Ment. Defic. Res* **12**, 22–35.
COMERFORD, J. B. (1965). Pregnancy with anencephaly. *Lancet* **i**, 679–80.
COMMITTEE ON SAFETY OF MEDICINES (1975). Hormonal pregnancy tests: a possible association with congenital abnormalities. *Adverse Reaction Series No 13.*
COMPTON, P. A., GOLDSTROM L., AND GOLDSTROM, J. M. (1974). Religion and legal abortion in Northern Ireland. *J. biosoc. Sci.* **6**, 493–500.
COOK, L. N., SHOTT, R. J., AND ANDREWS, B. F. (1974). Fetal complications of diagnostic amniocentesis: A review and report of a case with pneumothorax. *Pediatrics* **53**, 421–4.
COOKE, W. (1822). Translation of *The seats and causes of diseases investigated by anatomy* by Morgagni (1761). Longman, London.
COOPERMAN, E. M. (1977). Meningomyelocele: to treat or not to treat. *Can. med. Ass. J.* **116**, 1339–40.
CORBETT, T. H., BEAUDOIN, A. R., CORNELL, R. G., ENDRES, J. L., AND PAGE, A. (1974). Effects of low concentrations of methoxyflurane on rat pregnancy. *Teratology* **9**, A-15-A-16.
——, CORNELL, R. G., ENDRES, J. L., AND LIEDING, K. (1974). Birth defects among children of nurse-anesthetists. *Anesthesiology* **41**, 341–4.
CORNFIELD, J. (1951). A method of estimating comparative rates from clinical data. Applications to cancer of the lung, breast and cervix. *J. Nat. Cancer Inst.* **11**, 1269–75.
—— (1962). Joint dependence of risk of coronary heart disease on serum cholesterol and systolic blood pressure; a discriminant function analysis. *Federation Proceedings* **21** (4), 58–61.
—— (1967). Discriminant functions. *Rev. Inter. Stat. Inst.* **35** (2), 142–53.
COX, A. E., AND LARGE, E. C. (1960). *Agricultural Handbook No. 174: Potato blight epidemics throughout the world*. U.S. Department of Agriculture, Agricultural Research Service, Washington.
COX, D. R. (1970). *The analysis of binary data*. Methuen, London.
CRANDALL, B. F., LEBHERZ, T. B., AND FREIHUBE, R. (1978). Neural Tube Defects. Maternal serum screening and prenatal diagnosis. *Pediat. Clin. N. Amer.* **25**, 619–29.
CRAWFORD, M. D., GARDNER, M. J., AND SEDGWICK, P. A. (1972). Infant mortality and hardness of local water supplies. *Lancet* **i**, 988–92.
CREASY, M. R., AND ALBERMAN, E. D. (1976). Congenital malformations of the central nervous system in spontaneous abortions. *J. Med. Genet.* **13**, 9–16.
CREW, F. A. E. (1936). A repetition of McDougall's Lamarkian experiment. *J. Genet.* **33**, 61–102.
CRIDLAND, M. D. (1961). Seasonal incidence of clinical onset of Hodgkin's disease. *Br. med. J.* **1**, 621–3.
CROSS, H. E. AND MAUMENEE, A. E. (1972). Ocular trauma during amniocentesis. *New Engl. J. Med.* **287**, 993–4.
CROSS, R. G. (1968). Anencephalus and spina bifida. (letter). *Lancet* **ii**, 253.
CRUZ-COKE, R. (1972). Birth control, sex-ratio, and anencephaly. (letter). *Lancet* **ii**, 1094–5.
CZEIZEL, A. (1974). Unexplainable demographic phenomena of multiple births in Hungary. *Acta. Genet. Med. Gemellol.* **22**, 214–18.
—— AND RÉVÉSZ, C. (1970). Major malformations of the nervous system in Hungary. *Br. J. prev. soc. Med.* **24**, 205–22.

—— and Bognar, Z. (1971). Mortality and morbidity of legal abortion. (letter) *Lancet* **ii**, 209–10.

Damme, C. (1978). Infanticide: the worth of an infant under law. *Med. Hist.* **22**, 1–24.

Damyanov, I. and Dutz, W. (1971). Anencephaly in Shiraz, Iran. (letter) *Lancet*, **i**, 82.

Danforth, C. H., and Center, E. (1954). Nitrogen mustard as a teratogenic agent in the mouse. *Proc. Soc. exp. Biol. (N.Y.)* **86**, 705–7.

Darroch, J. N. (1962). Interactions in multifactor contingency tables. *J. Roy. Stat. Soc., Series B* **24**, 251–63.

Darwin, C. (1859). *The origin of species — by means of natural selection or the preservation of favoured races in the struggle for life*. John Murray, London.

—— (1868). *The variation of animals and plants under domestication*. Two volumes, First Edition. John Murray, London.

—— (1871). *The descent of man and selection in relation to sex*. Two volumes, First Edition. John Murray, London.

David, H. A. and Newell, D. J. (1965). The identification of annual peak periods for a disease. *Biometrics* **21**, 645–50.

David, T. J. and Nixon, A. (1976). Congenital malformations associated with anencephaly and iniencephaly. *J. med. Genet.* **13**, 263–5.

Davidson, R. G. and Sheffield, L. J. (1978). Hazards of prenatal detection of neural-tube defects by screening maternal serum for α-fetoprotein. *Can. med. Ass. J.* **118**, 1187–91.

Davidson, S., Passmore, R., Brock, J. F., and Treswell, A. S. (1975). *Human nutrition and dietetics*, Sixth Edition. Churchill-Livingstone, London.

Dean, L., Abell, D. A., and Beischer, N. A. (1977). Incidence of anencephaly and other major malformations when oestriol excretion is very low. *Br. med. J.* **1**, 257–8.

De Bruijn, H. W. A., and Huisjes, H. J. (1975). Omphalocele and raised alpha-fetoprotein in amniotic fluid. *Lancet* **i**, 525–6.

De Grouchy, J., Brissaud, H. E., Repessé, G., and Lamy, M. (1964). Anencéphalie familiale et remaniement de deux chromosomes 13–15. *Compt. rend. Acad. Sci. (Paris)* **258**, 691.

Dekaban, A. S. (1963). Anencephaly in early human embryos. *J. Neuropath. exp. Neurol.* **22**, 533–48.

De Klerk, D. J. J. and De Villiers, J. C. (1973). Frontal encephaloceles. *S. Afr. med. J.* **47**, 1350–55.

Dellepiane, G. (1956). Personal Communication, viz Böök, J. A. and Fraccaro, M. Research on congenital malformations. *Étud. néo-natal* **5**, 39–54.

De Morsier, G. and Bamatter, F. (1952). Anencephalie (telencephaloschizis total) et rhomboschizis avec heterotopies cerebelleuses medianes. Servie de 32 jours. *Arch. Psicol. Neurol. Psichiat. (Milan)* **13**, 2.

De Myer, W. (1967). The median cleft face syndrome: differential diagnosis of cranium bifidum occultum, hypertelorism and median cleft nose, lip and palate. *Neurology (Minneap.)* **17**, 961–71.

De Watteville, H., Jürgens, R., and Pfaltz, H. (1954). Einfluss von Vitaminmangel auf Fruchtbarkeit, Schwangerschaft und Nachkommen. *Schweiz. med. Wschr.* **84**, 875–83.

Department of Health and Social Security (1973). *Care of the child with spina bifida.* HMSO, London.

Dexeus Trias de Bes, J. M. (1950). Anencephalia: (Consideraciones sobre una revision estadistica). *Rev. Esp. Obstet. Ginec.* **9**, 11–26.

DHEW Environmental Protection Agency (1975). *Scientific and Technical Assessment Report on vinyl chloride and polyvinyl chloride*. US Department of Health, Education and Welfare, Washington, DC.

Dickens, B. M. (1976). The Morgentaler case: criminal process and aboriton law. *Osgoods Hall Law Journal* **14**, 229–85.

Dinno, N. D., Shearer, L., and Weisskopf, B. (1976). Chondrodysplastic dwarfism, cleft palate and micrognathia in a neonate, a new syndrome? *Eur. J. Pediatr.* **123** (1), 39–42.

Dixon, W. J. (1977). *BMDP—77: Biomedical Computer Programs P-Series.* University of California Press, Los Angeles.

Dobbing, J. (1974). The later growth of the brain and its vulnerability. *Pediatrics* **53**, 2–6.

Doll, R., Hill, A. B., and Sakula, J. (1960). Asian influenza in pregnancy and congenital defects. *Br. J. prev. soc. Med.* **14**, 167–72.

Dominion Bureau of Statistics (1969). Publication 62–531: *Family food expenditure in Canada*. Volume 1, Ottawa. The Queen's Printer.

Donald, I. (1977). Further developments in diagnostic sonar in obstetrics and gynecology. In *Obstetrics and Gynecology Annual 1977*, edited by Wynn, R. M. Appleton-Century-Crofts, New York, p. 23–65.

Doran, T. A., Allen, L. C., Pirani, B. B. K., and Shumak, K. H. (1977). False positive amniotic fluid alpha fetoprotein levels resulting from contamination with fetal blood: results of an experiment. *Am. J. Obstet. Gynecol.* **127**, 759–62.

Dudgeon, J. A. (1976). Infective causes of human malformations. *Br. Med. Bull.* **32**, 77–83.

Duff, R. S. and Campbell, A. G. M. (1973). Moral and ethical dilemmas in the special-care nursery. *New Eng. J. Med.* **289**, 890–4.

Dumoulin, J. G. and Gordon, M. E. (1959). Anencephaly in twins. *J. Obstet. Gynaec. Brit. Emp.* **66**, 964–8.

Duncan, S. L. B. (1975). Antenatal misdiagnosis of neural-tube defects. (letter). *Lancet* **ii**, 709.

——, Ginz, B., Ward, A. M., and Hingley, S. M. (1977). Amniotic fluid in multiple pregnancy. (letter). *Br. Med. J.,* **1** (2), 1354.

Dunelm, J. (1978). Ethical problems of screening for neural-tube defects. (letter). *Lancet* **ii**, 148.

Dunn, H. G. and Salter, J. G. (1944). Recurrent anencephaly. *J. Obstet. Gynaec. Brit. Emp.* **51**, 529–36.

Du Plessis, J. P. G., Winship, W. S., and Kirstein, J. D. L. (1974). Fetus *in fetu* and teratoma. A case report and review *S. Afr. Med. J.* **48**, 2119–22.

Durkin, M. V., Kaveggia, E. G., Pendleton, E., and Opitz, J. M. (1976). Sequential fetus-fetus interaction and C.N.S. defects. (letter). *Lancet* **ii**, 43.

Dyson, J. L. and Kohler, H. G. (1973). Anencephaly and ovulation stimulation. (letter). *Lancet* **i** 1256–7.

Eckstein, H. B. and MacNab, G. H. (1966). Myelomeningocele and hydrocephalus. The impact of modern treatment. *Lancet* **i**, 842–5.

Ederer, F., Myers, M. H., and Mantel, N. (1966). A statistical problem in space and time: do leukaemia cases come in clusters? *Biometrics* **20**, 626–8.

Edmonds, L. D., Falk, H., and Nissim, J. E. (1975). Congenital malformations and vinyl chloride. (letter) *Lancet* **ii**, 1098.

——, Anderson, C. E., Flynt, W. J. Jr., and James, L. M. (1978). Congenital central nervous system malformations and vinyl chloride monomer exposure: a community study. *Teratology* **17**, 137–42.

Edwards, J. H. (1958). Congenital malformations of the central nervous system in Scotland. *Br. J. prev. soc. Med.* **12**, 115–30.

—— (1960). The simulation of Mendelism. *Acta Genetica* **10**, 63–70.

—— (1961). The recognition and estimation of cyclic trends. *Ann. Hum. Genet. (Lond.)* **25**, 83–6.

—— (1969). Familial predisposition in man. *Br. Med. Bull.* **25**, 58–64.

—— (1969*a*). *Judging the unborn*. Inaugural lecture. University of Birmingham.

—— (1973). Screening for chromosomal abnormalities. (letter). *Lancet* **i**, 542.

—— (1974). The application of genetics to man 1869–1969. In *Fifty years of genetics*, edited by Jinks, J. Oliver and Boyd, Edinburgh, pp. 67–79.

—— (1978). Problems posed by spina bifida. *The Times*, 13 January.

Edwards, R. P. and Balfour, R. P. (1976). The clinical diagnosis of major congenital abnormalities of the fetal central nervous system. *Br. J. Obstet. Gynaec.* **83**, 422–4.

Egley, C. C. (1973). Laceration of fetal spleen during amniocentesis. *Am. J. Obstet. Gynec.* **116**, 582–3.

Ehrat, R. (1948). *Die missbildungen der neugeborenen an der universitats frauenklinik Zurich 1921–44*. Inaugural Dissertation. Zurich University, pp. 1–112.

Ellis, J. R. and Penrose, L. S. (1961). Enlarged satellites and multiple malformations in the same pedigree. *Ann. Hum. Genet. (Lond.)* **25**, 159–62.

Elwood, J. H. (1969). An epidemiological investigation into some aspects of infant mortality in Belfast. MD Thesis. The Queen's University of Belfast, pp. 1–350.
—— (1970). Anencephalus in Belfast. Incidence and secular and seasonal variations, 1950–1966. *Br. J. prev. soc. Med.* **24**, 78–88.
—— (1970*a*). Anencephalus in the British Isles. *Develop. Med. Child Neurol.* **12**, 582–91.
—— (1972). Major central nervous system malformations notified in Northern Ireland 1964–1968. *Develop. Med. and Child Neurol.* **14**, 731–9.
—— (1973). Infant mortality in Belfast and Dublin 1900–1969. *Irish J. med. Sci.* **142**, 166–73.
—— (1973*a*). Epidemics of anencephalus and spina bifida in Ireland since 1900. *Inter. J. Epidemiol.* **2**, 171–5.
—— (1973*b*). Secular trends in the incidence of major malformations of the central nervous system reported from three Dublin maternity hospitals, 1900–1965. *Irish J. Med. Sci.* **142** (6), 346–57.
—— (1975). Secular trends in the incidence of anencephalus and spina bifida in Belfast and Dublin 1953–1973. *Irish J. Med. Sci.* **144** (10), 388–94.
—— (1976). Major central nervous system malformations notified in Northern Ireland, 1969–1973. *Develop Med. Child Neurol.* **18**, 512–20.
—— (1976*a*). Anencephalus and spina bifida in the British Isles. In *Birth defects: risks and consequences*, edited by Kelly, S., Hook, E. B., Janerich, D. T., and Porter, I. H. Academic Press, New York, pp. 21–39.
—— (1976*b*). Actiology of anencephaly and spina bifida. (letter). *Br. Med. J.* **i**, 218.
—— and MacKenzie, G. (1971). Comparisons of secular and seasonal variations in the incidence of anencephalus in Belfast and four Scottish cities, 1956–66. *Br. J. prev. soc. Med.* **25**, 17–25.
——, —— (1973). Associations between the incidence of neurological malformations and potato blight outbreaks over 50 years in Ireland. *Nature (London)* **243**, 467–77.
—— and Nevin, N. C. (1973) Factors associated with anencephalus and spina bifida in Belfast. *Br. J. prev. soc. Med.* **27**, 73–80.
——, —— (1973*a*). Anencephalus and spina bifida in Belfast (1964–1968). *Ulster med. J.* **42**, 213–22.
—— and Thompson, W. (1975). Fetal viability. (letter). *Lancet* **i**, 862.
——, MacKenzie, G., and Cran, G. W. (1971). The measurement and comparison of infant mortality risks by binary multiple regression analysis. *J. Chron. Dis.* **24**, 93–106.
——, ——, —— (1974). Observations on single births to women resident in Belfast 1962–1966 Part III. Distribution of perinatal and postperinatal deaths by sex, age and cause. *J. Chron. Dis.* **27**, 549–62.
——, ——, —— (1974*a*). Observations on single births to women resident in Belfast 1962–1966. Part 1. Factors associated with perinatal mortality. *J. Chron. Dis.* **27**, 517–35.
——, ——, —— (1974*b*). Observations on single births to women resident in Belfast 1962–1966. Part II. Factors associated with postperinatal mortality. *J. Chron. Dis.* **27**, 537–48.
——, ——, —— (1976). Birthweight and gestation of single births in Belfast. *Irish J. Med. Sci.* **145**, 285–91.
Elwood, J. M. (1973). Changes in the twinning rate in Canada 1926–70. *Br. J. prev. soc. Med.* **27**, 236–41.
—— (1973*a*). Anencephaly and potato blight in eastern Canada. (letter). *Lancet* **i**, 769.
—— (1974). Anencephalus in Canada 1943–1970. *Am. J. Epidem.* **100**, 288–96.
—— (1974*a*). Clomiphene and anencephalic births. (letter). *Lancet* **i**, 31.
—— (1974*b*). Anencephalus and legitimacy. (letter). *Lancet* **ii**, 899.
—— (1975). Seasonal variation in anencephalus in Canada. *Br. J. prev. soc. Med.* **29**, 22–6.
—— (1976). Twinning and anencephalus occurrence in relation to fetus-fetus interaction. *Br. J. prev. soc. Med.* **30**, 29–31.
—— (1976*a*). Anencephalus, spina bifida and potato blight in Canada. *Can. J. Pub. Hlth.* **67**, 122–6.
—— (1976*b*). An epidemiological study of anencephalus in Canada. M.D. Thesis, The Queen's University of Belfast, pp. 1–608.
—— (1976*c*). Anencephaly and spina bifida in North America. In *Birth defects: risks and consequences.* Edited by Kelly, S., Hook, E. B., Janerich, D. T., and Porter, I. H. Academic Press, New York, pp. 3–19.

—— (1977). Anencephalus and drinking water composition. *Am. J. Epidem.* **105**, 460–7.

—— (1978). Maternal and environmental factors affecting twin births in Canadian cities. *Br. J. Obstet. Gynaec.* **85**, 351–8.

—— AND McBRIDE, M. L. (1979). Contrasting effects of maternal fertility and birth rank on the occurrence of neural tube defects. *J. Epidem. Comm. Hlth.* **33**, 78–83.

—— AND MOUSSEAU, G. (1978). Geographical, secular and ethnic influences in anencephalus. *J. Chron. Dis.* **31**, 483–91.

—— AND ROGERS, J. R. (1975). The incidence of congenital abnormalities in B.C., Alberta, Manitoba and New Brunswick 1966–1969. *Can. J. Publ. Hlth.* **66**, 471–6.

——, —— (1977). Seasonal occurrence of congenital abnormalities in Canada. *Can. J. Publ. Hlth.* **68**, 233–6.

——, RAMAN, S., AND MOUSSEAU, G. (1978). Reproductive history in the mothers of anencephalics. *J. Chron. Dis.* **31**, 473–81.

——, COLE, P., ROTHMAN, K. J., AND KAPLAN, S. D. (1977). Epidemiology of endometrial cancer. *J. Nat. Cancer Inst.* **59**, 1055–60.

EMANUEL, I. (1972) Spina bifida, anencephaly and potato blight. (letter). *Lancet* **ii**, 1308–9.

—— AND SEVER, L. E. (1973). Questions concerning the possible association of potatoes and neural-tube defects, and an alternative hypothesis relating to maternal growth and development. *Teratology* **8**, 325–32.

——, HUANG, S-W., GUTMAN, L. T., YU, F-C., AND LIN, C-C. (1972). The incidence of congenital malformations in a Chinese population: The Taipei collaborative study. *Teratology* **5**, 159–70.

EMERSON, D. J. (1962). Congenital malformation due to attempted abortion with aminopterin. *Am. J. Obstet. Gynec.* **84**, 356–7.

EMERY, A. E. H. (1973). Biochemical analysis of amniotic fluid. In *Antenatal diagnosis of genetic disease.* Edited by Emery, A. E. H., Churchill Livingstone, Edinburgh and London, pp. 113–36.

——, BURT, D., NELSON, M. M., AND SCRIMGEOUR, J. B. (1970). Antenatal diagnosis and amino acid composition of amniotic fluid. *Lancet* **i**, 1307–8.

——, ECCLESTON, D., SCRIMGEOUR, J. B., AND JOHNSTON, M. (1972). Amniotic fluid composition in CNS malformations. *J. Obstet. Gynaec. Br. Commonw.* **79**, 154–8.

——, BROCK, D. J. H., BURT, D., AND ECCLESTON, D. (1974). Amniotic fluid composition in malformations of the fetal central nervous system. *J. Obstet. Gynaec. Br. Commonw.* **81**, 512–16.

ENVIRONMENTAL PROTECTION AGENCY (1975). *Scientific and technical assessment report on vinyl chloride and polyvinyl chloride.* United States Department of Health, Education and Welfare, Washington, DC.

EPSTEIN, B. S. AND KOLKER, P. (1965). Congenital variations in cephalobrachial vessels in anencephaly. *Am. J. Roentgenol.* **93**, 339–42.

EPSTEIN, C. J. (1978). Maternal serum screening for neural tube defects in California (discussion). In *Prevention of neural tube defects: the role of alpha-fetoprotein*, edited by Crandall, B. F., and Brazier, M. A. Academic Press, New York, pp. 249–50.

ERICKSON, J. D. (1976). Racial variations in the incidence of congenital malformations. *Ann. Hum. Genet., Lond.* **39**, 315–20.

ERIKSSON, A. W. AND FELLMAN, J. (1967). Twinning and legitimacy. *Hereditas (Lund).* **57**, 395–402

EVANS, E. E. (1973). *The personality of Ireland. Habitat, heritage and history.* Cambridge University Press, Cambridge.

FALCONER, D. S. (1965). The inheritance of liability to certain diseases estimated from the incidence among relatives. *Ann. hum. Genet., Lond.* **29**, 51–76.

FARQUHAR, J. W. (1965). The influence of maternal diabetes on the fetus and child. In *Recent Advances in Pediatrics.* Third edition. Edited by D. Gairdner. Little, Brown and Company, Boston, pp. 126–9.

FARREL, A. G. W. (1964). Twin pregnancy, a study of 1000 cases. *S. Afr. J. Obstet. Gynaec.* **2**, 35–41.

FEDRICK, J. (1970). Anencephalus and the local water supply. *Nature (London)* **227**, 176–7.

—— (1974). Anencephalus and maternal tea drinking: evidence for possible association. *Proc. Roy. soc. Med.* **67**, 6–10.
—— (1976). Anencephalus in the Oxford Record Linkage study area. *Develop Med. Child. Neurol.* **18**, 643–56.
—— (1976*a*). Anencephalus in Scotland 1961–72. *Br. J. prev. soc. Med.* **30**, 132–7.
—— AND ADELSTEIN, P. (1973). Influence of pregnancy spacing on outcome of pregnancy. *Br. med. J.* **iv**, 753–6.
——, —— (1976). Area differences in the incidence of neural tube defect and the rate of spontaneous abortion. *Br. J. prev. soc. Med.* **30**, 32–5.
——, —— (1977). Preceding pregnancy loss as an index of risk of stillbirth or neonatal death in the present pregnancy. *Biol. Neonat. (Basel)* **31**, 84–93.
—— AND BUTLER, N. (1972). Accuracy of registered causes of neonatal deaths in 1958. *Br. J. prev. soc. Med.* **26**, 101–5.
—— AND WILSON, T. S. (1971). Malformations of the central nervous system in Glasgow. An examination of the evidence for clustering in space and time. *Br. J. prev. soc. Med.* **25**, 210–15.
FEHRMANN, H., AND DIMOND, A. E. (1967). Studies on auxins in the phyophora disease of the potato tuber. *Phytopathol. Z.* **59**, 83–100.
FELDSTEIN, M. S. (1965). A method of evaluating perinatal mortality risk. *Br. J. prev. soc. Med.* **19**, 135–9.
—— (1966). A binary variable multiple regression method of analysing factors affecting perinatal mortality and other outcomes of pregnancy. *J. Roy. Stat. Soc., Series A* **129** (1), 61–73.
—— AND BUTLER, N. R. (1965). Analysis of factors affecting perinatal mortality—a multivariate statistical approach. *Br. J. prev. soc. Med.* **19**, 128–34.
FEREMBACH, D. (1963). Frequency of spina bifida occulta in prehistoric human skeletons. *Nature (Lond.)* **199**, 100–1.
FERGUSON-SMITH, M. A., FERGUSON-SMITH, M. E., VINCE, J. D., AND ROBINSON, H. P. (1976). Prenatal screening for congenital abnormalities in the West of Scotland. *Hlth. Bull. (Edinb.)* **34** (2), 105–11.
——, MAY, H. M., VINCE, J. D., ROBINSON, H. P., RAWLINSON, H. A., TAIT, H. A., GIBSON, A. A. M., AND RATCLIFFE, J. G. (1978). Avoidance of anencephalic and spina bifida births by maternal serum-alphafetoprotein screening. *Lancet* **i**, 1330–3.
FERM, V. H. (1958). Teratogenic effects of Trypan Blue on hamster embryos. *J. Embryol. exp. Morph.* **6**, 284–7.
—— AND CARPENTER, S. J. (1968). The relationship of cadmium and zinc in experimental mammalian teratogenesis. *Lab. Invest.* **18**, 429–32.
FIELD, B. (1976). Bovine congenital arthrogryphosis and hydranencephaly and human neural-tube malformations in New South Wales. *Aust. Vet. J.* **52**, 101–2.
—— AND KERR, C. (1973). Potato blight and neural-tube defects. (letter) *Lancet* **ii**, 507–8.
——, —— (1974). Twinning and neural-tube defects. (letter). *Lancet* **ii**, 964–5.
——, —— (1974*a*). Ovulation stimulation and defects of neural-tube closure. (letter). *Lancet* **ii**, 1511.
——, —— (1975). Antenatal diagnosis of neural-tube defects. (letter). *Lancet* **ii**, 324.
FIELDING, D. W. AND SMITHELLS, R. W. (1971). Anencephalus and water hardness in S. W. Lancashire. *Br. J. prev. soc. Med.* **25**, 217–19.
FISHER, R. A. (1918). The correlation between relatives on the supposition of Mendelian inheritance. *Trans. roy. Soc. Edinb.* **52**, 399–433.
—— (1936). The use of multiple measurements in taxonomic problems. *Ann. Eugen.* **7**, 179–88.
FITZGERALD, R. J. AND HEALY, B. (1974). The spina bifida problem. A longer term review with special reference to the quality of survival. *J. Irish med. Ass.* **67**, 565–7.
FITZSIMMONS, J. S., SMITH, N., HILLER, E. J., AND WYNNE, J. (1975). Serum α-fetoprotein in cystic fibrosis. (letter). *Br. med. J.* **ii**, 544.
——, FILSHIE, G. M., HILL, A. S., AND KIME, R. (1976). Antenatal diagnosis of trisomy 13 with unexpected increase in alpha-fetoprotein. *J. med. Genet.* **13**, 400–12.
FLATZ, G. AND SUKTHOMYA, C. (1970). Fronto-ethmoidal encephalomeningoceles in the population of Northern Thailand. *Humangenetik* **11**, 1–8.
FLETCHER, E. W. L. (1978). Is fetal radiography really necessary? *Lancet* **i**, 600.

FLYNT, J. W. (1970). An unusual incidence of central nervous system defects in a military population. (Abstract) *Teratology* **3**, 199.

FOGEL, B. J., NITOWSKY, H. M., AND GREUNWALD, P. (1965). Discordant abnormalities in monozygotic twins. *J. Pediat.* **66**, 64–72.

FONTAINE, G., AND VANKEMMEL, P. (1978). Craniorachischisis in a double headed female fetus. (letter). *Teratology* **18**, 289–90.

FÖRSTER, A. (1865). *Die Missbildungen des Menschen Systematisch Dargestellt.* Druck und Verlag von Friedrıch Mauke, Jena.

FOWLER, I. (1953). Responses of the chick neural tube in mechanically produced spina bifida. *J. exp. Zool.* **123**, 115–42.

FOY, H., KONDI, A., AND LINSELL, C. A. (1970). Fetoprotein in pregnant African women. *Lancet* **ii**, 663–4.

FRANDSEN, V. A. AND STAKEMANN, G. (1961). The site of production of oestrogenic hormones in human pregnancy. Hormone excretion in pregnancy with anencephalic foetus. *Acta endocr. (Kbl.)* **47**, 265–76.

——, —— (1964). The site of production of oestrogenic hormones in human pregnancy. III. Further observations in the hormone excretion in pregnancy with anencephalic foetus. *Acta endocr. (Kb.)* **47**, 265–76.

FRASER, F. C. (1959). Causes of congenital malformations in man. *J. chron. Dis.* **10**, 97–110.

—— (1976). The multifactorial/threshold concept—uses and misuses. *Teratology* **14**, 267–80.

—— AND NORA, J. J. (1975). *Genetics of man*. Lea and Febiger, Philadelphia.

—— AND SKELTON, J. (1978). Possible teratogenicity of maternal fever. (letter). *Lancet* **ii**, 634.

FRASER, G. R. (1972). The short-term reduction in birth incidence of recessive diseases as a result of genetic counselling after the birth of an affected child. *Hum. Hered.* **22**, 1–6.

—— (1972*a*). Selective abortion, gametic selection and the X chromosome. *Am. J. hum. Genet.* **24**, 359–70.

—— (1973). Genetical implications of ante-natal diagnosis. *Ann. Génét.* **16**, 5–10.

FRAUMENI, J. F. JR., LI, F. P., AND DALAGER, N. (1973). Teratomas in children: epidemiological features. *J. nat. Cancer Inst.* **51**, 1425–30.

FREED, D. L. (1977). Adherent amniotic-fluid cells and neural-tube defects. (letter). *Lancet* **i** 1099.

FREEMAN, J. M. (1974). The shortsighted treatment of myelomeningocele: a long-term case report. *Pediatrics* **53**, 311–13.

FREEMAN, M. V. R., WILLIAMS, D. W., SCHIMKE, R. N., TEMTAMY, S. A., VACHIER, E., AND GERMAN, J. (1974). The Robert's syndrome. *Clin. Genet.* **5**, 1–16.

FRENS, D. B., ZITER, F. A., AND BRAY, P. F. (1977). Bony and vascular anomalies of the head. *Arch. Neurol.* **34**, 508–10.

FRÉZAL, J. AND LAMY, M. (1956). Quoted in Penrose, L. S. (1957). Genetics of anencephaly. *J. ment. def. Res.* **1**, 4–15.

——, KELLEY, J., GUILLEMOT, M. L., AND LAMY, M. (1964). Anencephaly in France. *Am. J. hum. Genet.* **16**, 336–50.

FRIED, K. (1973). Relatively high prevalence of the Meckel syndrome among Jews. *Israel J. Med. Sci.* **9**, 1399.

——, LIBAN, E., LURIE, M., FRIEDMAN, S., AND REISNER, S. H. (1971). Polycystic kidneys associated with malformations of the brain, polydactyly, and other birth defects in newborn sibs. A lethal syndrome showing the autosomal-recessive pattern of inheritance. *J. med. Genet.* **8**, 285–90.

FRIGOLETTO, F. D. AND GRISCOM, N. T. (1974). Amniography tor the detection of fetal myelomeningocele. *Obstet. Gynec.* **44**, 286–90.

FROGGAT, P. AND NEVIN, N. C. (1971). The 'Law of Ancestral Heredity' and the Mendelian–Ancestrian controversy in England, 1889–1906. *J. Med. Genet.* **8**, 1–36.

FUCHS, F. (1966). Volumes of amniotic fluid at various stages of pregnancy. *Clin. Obstet. Gynecol.* **9** (2), 449–60.

FUHRMANN, W., SEEGER, W., AND BÖHM, R. (1971). Apparently monogenic inheritance of anencephaly and spina bifida in a kindred. *Humangenetik* **13**, 241–3.

GAJDUSEK, D. C. (1977). *Unconventional viruses and the origin and disappearance of kuru.* Nobel Foundation, Stockholm.

Gal, I. (1972). Risks and benefits of the use of hormonal pregnancy test tablets. *Nature, (Lond.).* **240**, 241–2.
——, Kirman, B., and Stern, J. (1967). Hormonal pregnancy tests and congenital malformation. *Nature, (Lond.).* **216**, 83.
——, Sharman, I. M., and Pryse-Davies, J. (1972). Vitamin A in relation to human congenital malformations. *Adv. Teratology* **5**, 143–59.
Gale, T. F. (1973). The interaction of mercury with cadmium and mammalian embryonic development. *Environ. Res.* **6**, 95–105.
Gallera, J. (1951). Influence d'l'atmosphère artificiellement modifée sur le developpement embryonnaire du poulet. *Acta Anat. (Basel)* **11**, 549–85.
Galton, F. (1865). Hereditary, talent and character. *Macmillan's Magazine* **12**, 318–27.
Gardiner, A., Clarke, C., Cowen, J., Finn, R., and McKendrick, O. M. (1978). Spontaneous abortion and fetal abnormality in subsequent pregnancy. *Br. Med. J.* **ii**, 1016–18.
Gardner, W. J. (1973). *The dysraphic states from syringomyelia to anencephaly.* Excerpta Medica, Amsterdam.
Garoff, L. and Seppälä, M. (1973). Alpha fetoprotein and human placental lactogen levels in maternal serum in multiple pregnancies. *J. Obstet. Gynaec. Br. Commonw.* **80**, 695–700.
Gart, J. J. (1970). Point and interval estimation of the common odds ratio in the combination of 2 × 2 tables with fixed margnials. *Biometrika* **3**, 471–5.

Gasking, E. B. (1959). Why was Mendel's work ignored? *Journal of the history of ideas* **20**, 60–84.
General Register Office, Edinburgh (1978). Unpublished data.
Geoffroy, Y., Denis, P., Colin, R., Sanger, F., Matray, F., and Fondimare, A. (1970). Présence d'alpha-1-foetoprotéine chez l'adulte au cours d'une hépatite virale traitée par corticothérapie. *Presse Méd.* **78**, 1107–8.
——, Boureille, J., Denis, P., Colin, R., and Metayer, P. (1971). Bilan d'une recherche systématique de l'alpha-1-foetoprotéine dans 224 hépatopathies. *Sem. Hôp. Paris* **47**, 1281–5.
Gilbert, E. S. (1968). On discrimination using qualitative variables. *J. Am. Stat. Ass.* **63**, 1399–1412.
—— (1969). The effect of unequal variance–covariance matrices on Fisher's linear discriminant function. *Biometrics* **25**, 505–15.
Giroud, A. (1952). Carences maternelles en acide pantothenique et an acide folique. *Étud. neo-natal* **1**, 5–23.
—— (1960). Causes and morphogenesis of anencephaly (and discussion). In *Ciba Foundation Symposium on Congenital Malformations, London, 1960*, edited by G. E. W. Wolstenholme and C. M. O'Connor. Churchill, London, pp. 199–240.
—— and Martinet, M. (1957). Morphogenesis de l'anencephalie. *Arch. Anat. Micr. Morph. Exp.* **46**, 247–64.
Gitlin, D. (1973). Ontogeny of fetal plasma proteins. *Tumor Res.* **8**, 1–6.
—— (1975). Normal biology of alpha-fetoprotein. *Ann. N.Y. Acad. Sci.* **259**, 7–16.
—— and Boesman, M. (1966). Serum α-fetoprotein, albumin, and YG-globulin in the human conceptus. *J. clin. Invest.* **45**, 1826–38.
——, —— (1967). Fetus-specific serum proteins in several mammals and their relation to human α-fetoprotein. *Comp. Biochem. Physiol.* **21**, 327–36.
Gittelsohn, A. M. and Milham, S. (1962). Declining incidence of central nervous system anomalies in New York State. *Br. J. prev. soc. Med.* **16**, 153–8.
—— and Mulham, S. (1965). Observations on twinning in New York State. *Br. J. prev. soc. Med.* **19**, 8–17.
Glatnz, L. H. (1975). The legal aspects of fetal viability. In *Genetics and the law* edited by Milunsky, A. and Anas, G. J. Plenum Press, New York.
Glaser, O. C. (1916). The theory of autonomous folding in embryogenesis. *Science* **44**, 505–9.
Glass, N. J. and Cove, A. R. (1978). Cost-effectiveness of screening for neural tube defects. In *Towards the prevention of fetal malformation* edited by Scrimgeour, J. B., Edinburgh University Press, Edinburgh, pp. 217–23.
Glasser, J. H. (1970). A stochastic model for industrial illness absenteeism. *Am. J. publ. Hlth.* **60**, 1936–44.

GLIETENBERG, H. (1967). Congenital malformations from the obstetricians point of view. *S. Afr. Med. J.* 161–4.
GOLBUS, M. S., CONTE, F. A., SCHNEIDER, E. L., AND EPSTEIN, C. J. (1974). Intrauterine diagnosis of genetic defects: Results, problems and follow-up of one hundred cases in a prenatal genetic detection center. *Am. J. Obstet. Gynecol.* **118**, 897–905.
GOLDFARB, A. F., MORALES, A., RAKOFF, A. E., AND PROTOS, P. (1968). Critical review of 160 clomiphene-related pregnancies. *Obstet. Gynec.* **31**, 342–5.
GOLDMAN, B., MASHIAH, S., SERR, D. M., BLANKENSTEIN, J., CHAKI, R., NAVON, R., AND PADEH, B. (1977). A survey of amniocentesis in 925 patients at high risk of fetal genetic disorder. *Br. J. Obstet. Gynaec.* **84**, 808–14.
GOLDSTEIN, H. AND BUTLER, N. R. (1977). Definition of perinatal mortality. (letter). *Lancet* **i**, 1254.
GORDON, Y. B., RATKY, S. M., LEIGHTON, P. C., KITAU, M. J., AND CHARD, T. (1976). Amniotic fluid levels of fibrin (ogen) degradation fragment E and alpha-fetoprotein in normal pregnancy and with fetal neural tube defect. *Br. J. Obstet. Gynaec.* **83**, 771–4.
GOSDEN, C. M., AND BROCK, D. J. H. (1977). Morphology of rapidly adhering amniotic fluid cells as an aid to the diagnosis of neural-tube defects. *Lancet* **i**, 919–22.
——, BROCK, D. J. H., AND EASON, P. (1977). The origin of the rapidly adhering cells found in amniotic fluids from foetuses with neural-tube defects. *Clin. Genet.* **12**, 193–201.
GOTTDIENER, J. S., ELLISON, R. C., AND LORENZO, R. L. (1975). Arteriovenous fistula after penetration at amniocentesis. *New Engl. J. Med.* **293**, 1302–3.
GOULD, J. (1978). Ethical problems of screening for neural-tube defects. (letter). *Lancet* **ii**, 265.
GRANROTH, G., HAKAMA, M., AND SAXÉN, L. (1977). Defects of the central nervous system in Finland I. Variations in time and space, sex distribution, and parental age. *Br. J. prev. soc. Med.* **31**, 164–70.
——, HAAPAKOSKI, J., AND HAKAMA, M. (1978). Defects of the central nervous system in Finland II. Birth order, outcome of previous pregnancies and family history. *Teratology* **17**, 213–22.
GREEN, H. P. (1975). The fetus and the law. In *Genetics and the law* edited by Milunsky, A. and Annas, G. J. Plenum Press, New York, pp. 19–28.
GREEN, R. C. (1964). The frequency of maldevelopment in man. *Am. J. Obstet. Gynec.* **90**, 994–1013.
GREENBERG, G., INMAN, W. H. W., WEATHERALL, J. A. C., ADELSTEIN, A. M., AND HASKEY, J. C. (1977). Maternal drug histories and congenital abnormalities. *Br. med. J.* **4**, 853–6.
GREENWOOD, M. (1935). *Epidemics and crowd-diseases. An introduction to the study of epidemiology.* MacMillan, New York.
GREGG, N. McA. (1941). Congenital cataract following German measles in the mother. *Trans Ophthalmol. Soc. Aust.* **3**, 35–46.
GREGOR, W. (1881). *Folk-lore of the north-east of Scotland.* Elliot Stock, London, pp. 214–15.
GRIFFIN, G. V. AND SORRIE, G. S. (1964). Congenital abnormalities in Reading 1958–63. *Med. Offr.* **112**, 197–9.
GRIFFIN, J. W., MATTHES, F. T., HAZLEWOOD, C. F., AND NICHOLS, B. L. (1967). The conjoined twins of Port Lavaca. *Birth Defects, Original Article Series* **3** (1), 139–40.
GRIMES, L. D. AND CASSADY, G. (1970). Fetal gastrointestinal obstruction. Prenatal diagnosis based on amniotic fluid analysis. *Am. J. Obstet. Gynec.* **106**, 1196–200.
GRUBER, G. B. (1934). Vorweisungen zur frage der entstehung einiger missbildungen. *Verh. dtsch. path. Ges. (Jena).* **27**, 303–9.
GRUENWALD, P. (1941). Tissue anomalies of probable neural crest origin in a 20mm human embryo with myeloschisis. *Arch. Path.* **31**, 489–500.
GRUNBERG, F. (1973). Screening for chromosomal abnormalities. (letter). *Lancet* **i**, 543.
GRUNEBERG, H. (1952). Genetical studies on the skeleton of the mouse IV. Quasi-continuous variations. *J. Genet.* **51**, 95–114.
GRUYS, E. AND BETHLEHEM, M. (1976). The dysraphic state in the calf, lamb and piglet. *Zbl. Vet. Med. A.* **23**, 811–18.
GUHA-RAY, D. (1975). Obstetric problems in association with anencephaly. A survey of 60 cases. *Obstet. Gynecol.* **46**, 569–72.
GUINEY, E. J., FITZGERALD, R. J., MEHIGAN, D., PURI, P., AND SUNDAR, B. (1977). Surgical closure of myelomeningocele: problems and consequences of the introduction of a policy of selection. *Irish J. Med. Sci.* **146**, 260–2.

GUTHKELCH, A. N. (1962). Studies in spina bifida cystica: III. Seasonal variation in the frequency of spina bifida births. *Br. J. prev. soc. Med.* **16**, 159–62.
GUTTMACHER, A. F. AND NICHOLS, B. L. (1967). Teratology of conjoined twins. *Birth Defects, Original Articles Series* **3** (1), 3–9.

HACK, M., BRISH, M., SERR, D. M., INSLER, V., SALMONY, M., AND LUNENFELD, B. (1972). Outcome of pregnancy after induced ovulation. *J. Am. med. Ass.* **220**, 1329–33.
HADDOW, J. E. (1978). Ethical problems of screening for neural-tube defects. (letter). *Lancet* **ii**, 527.
HAGARD, S., CARTER, F., AND MILNE, R. C. (1976). Screening for spina bifida cystica: a cost-benefit analysis. *Br. J. prev. soc. Med.* **30**, 40–53.
HALEVI, H. S. (1967). Congenital malformations in Israel. *Br. J. prev. soc. Med.* **21**, 66–77.
HALL, M. H. (1972). Folic acid deficiency and congenital malformation. *Br. J. Obstet. Gynaec.* **79**, 159–61.
—— (1977). Folates and the fetus. (letter). *Lancet* **i**, 648–9.
HALPERIN, L. R. AND WILROY, R. S. JR. (1978). Maternal hyperthermia and neural-tube defects. (letter). *Lancet* **ii**, 212–13.
HALPERIN, M., BLACKWELDER, W. C., AND VERTER, J. (1971). Estimation of the multivariate logistic risk function: a comparison of the discriminant function and maximum likelihood approaches. *J. Chron. Dis.* **24**, 125–58.
——, WARE, J. H., BYAR, D. P., MANTEL, N., BROWN, C. C., KOZIOL, J., GAIL, M., AND GREEN, S. B. (1977). Testing for interaction in a $I \times J \times K$ contingency table. *Biometrika* **64**, 271–5.
HAMBURGER, V. AND HABEL, K. (1947). Teratogenic and lethal effects of influenza A and mumps viruses on early chick embryos. *Proc. Soc. Exp. Biol. Med.* **66**, 608–17.
HAMMOND, E. C. (1964). Smoking in relation to mortality and morbidity. Findings in first thirty-four months of follow up in a prospective study started in 1959. *J. Nat. Cancer Inst.* **32**, 1161–88.
HANAWAY, J. AND WELCH, G. (1970). Anencephaly: a review and interpretation in terms of modern experimental embryology. *Dis. Nerv. System* **31**, 527–33.
HARDY, J. M. B., AZAROWICZ, E. N., MANNINI, A., MEDEARIS, D. N., AND COOKE, R. E. (1961). The effect of Asian influenza on the outcome of pregnancy, Baltimore, 1957–58. *Am. J. publ. Hlth.* **51**, 1182–8.
HARE, E. H. AND PRICE, J. S. (1968). Mental disorder and season of birth: comparison of psychosis with neurosis. *Br. J. Psych.* **115**, 533–40.
HARPER, P. S. (1977). Mendelian inheritance or transmissible agent?—the lesson of kuru and the Australia antigen. *J. Med. Genet.* **14**, 389–98.
HARRIS, H. (1974). *Prenatal diagnosis and selective abortion.* The Nuffield Provincial Hospitals Trust, London, p. 76.
HARRIS, L. E. AND STEINBERG, A. G. (1954). Abnormalities observed during the first six days of life in 8,716 liveborn infants. *Pediatrics* **14**, 314–26.
HARRIS, R. (1978). Inadequate prenatal diagnosis of Down's syndrome. (letter). *Br. med. J.* **3**, 199–200.
——, JENNISON, R. F., BARSON, A. J., LAURENCE, K. M., RUOSLAHTI, E., AND SEPPÄLÄ, M. (1974). Comparison of amniotic fluid and maternal serum alpha-fetoprotein levels in the early antenatal diagnosis of spina bifida and anencephaly. *Lancet* **i**, 429–33.
HARRIS, W. J. AND TUPPER, L. S. (1977). A study of therapeutic abortion committees in British Columbia. *UBC Law Review* **11**, 101–18.
HAY, S. (1971). Incidence of selected congenital malformations in Iowa. *Am. J. Epidem.* **94**, 572–84.
—— AND WEHRUNG, D. A. (1970). Congenital malformations in twins. *Am. J. Hum. Genet.* **22**, 662–78.
HAYES, D. M. (1961). The seasonal incidence of acute leukaemia. *Cancer* **14**, 1301–5.
HAYNES, S. G., GIBSON, J. B., AND KURLAND, L. T. (1974). Epidemiology of neural-tube defects and Down's syndrome in Rochester, Minnesota, 1935–1971. *Neurology* **24**, 691–700.
HEASMAN, M. A. (1968). The use of record linkage in long-term prospective studies. In *Record linkage in medicine*, Acheson, E. D. editor. E & S Livingstone Ltd., Edinburgh, pp. 251–9.
HEGNAUER, H. (1951). Missbildungshaüfigkeit und Gebäralter. *Geburtsh. U. Frauenheilk* **11**, 777–92.

HELMHOLZ, R. H. (1974). Infanticide in the Province of Canterbury during the fifteenth century. *Hist. Childhood Q.* **2**, 379–90.
HENRION, R. (1976). Amniocentesis: 300 observations. In *Prenatal diagnosis*. INSERM, Paris, edited by Boué, A., Vol. **61**, pp. 45–52.
HENRY, A. P. J. AND MICKEL, R. E. (1974). Spina bifida in African and Indian babies. *J. Bone Jt Surg.* **56B**, 650–8.
HENRY, G. P., AND ROBINSON, A. (1977). Equivocal amniotic fluid levels of alpha fetoprotein in prenatal diagnosis of neural tube defects. *Am. J. Obstet. Gynecol.* **127**, 204.
——, PEAKMAN, D. C., AND ROBINSON, A. (1978). Prenatal genetic diagnosis: nine years' experience. *Obstet. Gynec. Survey.* **33**, 569–77.
HENZL, M. R. (1971). Mortality of abortion. (letter). *Lancet* **ii**, 368.
HERBST, A. L., ULFELDER, H., AND POSKANZER, D. C. (1971). Adenocarcinoma of the vagina. Association of maternal stilbestrol therapy with tumor appearance in young women. *New Engl. J. Med.* **284**, 878–81.
HEUSER, R. L. (1966). Multiple Births 1964. *U.S. Vital and Health Statistics Series* **21**, 8–15.
HEWITT, D. (1963). Geographical variations in the mortality attributed to spina bifida and other congenital malformations. *Br. J. prev. Soc. Med.* **17**, 13–22.
——, MILNER, J., CISIMA, A., AND PAKULA, A. (1971). On Edward's criterion of seasonality and a non-parametric alternative. *Br. J. prev. soc. Med.* **25**, 174–6.
HIBBARD, E. D. AND SMITHELLS, R. W. (1965). Folic acid metabolism and human embryopathy. *Lancet* **i**, 1254.
HICKS, S. P. (1953). Development of malformations produced by radiation. *Am. J. Roentgenol.* **69**, 272–93.
—— (1954). Effects of ionizing radiation, certain hormones, and radiometric drugs on the developing nervous system. In *Symposium on effects of radiation and other deleterious agents on embryonic development. J. cell. comp. Physiol.* **43**, suppl. 1, pp. 151–78.
—— AND D'AMATO, C. J. (1966). Effects of ionizing radiation on mammalian development. In *Advances in teratology.* Logos Press and Academic Press, London.
HIDE, D. W., WILLIAMS, H. P., AND ELLIS, H. L. (1972). The outlook for a child with myelomeningocele for whom early surgery was considered inadvisable. *Develop. Med. Child. Neurol.* **14**, 304–7.
HIGA, Y., SASAZUKI, T., NAKAJUNA, H., TAKAYAMA, M., TADA, M., AND SOMA, H. (1974). Amniotic fluid proteins in the antenatal diagnosis of some fetal abnormalities. *Am. J. Obstet. Gynecol.* **119**, 932–8.
HIILESMAA, V. (1945). A study of anencephalus and hydrocephalus deliveries. *Acta. Obst. Gyn. Scand. Suppl.* **25** (2), 27–50.
HILDEBRAND, I. (1893). Pathologisch-anatomische und klinische Untersuchungen zur Lehre von der spina bifida und den Hirnbrüchen. *Deutsche Ztschr. f. Chir., Leipzig* **36,** 433–535.
HILL, A. B. (1966). *Principles of medical statistics.* Eighth Edition. Oxford University Press, New York.
HINDSE-NIELSEN, S. (1938). Spina bifida-prognose: Erblichkeit. ein. klinische studie. *Acta Chir. Scand.* **80**, 525–78.
HOBBINS, J. C. AND MAHONEY, M. J. (1976). Clinical experiences with fetoscopy and fetal blood sampling. In *Intrauterine fetal visualization. A multidisciplinary approach.* Edited by Kaback, M. M and Valenti, C. Excerpta Medica, Amsterdam, pp. 164–70.
HOBBS, F. S. (1966). Anencephaly and hydrocephaly in a twin pregnancy. *Can. Med. Ass. J.* **94**, 1184.
HOBBS, M. S. T. (1969). Risk of anencephaly in migrant and non-migrant women in the Oxford area. *Br. J. prev. soc. Med.* **23**, 174–8.
HOFMANN, D. AND DIETZEL, F. (1966). Aborte und Missbildungen nach Kurzwellendurch flutung in der Schwangerschaft. *Geburtshilfe Frauenheilkd.* **26**, 378–90.
HOLLAND, E. L. AND LANE-CLAYPON, J. E. (1926). *Child life investigations. A clinical and pathological study of 1673 cases of dead-births and neonatal deaths.* MRC Special Report Series, No. 109. HMSO, London.
HOLLAND, W. W. (1974). Screening for disease. Taking stock. *Lancet* **ii** 1494–7.
HOLMES, L. B., DRISCOLL, S. G., AND ATKINS, L. (1976). Etiologic heterogeneity of neural-tube defects. *New Engl. J. Med* **294**, 365–9.

Hook, E. B. (1973). Behavioral implications of the human XYY genotype. *Science* **179**, 139.
—— (1975). Rates of XYY genotype in penal and mental settings. *Lancet* **i**, 98.
Horne, H. W. (1958). Anencephaly in four consecutive pregnancies. Report of a case. *Fertil. Steril.* **9**, 67.
Horner, R. and Lanzkowsky, P. (1966). Incidence of congenital abnormalities in Cape Town. *S. Afr. Med. J.* **40**, 171.
Horowitz, I. and McDonald, A. D. (1969). Anencephaly and spina bifida in Quebec. *Can. Med. Ass. J.* **100**, 748–55.
Horsley, R. J. and Peters, V. G. (1976). Radiation exposure from EMI-scanner-multiple scans. *Br. J. Radiol.* **49**, 810–11.
Hsia, Y. E., Bratu, M., and Herbordt, A. (1971). Genetics of the Meckel syndrome (dysencephalia splanchnocystica). *Pediatrics* **48**, 237–47.
Hull, E. W., Carbone, P. P., Moertel, C. G., and O'Conor, G. T. (1970). Serum alpha-fetoprotein in the USA. *Lancet* **i**, 779–80.
Humphry, G. M. (1885). The anatomy of spina bifida. *J. Anat Physiol.* **19**, 500–8.
Hungerford, P. (1971). Mortality and morbidity of abortion. (letter). *Lancet* **i**, 1012.
Hurley, L. S. (1974). Zinc deficiency, potatoes, and congenital malformations in man. *Teratology* **10** (2), 205–6.
—— and Swenerton, H. (1966). Congenital malformations resulting from zinc deficiency in rats. *Proc. Soc. exp. Biol. (N.Y.)* **123**, 692–7.
Hurwitz, C. H. (1955). Anencephalus. *Obstet. Gynecol.* **6**, 303–8.
Huxley, J. (1962). Eugenics in evolutionary perspective. *Eugen. Rev.* **54**, 123–41.

Iffy, L. (1963). Thrice recurring anencephalus. *Br. J. Clin. Pract.* **17**, 83.
——, Shepard, T. H., Jakobovits, A., Lemire, R. J., and Kerner, P. (1967). The rate of growth in young embryos of Streeter's horizons, XIII to XXIII. *Acta Anat. (Basel)* **66**, 178–86.
Illich, I. (1975). *Medical nemesis. The expropriation of health.* Calder & Boyars, London.
Illingworth, R. S. (1974). Some ethical problems in paediatrics. In *Modern trends in paediatrics—4*, edited by Apley, J. Butterworths, London, pp. 329–57.
Imaizumi, Y. (1974). Statistical analysis on anencephaly, spina bifida and congenital hydrocephaly in Japan. *Jap. J. hum. Genet.* **19** (2), 115–35.
Infante, P. (1976). Ontogenic and mutagenic risks in communities with polyvinyl chloride production facilities. *Ann. N.Y. Acad. Sci.* **271**, 49.
Ingalls, T. H. and Klingberg, M. A. (1965). Congenital malformations: clinical and community considerations. *Am. J. med. Sci.* **249**, 316–44.
——, Curley, F. J., and Prindle, R. A. (1950). Anoxia as a cause of fetal death and congenital defect in the mouse. *Am. J. Dis. Child.* **80** 34–45.
——, Pugh, T. F., and MacMahon, B. (1954). Incidence of anencephalus, spina bifida, and hydrocephalus related to birth rank and maternal age. *Br. J. prev. soc. Med.* **8**, 17–23.
Ingraham, F. D. (1944). *Spina bifida and cranium bifidum—papers reprinted from the* New England Journal of Medicine *with the addition of a comprehensive bibliography.* Massachusetts Medical Society, Cambridge, Massachusetts.
Ishiguro, T. (1973). Alpha-fetoprotein in pregnancy. (letter). *Lancet* **i**, 1509.
—— and Nishimura, T. (1973). Radioimmunoassay of maternal serum α-fetoprotein associated with pregnancy. *Am. J. Obstet. Gynec.* **116**, 27–33.
Ivemark, B. I. (1958). Implications of agenesis of the spleen on the pathogenesis of conotruncus anomalies in childhood. *Acta Paediatr. Scand. Suppl.* **44**, 1–100.

Jacobson, C. O. (1962). Cell migration in the neural plate and the process of neurulation in the axolotl larva. *Zool. Bidr. Uppsala* **35**, 433–49.
James, C. C. M. and Lassman, L. P. (1972). *Spinal dysraphisin*. Butterworths, London.
——, —— and Tomlinson, B. E. (1969). Congenital anomalies of the lower spine and spinal cord in Manx cats. *J. Path.* **97**, 269–76.
James, W. H. (1968). Stillbirth, neonatal death and birth interval. *Ann. Hum. Genet. (Lond).* **32**, 163–72.
—— (1969). Central nervous system malformation stillbirths, maternal age and birth order. *Ann. Hum. Genet. (Lond).* **32**, 223–36.
—— (1972). Secular changes in dizygotic twinning rates. *J. Biosoc. Sci.* **4**, 427–34.

—— (1973). Anencephaly, ovulation stimulation, subfertility and illegitimacy. (letter). *Lancet* **ii**, 916.

—— (1976). Twinning and anencephaly. *Ann. Hum. Biol.* **3**, 401–9.

—— (1976*a*). The power of a test for seasonality of birth with reference to schizophrenia. *Br. J. Psych.* **129**, 94–5.

—— (1977). Clomiphene, anencephaly and spina bifida. (letter). *Lancet* **i**, 603.

—— (1978). Recurrence rates in sibships and concordance rates in twins for anencephaly. *Ann. Hum. Biol.* **5**, 79–81.

—— (1978*a*). Hyperthermia and meningomyelocele and anencephaly. (letter). *Lancet* **i**, 770.

Jandial, W., Thom, H., and Gibson, J. (1976). Raised alpha-fetoprotein levels associated with minor congenital defects. *Br. Med. J.* **ii**, 22.

Janerich, D. T. (1972). Anencephaly and maternal age. *Am. J. Epidemiol.* **95,** 319–26.

—— (1972*a*). Maternal age and spina bifida: longitudinal versus cross-sectional analysis. *Am. J. Epidemiol.* **96**, 389–96.

—— (1972*b*). Maternal factors in C.N.S. malformations: a cohort approach. In *Congenital defects—new directions in research* edited by D. T. Janerich, R. G. Skalko, and I. H. Porter. Academic Press, New York, pp. 73–93.

—— (1973). Epidemic waves in the prevalence of anencephaly and spina bifida in N.Y. State. *Teratology* **8**, 253–6.

—— (1974). Endocrine dysfunction and anencephaly and spina bifida—an epidemiologic hypothesis. *Am. J. Epidem.* **99**, 1–6.

—— (1975). Female excess in anencephaly and spina bifida: possible gestational influences. *Am. J. Epidem.* **101**, 70–6.

—— (1977). Personal communication.

—— and Piper, J. (1978). Shifting genetic patterns in anencephaly and spina bifida. *J. Med. Genet.* **15**, 101–5.

——, ——, and Glebatis, D. M. (1974). Oral contraceptives and congenital limb-reduction defects. *New Engl. J. Med.* **291**, 697–700.

——, ——, —— (1975). Congenital limb-reduction deformities. (letter). *Lancet* **i**, 931.

Janz, D. and Fuchs, U. (1964). Sind antiepileptische Medikamente während der Schwangerschaft schädlich? *Dtsch. Med. Wochenschr.* **89**, 241–8.

Jeffcoate, T. N. A., Fliegner, J. R. H., Russell, S. H., Davis, J. C., and Wade, A. P. (1965). Diagnosis of the adrenogenital syndrome before birth. *Lancet* **ii**, 553–5.

Jelinek, R. (1960). Development of the experimental exencephaly in the chick. *Cs. Morfol.* **8**, 363–78.

Jepson, A. M. (1969). The problems of congenital defects of the central nervous system in a London borough. *Med. Offr.* **121**, 15–17.

Jick, H., Miettinen, O., Neff, R. K., Shapiro, S., Heinonen, O. P., and Slone, D. (1973). Coffee and myocardial infarction. *New Engl. J. Med.* **289**, 63–7.

Johnansson, S. G. O., Kjessler, B., and Sherman, M. S. (1976). Determination of α-fetoprotein by a new paper disc radioimmunoassay of the sandwich type. *Int. Archs. Allergy. Appl. Immun.* **52**, 384–91.

——, ——, ——, and Wahlström, J. (1977). Alpha-fetoprotein (AFP) levels in maternal serum and amniotic fluid in singleton pregnant women in their 10th-25th weeks post last menstrual period. *Acta Obstet. Gynecol. Scand. Suppl.* **69**, 20–4.

——, ——, ——, and Bennich, H. (1977). Quantitative determination of alpha-fetoprotein (AFP) in biological fluids by a direct and rapid radio-immunoassay, PRIST. *Acta Obstet. Gynecol. Scand. Suppl.* **69**, 15–19.

Johnson, A. F. (1971). Design of experiments: the single cycle sine wave model. *Biometrics* **27**, 730–4.

Johnston, J. (1963). *Econometric methods.* McGraw-Hill, New York, p. 207.

Johnston, K. P., Klasnja, R., and Johnston, R. T. (1971). Neural-tube defects of chick embryos: an indirect result of influenza–A virus infection. *J. Neuropathol. Exp. Neurol.* **30**, 68–74.

Jones, K. L., Smith, D. W., Ulleland, C. N., and Streissguth, A. P. (1973). Pattern of malformation in offspring of chronic alcoholic mothers. *Lancet* **i**, 1267–71.

——, ——, Hall, B. D., Hall, J. G., Ebbin, A. J., Massoud, H., and Golbus, M. S. (1974). A

pattern of craniofacial and limb defects secondary to aberrant tissue bands. *J. Pediat.* **84**, 90–5.
JONES, W. R. (1967). Anencephalus: a 23 year survey in a Sydney hospital. *Med. J. Aust.* **1**, 104–6.
JOSEPHSON, J. E. AND WALLER, K. B. (1933). Anencephaly in identical twins. *Can. med. Ass. J.* **29**, 34–7.

KAHN, E. (1956). Personal communication. *See* Penrose, L. S. (1957).
KALBACH, W. E. (1970). *The impact of immigration on Canada's population*. 1961 Census Monograph, The Queen's Printer, Ottawa.
KÄLLÉN, B. (1968). Early embryogenesis of the central nervous system with special reference to closure defects. *Dev. Med. Child. Neurol. suppl.* **16**, 44–53.
——, AND WINBERG, J. (1968). A Swedish Register of congenital malformations. Experience with continuous registration during two years with special reference to multiple malformations. *Pediatrics* **41**, 765–76.
KARP, L. E. AND HAYDEN, P. W. (1977). Fetal puncture during midtrimester amniocentesis. *Obstet. Gynec.* **49** (1), 115–17.
KARVOUNTZIS, G. G. AND REDEKER, A. G. (1974). Relation of alpha-fetoprotein in acute hepatitis to severity and prognosis. *Ann. Int. Med.* **80**, 156–60.
KATZEN, M. (1975). The results of a policy of 'selecting out' in children with myelomeningocele. *S. Afr. J. Surg.* **13**, 215–18.
KAZARIAN, E. AND GOLDSTEIN, P. (1977). Ankyloblepharon filiforme adnatum with hydrocephalus, meningomyelocele and imperforate anus. *Am. J. Ophthalm.* **84**, 355–7.
KEEN, J. A. (1962). The morphology of the skull in anencephalic monsters. *S. Afr. J. lab. clin. Med.* **8**, 1–9.
KEKOMAKI, M., SEPPALA, M., ENHOLM, C. C., SCHWARTZ, A. L., AND RAIVIO, K. (1971). Perfusion of isolated human fetal liver synthesis and release of α-fetoprotein and albumin. *Int. J. Cancer.* **8**, 250–8.
KEILANI, Z., CLARKE, P. C., KITAU, M. J. AND CHARD, T. (1978). The significance of raised maternal plasma alpha-fetoprotein in twin pregnancy. *Br. J. Obstet. Gynaec.* **85**, 510–11.
KELLUM, B. A. (1974). Infanticide in England in the later middle ages. *Hist. childhood Q.*, **1**, 367–88.
KELSEY, J. L., DWYER, T., HOLFORD, T. R., AND BRACKEN, M. B. (1978). Maternal smoking and congenital malformations: an epidemiological study. *J. Epidem. Community Hlth.* **32**, 102–7.
KENDALL, M. G. (1973). *Time series.* Hafner Press, New York.
——, AND STUART, A. (1976). *The advanced theory of statistics*. Volume 3, Third Edition. Charles Griffin, London.
KHERA, K. S. (1973). Ethylenethiorea: teratogenicity study in rats and rabbits. *Teratology* **7**, 243–52.
KILPATRICK, S. J., MATHERS, J. D., AND STEVENSON, A. C. (1955). The importance of population fertility and consanguinity data being available in medico-social studies. *Ulster Med. J.* **24**, 113–22.
KILNEN, L. AND HEWITT, A. (1973). Potato blight and anencephalus in Scotland. *Br. J. prev. soc. Med.* **27**, 208–13.
KIRKPATRICK, T. P. C., (1973). *The book of the Rotunda Hospital*. Bartholomew Press, London.
KITHIER, K., MASOPUST, J., AND RÁDL, J. (1968). Fetal alpha-globulin of bovine serum differing from fetuin. *Biochim. Biophys. Acta.* **160**, 135–7.
KJESSLER, B., JOHANSSON, S. G. O., SHERMAN, M., GUSTAVSON, K. H., AND HULTQUIST, G. (1975). Alpha-fetoprotein in antenatal diagnosis of congenital nephrosis. *Lancet* **i**, 432–3.
——, ——, LIDBJORK, G., AND SHERMAN, M. S. (1977). Alpha-fetoprotein (AFP) levels in maternal serum in relation to pregnancy outcome in 7158 pregnant women prospectively investigated during their 14th–20th week post last menstrual period. *Acta. Abstet. Gynec. Scand. Suppl.* **69**, 25–44.
——, HEMMINGSSON, A., NILSSON, B. A. AND JOHANSSON, S. G. O. (1977). Early diagnosis of trophoblastic disease and fetal maldevelopment by determination of alpha-fetoprotein (AFP), human chorionic gonadotrophin (LCG) and amniography. *Acta Obstet. Gynecol. Scand. Suppl.* **69**, 83–93.

KLEIJER, W. J., DE BRUIJN, H. W. A., AND LESCHOT, N. J. (1978). Amniotic fluid alpha-fetoprotein levels and the prenatal diagnosis of neural tube defects: a collaborative study of 2180 pregnancies in the Netherlands. *Br. J. Obstet. Gynaec.* **85**, 512–17.

KLEINMAN, H., PRINCE, J. T., MATHEY, W. E., ROSENFIELD, A. B., BEARMAN, J. E., AND SYVERTON, J. T. (1962). Echo 9 virus infections and congenital abnormalities: a negative report. *Pediatrics* **29**, 261–9.

KLINGBERG, M. A., CHEMKE, R. C. J., AND LEVIN, S. (1971). An epidemologic study of congenital malformations among different ethnic and social groups in Israel. *Develop. Med. Child Neurol.* **13**, 735–45.

KNILL-JONES, R. P., RODRIGUES, L. V., MOIR, D. D., SPENCE, A. A. (1972). Anaesthetic practice and pregnancy. Controlled survey of women anaesthetists in the United Kingdom. *Lancet* **i**, 1326–28.

——, NEWMAN, B. J., AND SPENCE, A. A. (1975). Anaesthetic practice and pregnancy. *Lancet* **ii**, 807–9.

KNOBLOCH, W. H. AND LAYER, J. M. (1971). Retinal detachment and encephalocele. *J. ped. Ophthal.* **8**, 181–4.

KNOX, E. G. (1963). Detection of low intensity epidemicity. Application to cleft lip and palate. *Br. J. prev. soc. Med.* **17**, 121–7.

—— (1964). Epidemiology of childhood leukaemia in Northumberland and Durham. *Br. J. prev. soc. Med.* **18**, 17–24.

—— (1967). Spina bifida in Birmingham. *Develop. med. Child Neurol., suppl.* **13**, 14–22.

—— (1970). Fetus-fetus interaction—a model aetiology for anencephalus. *Dev. med. Child Neurol.* **12**, 167–77.

—— (1972). Anencephalus and dietary intakes. *Br. J. prev. soc. Med.* **26**, 219–23.

—— (1974). Twins and neural tube defects. *Br. J. prev. soc. Med.* **28**, 73–80.

KOHN, J. (1975). Antenatal misdiagnosis of neural-tube defects. (letter). *Lancet* **ii**, 663.

KOSKIMIES, O., LAPINLEIMU, K., AND SAXÉN, L. (1978). Infections and other maternal factors as risk indicators for congenital malformations: a case-control study with paired serum samples. *Pediatrics* **61**, 832–7.

KOZOWER, M., FAWAZ, K. A., AND MILLER, H. M. (1971). Positive alpha-fetoglobulin in a case of gastric carcinoma. *New Engl. J. Med.* **285**, 1059–60.

KRESNO, S. B., GANDASOEBRATA, R., AND RÜMKE, P. (1970). Serum alpha-fetoprotein in Indonesia. (letter). *Lancet* **i**, 1178.

KUČERA, J. (1965). Die Erfassung der angeborenen Missbildungen in der CSSR. *Ann. Pediat.* **204**, 141–51.

—— (1971). Rate and type of congenital amonalies among offspring of diabetic women. *J. Reprod. Med.* **7**, 73–82.

KUHR, M. D. (1977). Neural-tube defects and mid-cycle abstinence: a test of the 'over-ripeness' hypothesis in man. *Develop. Med. Child Neurol.* **19**, 589–92.

KURENT, J. AND SEVER, J. L. (1973). Perinatal infections and epidemiology of anencephaly and spina bifida. *Teratology* **8**, 359–62.

KURTZKE, J. F., GOLDBERG, I. D., AND KURLAND, L. T. (1973). Congenital malformations of the nervous system. In *Epidemiology of neurologic and sense disorders* edited by Kurland, L. T., Kurtzke, J. F. and Goldberg, I. D. Harvard University Press, Cambridge, Massachusetts, pp. 169–209.

LAI, P. C. W., PETERS, E. H., AND LORSCHEIDER, F. L. (1978). Bovine fetus-specific serum proteins. Purification and characterization of α_1-fetoprotein and immunological identification of α_2 and β-fetoproteins. *Biochim. Biophys. Acta* **535**, 138–49.

LAKDAWALA, D. R. AND WIDDOWSON, E. M. (1977). Vitamin D in human milk. *Lancet* **i**, 167–8.

LAMB, M. P. (1975). Gangrene of a fetal limb due to amniocentesis. *Br. J. Obstet. Gynaec.* **82**, 829–30.

Lancet (1971). How safe is abortion? (editorial). *Lancet* **ii**, 1239–40.

—— (1975). Zinc in human medicine. (editorial). *Lancet* **ii**, 351–2.

—— (1975*a*). Ethics of selective treatment of spina bifida. Report of a working-party. *Lancet* **i**, 85–8.

—— (1978). Neural-tube defects (editorial). *Lancet* **i**, 312–3.

—— (1978*a*). Hyperthermia and the neural tube (editorial). *Lancet* **ii**, 560–1.

—— (1978*b*). The Braine Bill. *Lancet* **i**, 511.

LANGE, K. AND ELSTON, R. C. (1975). Extensions to pedigree analysis. *Hum. Hered.* **25**, 95–105.

LANGMAN, J. AND WELCH, G. (1967). Excess vitamin A and development of the cerebral cortex. *J. comp. Neurol.* **131**, 15–26.

LARDINOIS, R., ANAGHOSTAKIS, A., ORITZ, M. A., AND DELISLE, M. (1972). Human α_1-fetoglobulin during the last trimester of gestation. *Clin. Chim. Acta* **37**, 81–90.

LARSSON, K. S. (1974). Data banks. In *Birth defects*. Edited by Motulsky, A. G. and Lenz, W. Excerpta med. (Amst.)., pp. 187–90.

LAU, H. L. AND LINKINS, S. E. (1976). Alpha-fetoprotein. *Am. J. Obstet. Gynecol.* **124**, 533–54.

LAURENCE, K. M. (1964). The natural history of spina bifida cystica. Detailed analysis of 407 cases. *Arch. Dis. Child.* **39**, 41–57.

—— (1976). Prenatal diagnosis in anencephaly and spina bifida. In *Birth defects—risks and consequences*. Edited by Kelly, S., Hook, E. B., Janerich, D. T., and Porter, I. H. Academic Press, New York, pp. 63–89.

—— AND TEW, B. J. (1971). Natural history of spina bifida cystica and cranium bifidum cysticum. *Arch. Dis. Childh.* **46**, 127–38.

——, CARTER, C. O., AND DAVID, P. A. (1967). Major central nervous system malformations in South Wales. I. Incidence, local variation and geographical factors. *Br. J. prev. soc. Med.* **21**, 146–60.

——, ——, —— (1968). Major central nervous system malformations in South Wales. II. Pregnancy factors, seasonal variation, and social class effects. *Br. J. prev. soc. Med.* **22**, 212–22.

——, MILLER, M., VOWLES, M., EVANS, K., AND CARTER, C. (1971). Hormonal pregnancy tests and neural tube malformations. *Nature, (Lond.)* **233**, 495–6.

——, TURNBULL, A. C., HARRIS, R., JENNISON, R. F., RUOSLAHTI, E., AND SEPPÄLÄ, M. (1973). Antental diagnosis of spina bifida (letter). *Lancet* **ii**, 860.

——, PEARSON, J. F., PROSSER, R., RICHARDS, C., AND ROCKER, I. (1974). Fetoscopy followed by live birth. (letter). *Lancet* **i**, 1120.

——, WALKER, S. M., LLOYD, M., AND GRIFFITHS, B. L. (1975). Equivocal amniotic AFP levels associated with open spina bifida (letter). *Lancet* **ii**, 81.

——, EVANS, R. C., WEEKS, R. D., THOMAS, M. D., FRAZER, A. K., AND TEW, B. J. (1976). The reliability of prediction of outcome in spina bifida. *Develop. Med. Child Neurol.* **18**, suppl. **37**, 150–6.

LECK, I. (1963). Incidence of malformations following influenza epidemics. *Br. J. prev. soc. Med.* **17**, 70–80.

—— (1966). Changes in the incidence of neural tube defects. *Lancet* **ii**, 791–2.

—— (1966*a*). Incidence and epidemicity of Down's syndrome. *Lancet* **ii**, 457–60.

—— (1969). Ethnic differences in the incidence of malformations following migration. *Br. J. prev. soc. Med.* **23**, 166–73.

—— (1971). Further tests of the hypothesis that influenza in pregnancy causes malformations. *HSMHA Health Report* **86**, 265–9.

—— (1972). The etiology of human malformations: insights from epidemiology. *Teratology* **5**, 303–14.

—— (1974). Causation of neural tube defects: clues from epidemiology. *Br. med. Bull.* **30**, 158–63.

—— (1977). Correlations of malformation frequency with environmental and genetic attributes in man. In *Handbook of teratology*, Vol. 3, edited by Wilson, J. G. and Fraser, F. C. Plenum Publishing Co., New York, 243–323.

—— AND RECORD, R. G. (1966). Seasonal incidence of anencephalus. *Br. J. prev. soc. Med.* **20**, 67–75.

—— AND ROGERS, S. C. (1967). Changes in the incidence of anencephalus. *Br. J. prev. soc. Med.* **21**, 177–80.

——, RECORD, R. G., MCKEOWN, T., AND EDWARDS, J. H. (1968). The incidence of malformations in Birmingham, England, 1950–59. *Teratology* **1**, 263–80.

——, ILES, C. A., SHARMAN, I. M., TOE, T., AND WADSWORTH, G. R. (1974). A study of the extent to which maternal nutrition after delivery reflects the situation in early pregnancy (sum-

mary). Paper presented at the XVII Annual Meeting of the Society for Social Medicine, Southampton. *Br. J. prev. soc. Med.* **28**, 66.
LEE, J. A. H. (1962). Seasonal variation in the clinical onset of leukaemia in young people. *Br. med. J.* **ii**, 1737–38.
LEE, H.-Y. HIKIDA, R. S. AND LEVIN, M. A. (1976). Neural-tube defects caused by 5 Bromodeoxyuridine in chicks. *Teratology* **14**, 89–98.
LEE, T. Y. AND WEI, P. Y. (1970). Spectrophotometric analysis of amniotic fluid in anencephalic pregnancies. *Am. J. Obstet. Gynecol.* **107** (2), 917–20.
LEEK, A. E., RUOSS, C. F., KITAU, M. J., AND CHARD, T. (1975). Maternal plasma alphafetoprotein levels in the second half of normal pregnancy: relationship to fetal weight, and maternal age and parity. *Br. J. Obstet. Gynaec.* **82**, 669–73.
LEFEBVRES-BOISSELOT, J. (1951). Rôle teratogène de la déficience en acid pantothénique chez le rat. *Ann. Méd. (Paris)* **52**, 225–98.
LEICHTY, E. (1970). *Texts from Cuneiform Sources, Vol IV. The Omen series Shumma Izbu.* Augustin, J. J., Locust Valley, New York.
LEIGHTON, P. C., GORDON, Y. B., KITAU, M. J., LEEK, A. E., AND CHARD, T. (1975). Levels of alpha-fetoprotein in maternal blood as a screening test for fetal neural tube defect. *Lancet* **ii**, 1012–15.
LELEK, K., LIMANOWSKI, J., AND HAGER-MALECKA, B. (1973). A three-month old infant with birth weight 450 g. *Pediatr. Pol.* **48**, 221–6.
LEJEUNE, J. (1970). The William Allen Memorial Award Lecture. On the nature of man. *Am. J. hum. genet.* **22**, 121–8.
LEMIRE, R. J., BECKWITH, J. B., AND WARKANY, J. (1978). *Anencephaly*. Raven Press, New York.
——, SHEPHARD, T. H. AND ALVORD, E. D. JR. (1965). Caudal myeloschisis (lumbosacral spina bifida cystica) in a five millimeter (horizon XIV) human embryo. *Anat. Rec.* **152**, 9–16.
LENORMANT, F. (1875). *La divination et la Science des présages chez les chaldéens?*. Maisonneuve et Cie, Paris.
LENZ, W. (1961). Kindliche Missbildungen nach medikament wahrend der Draviditat? *Deutsch. Med. Wochenschr.* **86**, 2555–6.
LENZ, W. (1965). Epidemiology of congenital malformations. *Ann. N.Y. Acad. Sci.* **123**, 228–36.
LESCHOT, N. J. AND TREFFERS, P. E. (1975). Elevated amniotic-fluid alpha-fetoprotein without neural-tube defects (letter). *Lancet* **ii**, 1141.
LETCHWORTH, A. T., GORDON, Y. B., AND LEIGHTON, P. C. (1977). Raised amniotic fluid concentrations of alpha-fetoprotein in a twin pregnancy. *Br. med. J.* **1**, 689.
LEVINE, M. P., MCNEIL, D. E., KABACK, M. M., FRAZER, R. E., OKADA, D. M., AND HOBEL, C. J. (1976). Human fetoscopy and fetal blood sampling in the second trimester. In *Intrauterine fetal visualization. A multidisciplinary approach*. Edited by Kaback, M. M. and Valenti, C. Excerpta Medica, Amsterdam p. 171–8.
LEVY, E. P., COHEN, A., AND FRASER, F. C. (1973). Hormone treatment during pregnancy and congenital heart defects (letter). *Lancet* **i**, 611.
LEWIS, D. M. AND WILLIAMS, G. F. (1977). Definition of perinatal mortality (letter). *Lancet* **ii**, 86.
LIGHTOWLER, C. D. R. (1971). Meningomyelocele: the price of treatment. *Br. med. J.* **2**, 385–7.
LILEY, A. W. (1961). Liquor amnii analysis in the managment of the pregnancy complicated by rhesus sensitization. *Am. J. Obstet. Gynec.* **62**, 1359–70.
—— (1963). Errors in the assessment of hemolytic disease from amniotic fluid. *Am. J. Obstet. Gynec.* **86**, 485–94.
LINDER, E. AND SEPPÄLÄ, M. (1968). Localisation of the α-fetoprotein in the human fetus and placenta. *Acta path. microbiol. scand.* **73**, 565–71.
LINVILLE, G. P. AND SHEPARD, T. H. (1972). Neural tube closure defects due to cytochalasin B. *Nature New Biol.* **236**, 246–7.
LISTER, J., ZACHARY, R. B., AND BRERETON, R. (1977). Open myelomeningocele—a ten-year review of 200 consecutive closures. *Prog. ped. Surg.* **10**, 161–76.
LITT, S. AND STRAUSS, H. A. (1935). Monoamniotic twins, one normal, other anencephalic; multiple true knots in cord. *Am. J. Obstet. Gynec.* **30**, 728–30.
LORBER, J. (1965). The family history of spina bifida cystica. *Pediatrics* **35**, 589–95.
—— (1968). The problem of spina bifida. *Med. Offr.* **120**, 213–15.

—— (1971). Results of treatment of myelomeningocele. An analysis of 524 unselected cases with special reference to possible selection for treatment. *Develop. Med. Child Neurol.* **13**, 279–303.

—— (1971*a*). What are the chances for the second generation? *Link* **1**, 10–11.

—— (1972). Spina bifida cystica. Results of treatment of 270 consecutive cases with criteria for selection for the future. *Arch. Dis. Childh.* **47**, 854–73.

—— (1974). The potato trial. *Link* **30**, 7.

—— (1974a). Selective treatment of myelomeningocele: To treat or not to treat? *Pediatrics* **53**, 307–8.

—— (1977). Spina bifida cystica. Incidence, causes and prevention. In *Neurodevelopmental problems in early childhood; assessment and management*, edited by Drillien, C. M. and Drummond, M. B. Blackwell, Oxford, p. 371–82.

—— AND ROGERS, S. C. (1977). Spina bifida cystica and anencephalus in twins. *Z. Kindchir.* **22**, 565–71.

——, STEWART, C. R., AND WARD, A. M. (1973). Alphafetoprotein in antenatal diagnosis of anencephaly and spina bifida (letter). *Lancet* **i**, 1187.

LOUROS, N. AND KYRIAKIS, L. (1956). Quoted by Penrose, L. S. (1957) *see* p. 5.

LOWE, C. R., ROBERTS, C. L., AND LLOYD, S. (1971). Malformations of the central nervous system and softness of local water supplies. *Br. Med. J.* **2**, 357–61.

LOWE, C. U. (1978). The national amniocentesis registry. In *Genetic issues in public health and medicine*. Edited by Cohen, B. H., Lilienfeld. A. M., and Huang, P. C. Charles C. Thomas, Springfield, Illinois, p. 130–44.

LOWRY, R. B. AND ALLEN, A. B. (1977). Herbicides and spina bifida. *Can. med. Ass. J.* **117**, 580.

——, MILLER, J. R., SCOTT, A. E., AND RENWICK, D. H. G. (1975). The British Columbia Registry for handicapped children and adults: evolutionary changes over twenty years. *Can. J. publ. Hlth.* **66**, 322–6.

LUCEY, J. F., MANN, R. W., SIMMONS, G. M., AND FRIEDMAN, E. (1964). An increased incidence of spina bifida in Vermont in 1962. *Pediatrics* **33**, 981–4.

LUDUENNA, M. A. AND WESSELLS, N. K. (1973). Cell locomotion nerve elongation and microfilaments. *Develop. Biol.* **30**, 427–40.

LUTZ, N. AND LUTZ-OSTERTAG, Y. (1958). Actée encéphalie expérimentale *in vitro*. *J. Embryol. exp. Morph.* **6**, 504–8.

LYCOSTHENES, C. (1557). *Prodigiorum ac Ostentorum Chronicon.* H. Petrie, Basel.

MACAFEE, C. A. J. (1973). Maternal urinary estriol excretion when the fetus is malformed. (summary). In: *Fourth International Conference on Birth Defects*, ed. Motulsky, A. G. Excerpta med. (Amst.)., p. 55.

——, BEISCHER, N. A., AND FORTUNE, D. W. (1973). Feto-placental function and antenatal complications when the fetus has Hydrocephalus. *Aust. N.Z.J. Obstet. Gynaec.* **13**, 153–8.

——, ——, BROWN, J. B., AND FORTUNE, D. W. (1972). Fetoplacental function and antenatal complications when the fetus is malformed. *Aust. N.Z.J. Obstet. Gynaec.* **12**, 71–85.

MACAFEE, C. H. G. (1950). Hydramnios. *J. Obstet. Gynaec. Br. Emp.* **57**, 171–82.

MCBRIDE, M. L. (1978). Familial risks of anencephaly and spina bifida in British Columbia. MSc. thesis, University of British Columbia.

—— (1979). Sib risks of anencephaly and spina bifida in British Columbia. *Am. J. med. Genet.* In press.

MCBRIDE, W. G. (1961). Thalidomide and congenital abnormalities. (letter). *Lancet* **ii**, 1358.

MCCORMICK, W. F. (1971). Is anencephaly a single entity? A brief note on the morphologic heterogeneity of anencephaly. *Birth Defects: Original Articles Series* **3** (1), 94–6.

MCDONALD, A. D. (1958). Maternal health and congenital defect. *New Engl. J. Med.* **258**, 767–73.

—— (1961). Maternal health in early pregnancy and congenital defect. *Br. J. prev. soc. Med.* **15**, 154–66.

—— (1971). Seasonal distribution of abortions. *Br. J. prev. soc. Med.* **25**, 222–4.

—— (1971a). Abortion in neural tube defect fraternities. *Br. J. prev. soc. Med.* **25**, 220–1.

MACDONALD, P. C. AND SIITERI, P. K. (1965). Origin of estrogen in women pregnant with an anencephalic fetus. *J. Clin. Invest.* **44**, 465–74.

McDougall, W. (1927). An experiment for the testing of the hypothesis of Lamark. *Br. J. Psych.* **17**, 267–304.
—— (1930). Second report of Lamarkian experiment. *Br. J. Psych.* **20**, 201–18.
MacGillivray, I. and Horobin, G. (1973). *Experience with abortion*. Cambridge University Press, London, p. 4.
McKay, R. (1957). A retrospect of fifty years outbreaks of potato blight in Ireland 1907–56. *J. Dept. Agric. Tech. Instruct. Ire.* **53**, 3–10.
McKeown, T. and Lowe, C. R. (1951). Sex ratio of stillbirths related to birth weight. *Br. J. Soc. Med.* **5**, 229–35.
—— and Record, R. G. (1951). Seasonal incidence of congenital malformations of the CNS. *Lancet* **i**, 192–6.
McKusick, V. A. (1969). On lumpers and splitters, or the nosology of genetic disease. *Birth Defects, Original Article Series* **5**, 23–30.
MacLeod, S. C., Brown, J. B., Beischer, N. A., and Smith, M. A. (1967). The value of urinary oestriol measurements during pregnancy. *Aust. N. Z. J. Obstet. Gynaecol.* **7**, 25–38.
MacMahon, B. and McKeown, T. (1952). A note on the sex ratio of anencephalus. *Br. J. soc. Med.* **6**, 265–6.
—— and Pugh, T. F. (1970). *Epidemiology: principles and methods*. Little, Brown and Company, Boston.
—— and Yen, S. (1971). Unrecognised epidemic of anencephaly and spina bifida. *Lancet* **i**, 31–3.
——, —— (1971a). Influenza and neural tube defects. *Lancet* **ii**, 260–1.
——, Record, R. G., and McKeown, T. (1951). Secular changes in the incidence of malformations of the central nervous system. *Br. J. prev. soc. Med.* **5**, 254–8.
——, Pugh, T. F., and Ingalls, T. H. (1953). Anencephalus, spina bifida and hydrocephalus. Incidence related to sex, race and season of birth and incidence in siblings. *Br. J. prev. soc. Med.* **7**, 211–19.
——, Yen, S. and Rothman, K. J. (1973). Potato blight and neural tube defects. (letter). *Lancet* **1**, 598–9.
McNeil, J. R. and Gainer, H. M. (1938). *Medieval handbooks of penance*. Translation. Columbia University Press, New York, p. 197.
McPherson, K., Smith, P., and Vessey, M. (1978). Teratogenic effects of waste anaesthetic gases. (letter). *Br. med. J.* **1**, 437–8.
Macri, J. N., Weiss, R. R., and Joshi, M. S. (1974*a*). Beta-trace protein and neural-tube defects. *Lancet* **i**, 1109–10.
——, ——, —— and Evans, M. I. (1974). Antenatal diagnosis of neural-tube defects using cerebrospinal-fluid proteins. *Lancet* **i**, 14–15.
——, ——, Elligers, K. W., and Federgreen, W. R. (1976). Racial differences in maternal serum-alpha-fetoprotein. (letter). *Lancet* **i**, 207–8.
MacVicar, J. (1976). Antenatal detection of fetal abnormality—physical methods. *Br. med. Bull.* **32**, 4–8.
Maksymiuk, J. P. (1974–75). The Abortion Law. A study of R v Morgentaler. *Sask. Law. Rev.* **39**(2), 259–84.
Malpas, P. (1937). Incidence of human malformations and significance of changes in maternal environment in their causation. *J. Obstet. Gynaec. Br. Emp.* **44**, 434–54.
Mann, J. R., Lakin, G. E., Leonard, J. C., Rawlinson, H. A., Richardson, S. G. N., Corkery, J. J., Cameron, A. H., and Shah, K. J. (1978). Clinical applications of serum carcinoembryonic antigen and alpha-fetoprotein levels in children with solid tumours. *Arch. Dis. Childh.* **53**, 366–74.
Manson, M. M., Logan, W. P. D., and Loy, R. M. (1960). *Rubella and other virus infections during pregnancy*. Ministry of Health Reports on Public Health and Medical Subjects, No. 101. HMSO, London.
Mantel, N. (1963). Chi-square tests with one degree of freedom; extensions of the Mantel–Haenszel procedure. *J. Am. Statist. Ass.* **58**, 690–700.
—— (1967). The detection of disease clustering and a generalized regression approach. *Cancer Res.* **27**, 209–20.
—— and Haenszel, W. (1959). Statistical aspects of the analysis of data from retrospective studies of disease. *J. Nat. Cancer Inst.* **22**, 719–48.

——, Brown, C., and Byar, D. P. (1977). Tests for homogeneity of effect in an epidemiological investigation. *Am. J. Epidemiol.* **106**, 125–9.

Marin-Padilla, M. (1965). Study of the skull in human cranioschisis. *Acta Anat.* **62**, 1–20.

—— (1966). Mesodermal alterations induced by hypervitaminosis A. *J. Embryol. exp. Morph.* **15**, 261–9.

—— (1970). Morphogenesis of anencephaly and related malformations, in *Current Topics in Pathology*. Springer-Verlag, Berlin, **51**, pp. 145–74.

—— (1970*a*). The closure of the neural tube in the golden hamster. *Teratology* **3**, 39–46.

Marsh, H., Gould, A. P., Clutton, H. H., and Parker, R. W. (1885). Report of a Committee of the Society nominated November 10, 1882 to investigate spina bifida and its treatment by the injection of Dr. Morton's iodo-glycerine solution. *Trans. clin. Soc. Lond.* **18**, 339–85.

Marshall, R., Newnham, R. E., Rawstron, J. R., Ellis, J. R., and Stevens, L. J. (1964). Features of 13–15 trisomy syndrome with normal karotype. (letter). *Lancet* **i**, 556.

Marshall, V. F. and Muecke, E. C. (1962). Variations in exstrophy of the bladder. *J. Urol.* **88**, 766–96.

Martin, A. H. (1971). A congenital defect in the spinal cord of the Manx cat. *Vet. Path.* **8**, 232–8.

Martin, J. (1840). Succession of monstrous births occurring in the same female. *Med. Exam.* **5**, 23.

Masopust, J., Kithier, K., Rádl, J., Koutecký, J., and Kotál, L. (1968). Occurrence of fetoprotein in patients with neoplasms and non-neoplastic diseases. *Int. J. Cancer* **3**, 364–73.

——, Zizkovsky, V., and Kithier, K. (1970). Fetoproteins in different species of mammals. *Protides Biol. Fluids* **18**, 63–73.

Masseyeff, R. (1972). Human alpha-feto-protein. *Path. et Biol.* **20**, 703–25.

——, Cassuto, J. P., Krebs, B. P., Audoly, P., and Dujardin, P. (1968). Alpha-fetoprotein radioimmunoassay in blood diseases. *New Engl. J. Med.* **291**, 532.

——, Sankale, M., Onde, M., Menye, A., Camain, R., Quenum, C., Maydat, L., Mattern, P., Ancelle, P., and Leblanc, L. (1968*a*). Valeur de la recherche de l'alpha-1-fetoprotéine sérique pour le diagnostic du cancer primitif du foie. *Bull. Soc. méd. Afr. noire Langue franc.* **13**, 537–48.

Master-Notani, P., Kolah, P., and Sanghvi, L. D. (1968). Congenital malformations in the new born in Bombay, Part I. *Acta genet. (Basel)* **18**, 97–108.

Masterson, J. G. (1970). Consanguinity in Ireland. *Hum. Heredity* **20**, 371–82.

——, Frost, C., Bourke, G. J., Joyce, N. M., Herity, B., and Wilson-Davis, K. (1974). Anencephaly and potato blight in the Republic of Ireland. *Br. J. prev. soc. Med.* **28**, 81–4.

Mathen, K. K. (1963). Matching in comparative studies in public health. *Indian J. Publ. Hlth.* **7**, 161–9.

Mawas, C., Kohen, M., Lemerle, J., Buffé, D., Schweisguth, O., and Burtin, P. (1969). Serum alpha-1-fetoprotein in children with malignant ovarian or testicular teratomas. Preliminary results. *Int. J. Cancer* **4**, 76–9.

Meadow, S. R. (1968). Anticonvulsant drugs and congenital abnormalities. (letter). *Lancet* **ii**, 1296.

Meckel, J. F. (1822). Beschreibung zweler durch sehr ähnliche Bildungsabweichung entstellter Geschwister. *Dtsch. Arch. Physiol.* **7**, 99–172.

Medical Journal of Australia (1971). Editorial—Selection in treatment of spina bifida. *Med. J. Aust.* **2** (23), 1151–2.

Medical Research Council of Canada (1977). *Diagnosis of genetic disease by amniocentesis during the second trimester of pregnancy.* Report no. 5, Ottawa. The Queen's Printer.

Medical Research Council of the United Kingdom (1978). Report of the working party on amniocentesis. An assessment of the hazards of amniocentesis. *Br. J. Obstet. Gynaec.* Suppl. No. 2, pp. 1–14.

Mehlman, D. J., Bulkley, B. H., and Wiernik, P. H. (1971). Serum alpha$_1$-fetoprotein with gastric and prostatic carcinomas. *New Engl. J. Med.* **285**, 1060–1.

Meire, H. B., Farrant, P., and Wilkins, R. A. (1978). Place of ultrasound and radiography in obstetrics *Br. med. J.* **2**, 882.

Melzer, H. J. (1956). Congenital anomalies due to attempted abortion with 4-aminopteroglutamic acid. *J. Am. med. Ass.* **161**, 1253.

MENASHI, M., ORNOY, A., AND COHEN, M. M. (1977). Anencephaly in trisomy 18: related or unrelated? *Teratology* **15**, 325–8.

MENELAUS, M. B. (1971). *The orthopaedic management of spina bifida cystica.* E. & S. Livingstone, Edinburgh.

MENNUTI, M. T., MORANZ, J. G., SCHWARZ, R. H., AND MELLMAN, W. J. (1977). Amniography for the early detection of neural tube defects. *Obstet. Gynecol.* **49**, 25–30.

MIETTINEN, O. S. (1970). Matching and design efficiency in retrospective studies. *Am. J. Epidemiol.* **91**, 111–17.

—— (1972). Components of the crude risk ratio. *Am. J. Epidemiol.* **96**, 168–72.

—— (1972*a*). Standardization of risk ratios. *Am. J. Epidemiol.* **96**, 383–8.

—— (1974). Confounding and effect modification. *Am. J. Epidemiol.* **100**, 350–3.

—— (1976). Stratification by a multivariate confounder score. *Am. J. Epidemiol.* **104**, 609–20.

MIKAKHUR, R. K. (1978). Teratogenic effects of waste anaesthetic gases. (letter). *Br. Med. J.* **1**, 300–1.

MILHAM, S. JR. (1964). Pituitary gonadotrophin and dizygotic twinning. *Lancet* **ii**, 566.

—— AND GITTELSOHN, A. M. (1965). Parental age and malformations. *Hum. Biol.* **37**, 13–22.

MILIC, A. B. AND ADAMSONS, K. (1969). The relationship between anencephaly and prolonged pregnancy. *J. Obstet. Gynaec. Br. Commonw.* **76**, 102–11.

MILLER, J. R. (1964). The Use of Registries and vital statistics in the study of congenital malformations. In *Second International Conference on Congenital Malformations.* Edited by Fishbein, M. International Medical Congress Ltd., New York, pp. 334–40.

—— (1976). Description of a handicapped population: The British Columbia Health Surveillance Registry. *Birth Defects: Original Article Series* **12** (4), 1–11.

—— (1977). Birth defects monitoring systems: An overview. *Cong. Anom.* **17**, 1–12.

—— AND LOWRY, R. B. (1977). Birth Defects Registries and surveillance. In *Handbook of teratology.* Vol. 3. *Comparative, maternal and epidemiological aspects.* Edited by J. G. Wilson and F. C. Fraser. Plenum Press, New York, pp. 227–42.

MILLER, J. Q. AND SELDEN, R. F. (1967). Arhinencephaly, encephalocele and 13–15 trisomy syndrome with normal chromosomes. *Neurology* **17**, 1087–91.

MILLER, P., SMITH, D. W., AND SHEPARD, T. H. (1978). Maternal hyperthermia as a possible cause of anencephaly. *Lancet* **i**, 519–21.

MILLER, R. W. (1963). Down's syndrome (mongolism), other congenital malformations and cancers among the sibs of leukaemic children. *New Engl. J. Med.* **268**, 393–401.

MILUNSKY, A. (1973). *The prenatal diagnosis of hereditary disorders.* Charles C. Thomas, Springfield, Illinois.

—— (1977). Prenatal detection of neural tube defects: False positive and negative results. *Pediatrics* **59**, 782–3.

—— (1978). Prenatal detection of neural tube defects: experience with alpha-fetoprotein assays of amniotic fluid. In *Prevention of neural tube defects: the role of alpha-fetoprotein.* Edited by Crandall, B. F. and Brazier, M. A. Academic Press, New York, pp. 163–8.

—— AND ALPERT, E. (1974). The value of alpha-fetoprotein in the prenatal diagnosis of neural-tube defects. *J. Pediat.* **84**, 889–93.

—— —— (1976). Prenatal diagnosis of neural tube defects I. Problems and pitfalls: analysis of 2495 cases using the alpha-fetoprotein assay. *Obstet. Gynecol.* **48**(1), 1–12.

—— AND GAYNOR, M. F., JR. (1968). Methotrexate-induced congenital malformations, with a review of the literature. *J. Pediat.* **72**, 790–5.

——, MACRI, J. N., WEISS, R. R., ALPERT, E., MCISAAC, D. G., AND JOSHI, M. S. (1975). Prenatal detection of neural tube defects. Comparison between alpha-fetoprotein and beta-trace protein assays. *Am. J. Obstet. Gynec.* **122**, 313–15.

MINOGUE, M. (1974). A review of twin pregnancies at the National Maternity Hospital (1967 to 1971). *J. Irish med. Ass.* **67**, 181–6.

MIRAKHUR, R. K. (1978). Teratogenic effects of waste anaesthetic gases. (letter). *Br. med. J.* **1**, 300–1.

MOLSTED-PEDERSEN, L., TYGSTRUP, I., AND PEDERSEN, J. (1964). Congenital malformation in newborn infants of diabetic women: correlation with maternal diabetic vascular complications. *Lancet* **i**, 1124–6.

MONAHAN, E. T. (1956). Anencephalus. *Delaware Med. J.* **28**, 103–6.

MONTGOMERY, J. R., FLANDERS, R. W., AND YOW, M. D. (1973). Congenital Anomalies and Herpesvirus Infection. *Am. J. Dis. Child.* **126**, 364–6.

MOORE, J. E. (1905). Spina bifida, with a report of three hundred and eighty-five cases treated by excision. *Surg. Gynec. Obstet.* **1**, 137–40.

MORGAGNI, G. B. (1761). *De sedibus et causis morborum, per anatomen indigatis.* Translated by B. Alexander (1769). Millar and Cadell, London.

MORISON, J. E. (1970). *Foetal and neonatal pathology.* Third Edition, Butterworths, London.

MORTON, J. (1877). *Treatment of spina bifida by a new method.* J. Maclehose, Glasgow.

MORTON, M. S., ELWOOD, P. C., AND ABERNETHY, M. (1976). Trace elements in water and congenital malformations of the central nervous system in South Wales. *Br. J. prev. soc. Med.* **30**, 36–9.

MORTON, N. E. (1958). Empirical risks in consanguineous marriages; birth weight, gestation time and measurements of infants. *Am. J. hum. Genet.* **10**, 344–9.

—— (1967). The detection of major genes under additive continuous variation. *Am. J. hum. Genet.* **19**, 23–34.

——, CHUNG, C. S., AND MI, M. (1967). Genetics of inter-racial crosses in Hawaii. *Monogr. hum. Genet.* **3**, p. 124.

——, RAO, D. C, LANG-BROWN, H., MACLEAN, C. J., BART, R. D., AND LEW, R. (1977). Colchester revisited: a genetic study of mental defect. *J. Med. Genet.* **14**, 1–9.

MOSS, B. J. L. (1964). Congenital abnormalities in Leicester 1953–62. *Med. Offr.* **112**, 79–82.

MOSZKOWICZ, L. (1934). Zur Genese der Missbildungen. *Virchows Arch. path. Anat.* **293**, 78–96.

MOTULSKY, A. G. (1974). Brave New World? Ethical issues in prevention, treatment and research of human birth defects. In *Birth Defects. Proceedings of the Fourth International Conference, Vienna 1973*. Excerpta Medica Amsterdam, American Elsevier Publishing Co., Inc., New York, pp. 311–28.

——, FRASER, G. R., AND FELSENSTEIN, J. (1971). Public health and long-term genetic implications of intrauterine diagnosis and selective abortion. *Birth Defects, Original Article Series* **7**, 22–33.

MUDALIAR, A. L. (1930). Double monsters—a study of their circulatory system and some other anatomical abnormalities and the complications in labour. *J. Obstet. Gynaec. Br. Emp.* **37**, 753–68.

MUFARRIJ, I. K. AND KILEJIAN, V. O. (1963). Anencephaly. An analysis of anencephalic births and a report of a case of repeated anencephaly. *Obstet. Gynec.* **22**, 657–61.

MUKOJIMA, T., HATTORI, N., NAKAYAMA, N., HASEGAWA, H., OHKURA, H., AND KITAOKA, H. (1973). Elimination rate of AFP after surgical operation and prognosis of the patients with hepatoblastoma and hepatoma. *Tumor Res.* **8**, 194–7.

MUNROE, M. E. (1951). *Theory of probability*. McGraw-Hill, New York.

MURKEN, J. (1976). Investigations of children born after amniocentesis. In *Prenatal diagnosis* edited by Boué, A. Inserm, Paris, Vol. **61**, pp. 273–82.

MURPHY, D. P. (1940). *Congenital malformations.* Second edition. University of Pennsylvania Press, published by J. B. Lippincott & Co., Philadelphia.

MUSTACCHI, P., DAVID, F. N., AND FIX, E. (1967). Three tests for space–time interaction: a comparative evaluation. In *Proceedings of the Fifth Berkeley Symposium on Mathematical Statistics and Probability*, Vol. 4, pp. 229–235. University of California, Berkeley and Los Angeles.

MYERS, R. E. (1969). Brain pathology following fetal vascular occlusion: an experimental study. *Invest. Ophthal.* **8**, 41–50.

MYRIANTHOPOULOS, N. C. (1970). An epidemiologic survey of twins in a large, prospectively studied population. *Am. J. Hum. Genet.* **22**, 611–29.

NAEYE, R. L., MILIC, A. B., AND BLANC, W. A. (1970). Fetal endocrine and renal disorders: clues to the origin of hydramnios. *Am. J. Obstet. Gynec.* **108**, 1251–6.

NAGGAN, L. (1969). The recent decline in prevalence of anencephaly and spina bifida. *Am. J. Epidem.* **89**, 154–60.

—— (1971). Anencephaly and spina bifida in Israel. *Pediatrics* **47**, 577–86.

—— (1976). I. Methodology of ascertainment in international comparisons. II. Anencephaly and spina bifida in Israel. In *Birth defects: risks and consequences*, edited by Kelly, S., Hook, E. B., Janerich, D. T. and Porter, I. H. Academic Press Inc., New York, pp. 41–58.

—— AND MACMAHON. (1967). Ethnic differences in the prevalence of anencephaly and spina bifida in Boston, Massachusetts. *New Engl. J. Med.* **227**, 1119–23.

NAKONO, K. K. (1973). Anencephaly—a review. *Develop. Med. Child. Neurol.* **15**, 383–400.

NAÑAGAS, J. C. (1925). A comparison of the growth of the body dimensions of anencephalic human fetuses with normal fetal growth as determined by graphic analysis and empirical formulae. *Am. J. Anat.* **35**, 455–94.

NANCE, W. E. (1969). Anencephaly and spina bifida: a possible example of cytoplasmic inheritance in man. *Nature (Lond.)* **224**, 373–5.

NATHANSON, B. N. (1974). Sounding Board. Deeper into Abortion. *New Eng. J. Med.* **291**(2), 1189–90.

NATIONAL ACADEMY OF SCIENCES (1975). *Genetic screening programs: principles and research.* Report by the Committee for the Study of Inborn Errors of Metabolism. Washington, D.C., pp. 359–80.

NATIONAL INSTITUTE OF CHILD HEALTH AND HUMAN DEVELOPMENT NATIONAL REGISTRY FOR AMNIOCENTESIS STUDY GROUP (1976). Midtrimester amniocentesis for prenatal diagnosis. *J. Am. med. Ass.* **236**, 1471–6.

NEEL, J. V. (1958). A study of major congenital defects in Japanese infants. *Am. J. hum. Genet.* **10**, 398–445.

NELSON, M. M., RUTTIMAN, M. T., AND BROCK, D. J. H. (1974). Predictive value of amniotic-fluid macrophages in gross CNS defects. (letter). *Lancet* **i**, 504.

——, WRIGHT, H. V., ASLING, C. W., AND EVANS, H. M. (1955). Multiple congenital abnormalities resulting from transitory deficiency of pteroylglutamic acid during gestation in the rat. *J. Nutr.* **56**, 349–69.

——, BAIRD, C. D. C., WRIGHT, H. V., AND EVANS, H. M. (1956). Multiple congenital abnormalities in the rat resulting from Riboflavin deficiency induced by the antimetabolite galactoflavin. *J. Nutr.* **58**, 125–34.

NERI, L. C., JOHANSEN, H. L., AND TALBOT, F. D. F. (1977). *Chemical content of Canadian drinking water related to cardiovascular health.* University of Ottawa, Ottawa.

NEVIN, N. C. AND ARMSTRONG, M. J. (1975). Raised alpha-fetoprotein levels in amniotic fluid and maternal serum in a triplet pregnancy in which one fetus had an omphalocoele. *Br. J. Obstet. Gynaec.* **82**, 826–8.

—— AND HARLEY, J. M. G. (1976). Clomiphene and neural tube defects. *Ulster Med. J.* **45**, 59–64.

—— AND MERRETT, J. D. (1975). Potato avoidance during pregnancy in women with a previous infant with either anencephaly and/or spina bifida. *Br. J. prev. soc. Med.* **29**, 111–15.

——, NESBITT, S., AND THOMPSON, W. (1973). Myelocele and alpha-fetoprotein in amniotic fluid. (letter). *Lancet* **i**, 1383.

——, THOMPSON, W., AND NESBITT, S. (1974). Amniotic fluid alpha-fetoprotein in the antenatal diagnosis of neural tube defects. *J. Obstet. Gynaec. Br. Commonw.* **81**, 757–60.

——, RITCHIE, A., MCKEOWN, F., AND ROBERTS, G. (1978). Raised alpha-fetoprotein levels in amniotic fluid and maternal serum associated with distension of the fetal bladder caused by absence of urethra. *J. Med. Genet.* **15**, 61–3.

NEWCOMBE, H. B. (1964). Discussion of Miller, J. R. The use of registries and vital statistics in the study of congenital malformations. In *Second International Conference on Congenital Malformations*, edited by Fishbein, M. The International Medical Congress Ltd., New York, p. 347.

—— (1967). Present state and long-term objectives of the British Columbia population study. In *Proceeding of the Third International Congress of Human Genetics*, John Hopkins Press, Baltimore, pp. 291–313.

NICHOLS, J., LESCURE, O. L., AND MIGEON, C. J. (1958). Levels of 17-hydroxycorticosteroids and 17-ketosteroids in maternal and cord plasma in term anencephaly. *J. clin. Endocr.* **18**, 444–52.

NIE, N. H., HULL, C. H., JENKINS, J. G., STEINBRENNER, K., AND BENT, D. H. (1975). *SPSS: Statistical Package for the Social Sciences.* Second Edition. McGraw-Hill, New York.

NISHI, S. (1970). Isolation and characterisation of a human fetal α-globulin from the sera of fetuses and hepatoma patient. *Cancer Res.* **30**, 2507–13.

——, Watanabe, H., Tsukada, J., and Hirai, H. (1971). Purification and chemical characterisation of human alpha-fetoprotein. *Protides Biol. Fluids* **18**, 43–7.

Nishie, K., Gumbmann, M. R., and Keyl, A. C. (1971). Pharmacology of solanine. *Toxicol. appl. Pharmacol.* **19**, 81–92.

Nishimura, H. (1970). Incidence of malformations in abortions. In *Congenital malformations: Proceedings of the Third International Conference.* Excerpta med. (Amst.), pp. 275–83.

—— and Okamoto, N. (1976). Editors. *Sequential atlas of human congenital malformations.* University Park Press, Baltimore.

——, Takano, K., Tanimura, T., and Yasuda, M. (1968). Normal and abnormal development of human embryos: first report of the analysis of 1,213 intact embryos. *Teratology* **1**, 281–90.

——, Tanimura, T., Semba, R., and Uwabe, C. (1974). Normal development of early human embryos: observation of 90 specimens at Carnegie stages 7 to 13. *Teratology* **10**, 1–8.

Nora, A. H. and Nora, J. J. (1975). A syndrome of multiple congenital anomalies associated with teratogenic exposure. *Arch. environm. Hlth.* **30**, 17–21.

Nora, J. J. and Nora, A. H. (1973). Birth defects and oral contraceptives. (letter). *Lancet* **i**, 941–2.

Nørgaard-Pedersen, B. (1978). Interpreting amniotic fluid alpha-fetoprotein. (letter). *Lancet* **i**, 100.

—— and Lindholm, J. (1972). Quantitative of red cell carbonic anhydrases B and C and hemoglobin F in thyroid disorders. *Acta med. Scand.* **192**, 227–30.

Norio, R. (1966). Heredity in the congenital nephrotic syndrome. A genetic study of 57 Finnish families with a review of reported cases. *Acta paediat. Fenn.* **12**, (suppl. 27), 1–94.

Nulsen, F. E. and Spitz, E. B. (1951). Treatment of hydrocephalus by direct shunt from ventricle to jugular vein. *Surg. Forum* **2**, 399–403.

Nutrition Canada (1975). *Provincial survey reports: reports from Nutrition Canada by the Bureau of Nutritional Sciences, Department of National Health and Welfare.* Information Canada, Ottawa.

Oakley, G. P. (1975). The use of human abortuses in the search for teratogens. In *Methods for detection of environmental agents that produce congenital defects.* Edited by Shepard, T. H., Miller, J. R. and Marois, M. North Holland Publishing Co. Amsterdam, pp. 189–96.

O'Connor, G. T., Tatarinov, Y. S., Abelev, G. I., and Uriel, J. (1970). A collaborative study for the evaluation of a serologic text for primary liver cancer. *Cancer* **25**, 1091–8.

Office of Population Censuses and Surveys (1978). *Occupational mortality. Decennial Supplement 1970–1972.* HMSO, London.

Olmsted, J. M. D. (1946). *Charles Édouard Brown Séquard, a nineteenth century neurologist and endocrinologist.* The John Hopkins Press, Baltimore.

Olsson, J. E., Sherman, M. S., and Kjessler, B. (1974). Beta-trace protein and neural-tube defects. *Lancet* **ii**, 347–8.

Opitz, J. M. and Howe, J. J. (1969). The Meckel syndrome (dysencephalia splanchocystica, the Gruber syndrome). *Birth Defects: Original Article Series* **5**, 167–79.

——, Herrmann, J., and Dieker, H. (1969). The study of malformations syndromes in man. *Birth Defects; Original Article Series* **5**, 1–10.

Oppert, J. (1871). Tablettes Assyriennes. *J. Asiatique* **18**, 449–53.

Padget, D. H. (1968). Spina bifida and embryonic neuroschisis—a causal relationship. *Johns Hopkins med. J.* **123**, 233–52.

Page, M. (1973). α-fetoprotein: purification on sepharose-linked concanavalin-A. *Can. J. Biochem.* **51**, 1213–17.

Pagon, R. A., Chandler, J. W., Collie, W. R., Clarren, S. K., Moon, J., Minkin, S. A., and Hall, J. G. (1978). Hydrocephalus, agyria, retinal dysplasia, encephalocele (Hard ± E) syndrome: an autosomal recessive condition. *Birth Defects; Original Article Series* **14**, (6B), 233–41.

Pagniez, P., Plichet, A., Salles, P., and Laplane, R. (1934). Du rôle des poux dan l'épilepsie de Brown-Séquard du Cobaye. *C.R. Soc. de Biol.* **116**, 314–15.

Pantaleón-Mena, R., Díaz, H., Justiniano, R., Rudolph, A. J., and Nichols, B. L. (1967). The conjoined twins of Bayamon. *Birth Defects: Original Article Series* **3**(1), 137–8.

PARÉ, A. (1678). *Complete Works.* First French Edition, translated into English by Thomas Johnson. J. Clark, London.

PASSARGE, E., TRUE, C. W., SUEOKA, W. T., BAUMGARTNER, N. R., AND KEER, K. R. (1966). Malformations of the central nervous system in trisomy 18 syndrome. *J. Pediat.* **69**, 771–8.

PATTEN, B. M. (1953). Embryological stages in the establishing of myeloschisis with spina bifida. *Am. J. Anat.* **93**, 365–96.

PEARSON, K. (1930). *The life, letters and labours of Francis Galton.* Volume III A. The University Press, Cambridge.

PEDERSEN, K. (1944). Fetuin, a new globulin isolated from serum. *Nature (Lond.)* **154**, 575.

PEDLOW, R. (1961). Anencephaly in a mono-amniotic twin. *Br. med. J.* **2**, 997–8.

PENROSE, L. S. (1938). *A clinical and genetic study of 1,280 cases of mental defect.* Medical Research Council, Special Report Series, No. 229.

—— (1946). Familial data on 144 cases of anencephaly, spina bifida and congenital hydrocephaly. *Ann. Eugen.* **13**, 73–96.

—— (1957). Genetics of anencephaly. *J. ment. def. Res.* **1**, 4–15.

PERGAMENT, E. (1977). α-fetoprotein and the prenatal diagnosis of neural tube defects. In *Obstetrics and Gynecology Annual* edited by R. M. Wynn. Appleton-Century-Crofts, New York, pp. 173–89.

PERRY, B. J. AND BRIDGES, C. (1973). Computerised transverse axial scanning (tomography). Part. III: Radiation dose considerations. *Br. J. Radiol.* **46**, 1048–51.

PETTIFOR, J. M. AND BENSON, R. (1975). Congenital malformations associated with the administration of oral anticoagulants during pregnancy. *J. Pediat.* **86**, 459–62.

PHAROAH, P. O. D., ALBERMAN, E., AND CHAMBERLAIN, G. (1977). Outcome of pregnancy among women in anaesthetic practice. *Lancet* **i**, 34–6.

PHILIP, J. AND BANG, J. (1978). Outcome of pregnancy after amniocentesis for chromosome analysis. *Br. Med. J.* **4**, 1183–4.

PLACKETT, R. L. (1969). Multidimensional contingency tables: A survey of models and methods. *Bull. Inter. Stat. Inst.* **43**, 133–42.

PLEYDELL, M. J. (1960). Anencephaly and other congenital abnormalities. An epidemiological study in Northamptonshire. *Br. med. J.* **1**, 309–15.

POCOCK, S. J. (1972). Relationship between sickness absence and meteorological factors. *Br. J. prev. soc. Med.* **26**, 238–45.

—— (1974). Harmonic analysis applied to seasonal variations in sickness absence. *J.R. Stat. Soc., series C* **23**, 103–20.

POLAND, B. J. AND HARRIS, M. (1978). Personal communication.

POLANI, P. E. (1959). Nuclear chromatin of anencephalic foetuses. (letter). *Lancet* **ii**, 240–1.

—— AND CLAIREAUX, A. E. (1959). Sex in anencephalus. *Lancet* **ii**, 599–600.

POLITZER, G. (1952). Über Frühembryonale encephalomyeloschisis beim Menschen. *Wein. Ztschr. Nervenlk.* **5**, 1–22.

—— (1955). Über Spaltbindungen des Gehirns und Rückenmarks Menschlicher embryonen und ihre uterscheidung von Verlëtzungen. *Wein. Z. Nervenlk. Grenzgebiete* **10**, 18–34.

POLMAN, A. (1950). Anencephaly, spina bifida and hydrocephaly: a contribution to our knowledge of the causal genesis of congenital malformations. *Genetica* **25**, 29–78.

POOLE, T. R. (1960). Congenital malformations in West Virginia. *West Virginia Med. J.* **56**, 16–21.

POSWILLO, D. E., SOPHER, D., AND MITCHELL, S. J. (1972). Experimental induction of fetal malformation with 'blighted' potato. *Nature (Lond.)* **239**, 462–4.

——, ——, ——, COXON, D. T., CURTIS, R. F., AND PRICE, K. R. (1973). Investigations into the teratogenic potential of imperfect potatoes. *Teratology* **8**, 339–48.

POWERS, R. (1978). Personal communication.

PRITCHARD, J. A. (1965). Deglutition by normal and anencephalic fetuses. *Obstet. Gynec.* **25**, 289–97.

PURDIE, D. W., HOWIE, P. W., EDGAR, W., FORBES, C. D., AND PRENTICE, C. R. M. (1975). Raised amniotic-fluid F.D.P. in fetal neural tube anomalies. *Lancet* **i**, 1013–14.

PURTILO, D. T., CLARK, J. V., AND WILLIAMS, R. (1975). Primary hepatic malignancy in pregnant women. *Am. J. Obstet. Gynec.* **121**, 41–4.

RAAB, G. (1978). Screening for neural-tube defects. (letter). *Lancet* **ii**, 217.

RALIS, Z. A. (1975). Traumatizing effect of breech delivery on infants with spina bifida. *J. Pediat.* **87**, 613–16.
RECKLINGHAUSEN, F. D. VON (1886). Untersuchungen über die spina bifida, Virchows Archiv für pathologische Anatomie und Physiologie und für klinische Medizin, **105**, 243–330.
RECORD, R. G. (1961). Anencephalus in Scotland. *Br. J. prev. soc. Med.* **15**, 93–105.
—— (1978). Personal communication.
—— AND MCKEOWN, T. (1949). Congenital malformations of the central nervous system. I – A survey of 930 cases. *Br. J. soc. Med.* **4**, 183–219.
—— —— (1949*a*). Congenital malformations of the central nervous system. II – maternal reproductive history and familial incidence. *Br. J. soc. Med.* **4**, 26–50.
—— —— (1950). Congenital malformations of the central nervous system. III – Risk of malformation in sibs of malformed individuals. *Br. J. soc. Med.* **4**, 217–20.
—— —— (1951). Congenital malformations of the central nervous system, data on 69 pairs of twins. *Ann. Eugen. (Lond.)* **15**, 285–92.
Reich, T., JAMES, J. W., AND MORRIS, C. A. (1972). The use of multiple thresholds in determining the mode of transmission of semi-continuous tracts. *Ann. hum. Genet. (Lond.)* **36**, 163–84.
REID, R. (1977). Spina bifida: the fate of the untreated. *Hastings Centre Report* **7**, 16–19.
REILLY, P. R. (1975). Legislation on genetic screening. (letter). *Am. J. hum. Genet.* **27**, (1), 120.
—— (1975*a*). Genetic screening legislation. *Adv. Hum. Genet.* **5**, 319–76.
—— (1977). Mass neonatal screening in 1977. (letter). *Am. J. Hum. Genet.* **29** (3), 302–4.
RENKONEN, K. O. (1969). Fertility of mothers with twins. *Ann. Hum. Genet. (Lond.)* **32**, 383–9.
RENWICK, J. H. (1972). Hypothesis—anencephaly and spina bifida are usually preventable by avoidance of a specific but unidentified substance present in certain potato tubers. *Br. J. prev. soc. Med.* **26**, 67–88.
—— (1972*a*). Spina bifida and the potato. *New Scientist* **56**, 277–9.
—— (1972*b*). The risk of spina bifida. *New Society* 28 October, 212–13.
—— (1973). Prevention of anencephaly and spina bifida in man. *Teratology* **8**, 321–4.
—— (1974). The epidemiology of natural teratogens. In *Trace substances in environmental health* edited by Hemphill, D. D., University of Missouri, Columbia, pp. 3–8.
——, POSSAMI, A. M., AND MUNDAY, M. R. (1974). Potatoes and spina bifida. *Proc. Roy. Soc. Med.* **67**, 360–4.
REVILL, W. D. L. AND BARKER, D. J. P. (1972). Seasonal distribution of mycobacterial skin ulcers. *Br. J. prev. soc. Med.* **26**, 23–7.
RHODES, A. J. (1961). Virus infections and congenital malformations. In *First International Conference on Congenital Malformations.* Lippincott, Philadelphia, pp. 106–16.
RICCARDI, V. M. AND BERGMANN, C. A. (1977). Anencephaly with incomplete twinning (diprosopus). *Teratology* **16**, 137–40.
RICHARDS, I. D. G. (1969). Congenital malformations and environmental influences in pregnancy. *Br. J. prev. soc. Med.* **25**, 59–64.
—— (1973). Fetal and infant mortality associated with congenital malformations. *Br. J. prev. soc. Med.* **27**, 85–90.
—— AND LOWE, C. R. (1971). Incidence of congenital defects in South Wales 1964–66. *Br. J. prev. soc. Med.* **25**, 59–64.
——, MCINTOSH, H. T., AND SWEENIE, S. (1972). A genetic study of anencephaly and spina bifida in Glasgow. *Develop. Med. Child. Neurol.* **14**, 626–39.
——, ROBERTS, C. J., AND LLOYD, S. (1972). Area differences in prevalence of neural tube malformations in South Wales. *Br. J. prev. soc. Med.* **26**, 89–93.
RICKMAN, P. P. (1963). Nicholas Tulp and spina bifida. *Clin. pediat.* **2**, 40–2.
RICKHAM, P. P. (1976). The swing of the pendulum: the indications for operating on myelomeningoceles. *Med. J. Aust.* **2**, 743–6.
—— AND MAWDSLEY, T. (1966). The effect of early operation on the survival of spina bifida cystica. *Develop. Med. Child Neurol. Suppl.* **11**, 20–6.
RICKWOOD, A. M. K. (1977). A case of ileal atresia and ileocutaneous fistula caused by amniocentesis. *J. Pediat.* **91**, 312.
ROBARDS, M. F., THOMAS, G. G., AND ROSENBLOOM, L. (1975). Survival of infants with unoperated myeloceles. *Br. med. J.* **4**, 12–13.
ROBERTS, C. J. AND LLOYD, S. (1973). Area differences in spontaneous abortion rates in South Wales and their relation to neural tube defect incidence. *Br. med. J.* **4**, 20–2.

—— AND POWELL, R. G. (1975). Interrelation of the common congenital malformations—some aetiological implications. *Lancet* **ii**, 848–50.
——, LOWE, C. R., AND LLOYD, S. (1972). Cyclic variation in date of last menstrual period of mother of infants with congenital malformation in South Wales, 1964–66. *Br. J. prev. soc. Med.* **26**, 212–18.
——, REVINGTON, C. J., AND LLOYD, S. (1973). Potato cultivation and storage in South Wales and its relation to neural tube malformation prevalence. *Br. J. prev. soc. Med.* **27**, 214–16.
——, LAURENCE, K. M., AND LLOYD, S. (1975). An investigation of space and space-time clustering in a large sample of infants with neural tube defects born in Cardiff. *Br. J. prev. soc. Med.* **29**, 202–4.
ROBERTS, I. F. AND WEST, R. J. (1977). Teratogenesis and maternal progesterone. (letter). *Lancet* **ii**, 982.
ROBERTSON, E. G. (1953). Craniopagus parietalis: report of a case. *Arch. Neurol. Psychiat. (Chi.)* **70**, 189–205.
ROBERTSON, G. G., WILLIAMSON, A. P., AND BLATTNER, R. J. (1955). A study of abnormalities in early chick embryos inoculated with Newcastle disease virus. *J. Exp. Zool.* **129**, 5–43.
ROBERTSON, J. A. (1975). Discretionary non-treatment of defective newborns. In *Genetics and the law* edited by Milunsky, A. and Annas, G. J., Plenum Press, New York, pp. 451–65.
—— (1975*a*). Involuntary euthanasia of defective newborns: a legal analysis. *Stanford Law. Rev.* **27**, 213–69.
ROBSON, A. M. (1895). The treatment of spina bifida by a plastic operation with reports of twenty cases. *Ann. Surg. (Philad.)* **22**, 81–5.
RODECK, C. H. AND CAMPBELL, S. (1978). Early prenatal diagnosis of neural-tube defects by ultrasound-guided fetoscopy. *Lancet* **i**, 1128–9.
ROGER, J. H. (1977). A significance test for cyclic trends in incidence data. *Biometrika* **64**, 152–5.
—— (1977*a*). An explanation for the observed increase in mortality after a birthday in people over 75 years old. *Br. J. prev. soc. Med.* **31**, 62–4.
ROGERS, S. C. (1969). Epidemiology of stillbirths from congenital abnormalities in England and Wales, 1961–1966. *Develop. Med. Child Neurol.* **11**, 617–29.
—— (1976). Anencephalus, spina bifida, twins and teratoma. *Br. J. prev. soc. Med.* **30**, 26–8.
—— AND MORRIS, M. (1971). Infant mortality from spina bifida, congenital hydrocephalus, monstrosity and congenital diseases of the cardiovascular system. *Ann. Hum. Genet. (Lond.)* **34**, 295–305.
—— —— (1973). Anencephalus: a changing sex ratio. *Br. J. prev. soc. Med.* **27**, 81–4.
—— AND WEATHERALL, J. A. C. (1976). *Anencephalus, spina bifida and hydrocephalus—England and Wales 1964–1972.* Studies on Medical and Population Subjects No. 32. HMSO, London.
ROGOT, E., FABSITZ, R., AND FEINLEIB, M. (1976). Daily variation in USA mortality. *Am. J. Epidem.* **103**, 198–211.
ROMANES, G. J. (1895). *Darwin and after Darwin* Vol. 2 Post-Darwinism questions: heredity and utility. The Open Court Publishing Co., Chicago.
ROTHMAN, K. J. AND FYLER, D. C. (1974). Seasonal occurrence of complex ventricular septal defects. *Lancet* **i**, 193–7.
—— AND LOUIK, C. (1978). Oral contraceptives and birth defects. *New Engl. J. Med.* **299**, 522–4.
—— AND MONSON, R. R. (1973). Survival in trigeminal neuralgia. *J. Chron. Dis.* **26**, 303–9.
ROUX, C. (1959). Teratogenic action of prochlorpemazine. *Arch. franc. Pédiat.* **16**, 968–71.
RUDDICK, J. A., HARWIG, J., AND SCOTT, P. M. (1974). Nonteratogenicity in rats of blighted potatoes and compounds contained in them. *Teratology* **9**, 165–8.
RUGH, R. AND GRUPP, E. (1959). X-irradiation exencephaly. *Am. J. Roentgenol.* **81**, 1026–52.
RUNNER, M. N. (1959). Inheritance of susceptibility to congenital deformity: metabolic clues provided by experiments with teratogenic agents. *Pediatrics* **23**, 245–51.
RUOSLAHTI, E. AND SEPPÄLÄ, M. (1971). Studies of carcino-fetal proteins: physical and chemical properties of human α-fetoprotein. *Int. J. Cancer* **7**, 218–25.
—— —— (1972). α-fetoprotein in normal human serum. *Nature (Lond.)* **235**, 161.
RUSSELL, J. C. (1948). *British medieval population.* The University of New Mexico Press, Albuquerque, pp. 148–9.

Rushton, D. I. (1978). Teratogenic effects of waste anaesthetic gases. (letter). *Br. med. J.* **1**, 438.

Sachtleben, R. (1903). *Die in der chirurgischen Klinik zu Breslau beobachteten Fälle von Spina bifida aus den Jahren 1891–1903.* Inaugural Address, Breslau.

Safra, M. J. and Oakley, G. P., Jr. (1975). Association between cleft lip with or without cleft palate and prenatal exposure to diazepam. *Lancet* **ii**, 478–80.

Saint-Hilaire, E. G. (1826). Description d'un monstre humain ré avant l'ere chretienne, comparé à an pareil monstre de l'époque actuelle; et considerations zootomiques et physiologiques sur le caractère de ces monstruosltés, dites anencephales; sur l'independance de deformation de chique sexe; et sur l'existence de deux noyaux dan l'os basilaire. *Ann. Sci. Nat.* **7**, 357.

St Leger, A. S. (1976). Comparison of two tests for seasonality in epidemiological data. *J.R. Stat. Soc., Series C* **25**, 280–6.

Sandahl, B. (1977). Seasonal incidence of some congenital malformations of the central nervous system in Sweden. 1965–1972. *Acta Paed. Scand.* **66**, 65–72.

Sandler, B. (1973). Anencephaly and ovulation stimulation. (letter). *Lancet* **ii**, 379.

Sare, W. M. and Forbes, P. I. (1972). Possible dysmorphogenic effects of an agricultural chemical: 2.4.5–T. *N.Z. Med. J.* **75**, 37–8.

Saunders, R. L. de C. H. (1943). Combined anterior and posterior spina bifida in a living neonatal human female. *Anat. Rec.* **87**, 255–78.

Saxén, L., Hjelt, L., Sjostedt, J. E., Hakosalo, J., and Hakosalo, H. (1960). Asian influenza during pregnancy and congenital malformation. *Acta Path. Microbiol. Scand.* **49**(1), 114–26.

Say, B. and Coldwell, J. G. (1975). Hereditary defect of the sacrum. *Humangenetik* **27**, 231–4.

Schlesselman, J. J. and Spiers, P. S. (1975). Anencephaly, spina bifida and dizygotic twinning: A review of the data of Stevenson *et al. Am. J. Epidem.* **101**, 14–16.

Schmid, W. and Mühlethaler, J. P. (1975). High amniotic fluid alpha$_1$-fetoprotein in a case of fetal sacrococcygeal teratoma. *Humangenetik* **26**, 353–4.

—— ——, Briner, J., and Knechtli, H. (1975*a*). Ring chromosome 13 in a polymalformed anencephalic. *Humangenetik* **27**, 63–6.

Schull, W. J., Harburg, E., Schork, M. A., and Chakraborty, R. (1977). Heredity, stress and blood pressure, a family set method. *J. Chron. Dis.* **30**, 701–4.

Schwalbe, E. and Gredig, M. (1906). Über entwicklungsstörungen des Kleinhirns, Hirnstamms und Halsmarks bei spina bifida (Arnold'sche und Chiari'sche Missbildung). *Beitr. path. Anat. (Jena)* **40**, 182–94.

Scotsman (1977). Glasgow rate of birth defects now lowest in UK. 1 December, p. 8.

Scott, D. E., Whalley, P. J., and Pritchard, J. A. (1970). Maternal folate deficiency and pregnancy wastage. II. Fetal malformation. *Obstet. Gynec.* **36**, 26–8.

Scott, J. M. and Patterson, L. (1966) Monozygous anencephalic triplets—a case report. *J. Obstet. Gynaec. Br. Commonw.* **73**, 147–51.

Scott, M. J. (1975). Congenital malformations in children born in Belfast 1964–1968. M.D. thesis, The Queen's University of Belfast.

Scott, W. J., Butcher, R. E., Kindt, C. W., and Wilson, J. G. (1972). Greater sensitivity of female than male rat embryos to acetazolamide teratogenicity. *Teratology* **6**, 239–40.

Scrimgeour, J. B. (1974). Fetoscopy. In *Birth defects: Proceedings of the Fourth International Conference* ed. Motulsky, A. G. and Lenz, W. Excerpta Medica, Amsterdam, pp. 234–9.

—— (1976). Amniocentesis in early pregnancy: Technical aspects and complications. In *Prenatal diagnosis* edited by Boué, A. Inserm, Paris, Vol. **61**, pp. 39–44.

Searle, A. G. (1956). Quoted by Penrose, L. S. (1957), p. 5.

—— (1959). The incidence of anencephaly in a polytypic population. *Ann. hum. Genet. (Lond.)* **23**, 279–87.

Seller, M. J. (1975). Case report: Prenatal diagnosis of a neural tube defect: Meckel syndrome. *J. med. Genet.* **12**, 109–10.

—— and Adinolfi, M. (1975). α-fetoprotein and alternative markers for the antenatal diagnosis of neural tube defects. (letter). *Lancet* **ii**, 984–5.

——, Campbell, S., Coltart, T. M., and Singer, J. D. (1973). Early termination of anencephalic pregnancy after detection by raised alpha-fetoprotein levels. *Lancet* **ii**, 73.

——, Singer, J. D., Coltart, T. M., and Campbell, S. (1974). Maternal serum-alpha-fetoprotein levels and prenatal diagnosis of neural tube defects. *Lancet* **i**, 428–9.

——, Creasy, M. R., and Alberman, E. D. (1974). Alpha-fetoprotein levels in amniotic fluids from spontaneous abortions, *Br. med. J.* **2**, 524–5.

——, Dumon, J. E., and Vanderheyden, J. S. D. (1977). Amniotic fluid AFP in multiple pregnancy. (letter). *Br. med. J* **2**, 1600.

Seppälä, M. (1973). Increased alpha-fetoprotein in amniotic fluid associated with a congenital oesophageal atresia of the fetus. *Obstet. Gynecol.* **42**, 613–14.

—— (1975). Fetal pathophysiology of human α-fetoprotein. *Ann. N.Y. Acad. Sci.* **259**, 59–73.

—— and Ruoslahti. (1972). Radioimmunoassay of maternal serum alpha fetoprotein during pregnancy and delivery. *Am. J. Obstet. Gynec.* **112**, 208–12.

—— —— (1973). Alpha fetoprotein: physiology and pathology during pregnancy and application to antenatal diagnosis. *J. Perinatal Med.* **1**, 104–13.

—— —— (1973*a*). Alpha-fetoprotein in antenatal diagnosis. (letter). *Lancet* **i**, 155.

—— and Unnerus, H. A. (1974). Elevated amniotic fluid alpha fetoprotein in fetal hydrocephaly. *Am. J. Obstet. Gynec.* **119**, 270–2.

——, Tallberg, T., and Enholm, C. (1967). Studies on embryo-specific proteins. Physiological characteristics of embryospecific alpha-globulin. *Anns. Med. Exp. Biol. Fenn.* **45**, 16–19.

Sever, J. L. (1975). Infectious agents as teratogens. In *Methods for detection of environmental agents that produce congenital defects.* Edited by Shepard, T. H., Miller, J. R. and Marois, M. North-Holland Publishing Company, Amsterdam, pp. 221–32.

Sever, L. E. (1975). Zinc and human development: a review. *Human Ecology* **3**(1), 43–57.

—— and Emanuel, I. (1973). Is there a connection between maternal zinc deficiency and congenital malformations of the central nervous system in man? *Teratology* **7**, 117–18.

Shapiro, L. M., Skinner, L. G., Phillips, H. V., and Whitfield, C. R. (1975). Racial variation in maternal serum-alpha-fetoprotein. (letter). *Lancet* **ii**, 1142.

Sharrard, W. J., Zachary, R. B., Lorber, J., and Bruce, A. M. (1963). A controlled trial of immediate and delayed closure of spina bifida cystica. *Arch. Dis. Childh.* **38**, 18–22.

Shearman, R. P. and Garrett, W. J. (1963). Double-blind study of effect of 17-hydroxyprogesterone caproate on abortion rate. *Br. med. J.* **1**, 292–5.

Sheffield, L. J. (1978). Methodological aspects of the prenatal diagnosis of neural tube defects. MSc. thesis, McMaster University, Hamilton, Ontario, pp. 1–140.

Shenefelt, R. E. (1972). Morphogenesis of malformations in hamsters caused by retinoic acid: relation to dose and stage at treatment. *Teratology* **5**, 103–18.

Shepard, T. H. (1976). *Catalog of teratogenic agents.* Second Edition. The John Hopkins University Press, Baltimore.

——, Miller, J. R., and Marois, M. (1975). *Methods for detection of environmental agents that produce congenital defects.* North-Holland Publishing Company, Amsterdam.

Shrewsbury, J. F. D. (1949). A contribution to the historical record of monstrous births. *J. Obstet. Gynaec. Brit. Emp.* **56**, 67–85.

Siemiatycki, J. and McDonald, A. D. (1972). Neural tube defects in Quebec. A search for evidence of 'clustering' in time and place. *Br. J. prev. soc. Med.* **26**, 10–14.

Silberg, S. L., Watson, F. R., and Martin, J. C. (1968). Seasonal variation of congenital malformations. *Can. J. Publ. Hlth.* **59**, 239–43.

Simon, Von St (1932). Anencephalus bei Zwillingshevongerschaft. *Zbl. Gynäk (Leipzig)* **56**, 1536–9.

Simpson, J. Y. and Barth, D. C. (1869). A lecture on the Siamese and other viable united twins. *Br. med. J.* **13**, 6.

Simpson, J. L., Dische, R., and Morillo-Cucci, G. (1972). Triploidy (69, XXY) in a liveborn infant. *Ann. Genet. (Paris)* **15**, 103–6.

Sizaret, P. and Anderson, S. G. (1976). The International Reference Preparation for alpha-foetoprotein. *J. Biol. Stand.* **4**, 149.

Škreb, N. and Frank, Z. (1963). Developmental abnormalities in the rat induced by heat shock. *J. Embryol. exp. Morphol.* **11**, 445–57.

Slater, B. C. S., Watson, G. I., and McDonald, J. C. (1964). Seasonal variation in congenital abnormalities. *Br. J. prev. soc. Med.* **18**, 1–7.

Smart, J. L. and Dobbing, J. (1971). Vulnerability of developing brain. II: Effects of early

nutritional deprivation on reflex ontogeny and development of behavior in the rat. *Brain Res.* **28**, 85–95.
SMILKSTEIN, G. (1962). A ten year study of anencephaly. *California Med.* **96**, 350–3.
SMITH, A. (1966). Observations on the determinants of human multiple birth. In: *Annual Report of the Registrar General for Scotland, 1964.* HMSO, Edinburgh, p. 70.
SMITH, A. U. (1957). The effects on foetal development of freezing pregnant hamsters (mesocricetus auratus). *J. Embryol. exp. Morph.* **5**, 311–23.
SMITH, A. G., SHUSTER, S., CLARK, D., THODY, A. J., DAVISON, E. V., AND WARD, A. M. (1978). Neural tube defects and immunoreactive β-melanocyte-stimulating hormone in amniotic fluid. *Br. med. J.* **2**, 20–1.
SMITH, B. E., USUBIAGA, L. E., AND LEHRER, S. B. (1971). Cleft palate induced by halothane anesthesia in C-57 black mice. (Abstract). *Teratology* **4**, 242.
SMITH, C. (1975). Quantitative Inheritance. In *Textbook of human genetics*, edited by G. R. Fraser and O. Mayo. Blackwell Scientific Publications, Oxford, pp. 382–441.
——, WATT, M., BOYD, A. E. W., AND HOLMES, J. C. (1973). Anencephaly, spina bifida, and potato blight in the Edinburgh area. (letter). *Lancet* **i**, 269.
SMITH, C. A. (1947). Effects of wartime starvation in Holland on pregnancy and its products. *Am. J. Obstet Gynec.* **53**, 599–608.
SMITH, C. A. B. (1961). Note on the error variance. *Ann. Hum. Genet. (Lond.)* **25**, 86–7.
SMITH, D. W., CLARREN, S. K., AND HARVEY, M. A. S. (1978). Hyperthermia as a possible teratogenic agent. *J. Pediat.* **92**, 878–83.
SMITH, P. G. (1978). Current assessment of 'case clustering' of lymphomas and leukaemias. *Cancer* **42**, 1026–34.
SMITHBERG, M., SANCHEZ, H. W., AND RUNNER, M. N. (1956). Congenital deformity in the mouse induced by insulin. (abstract). *Anat. Rec.* **124**, 441.
SMITHELLS, R. W. (1968). Incidence of congenital abnormalities in Liverpool 1960–1964. *Br. J. prev. soc. Med.* **22**, 36–7.
—— (1976). Environmental teratogens in man. *Br. Med. Bull.* **32**, 27–33.
—— (1976*a*). See Lorber, J. and Rogers, S. C. (1977).
SMITHELLS, R. W. AND CHINN, E. R. (1965). Spina bifida in Liverpool. *Develop. Med. Child Neurol.* **7**, 258–68.
—— —— AND FRANKLIN, D. (1964). Anencephaly in Liverpool. *Develop. Med. Child Neurol.* **6**, 231–40.
——, D'ARCY, E. E., AND MCALLISTER. (1968). The outcome of pregnancies before and after the birth of infants with nervous system malformations. *Develop. Med. Child Neurol., Suppl.* **15**, pp. 6–10.
——, SHEPPARD, S., AND SCHORAH, C. J. (1975). Nutritional deficiencies and neural tube defects. *Arch. Dis. Childh.* **51**, 944–950.
SMYTH, B. T., PIGGOT, J., FORSYTHE, W. I., AND MERRETT, J. D. (1974). A controlled trial of immediate and delayed closure of myelomeningocele. *J. Bone Jt Surg.* **56–B**, 297–304.
SNELL, G. D. (1935). The induction by X-rays of hereditary changes in mice. *Genetics* **20**, 545–67.
SNOW, J. (1855). *On the mode of communication of cholera.* Second Edition. Churchill, London.
SOLER, N. G., WALSH, C. H., AND MALINS, J. M. (1976). Congenital malformations in infants of diabetic mothers. *Q. J. Med.* **45**, 303–13.
SOLOWY, M. K. AND SHEPHARD, F. M. (1971). Anencephaly in Central Virginia. *Clin. Pediat.* **10**, 43–5.
SOUTH, M. A., TOMPKINS, W. A. F., MORRIS, C. R., AND RAWLS, W. E. (1969). Congenital malformation of the central nervous system associated with genital type (type 2) herpesvirus. *J. Pediatrics* **75**, 13–18.
SPELLMAN, M. P. (1969). Anencephaly—a five year survey in Cork. *J. Irish med. Ass.* **62**, 316–320.
—— (1970). A five year survey in Cork of spina bifida and hydrocephaly. *J. Irish med. Ass.* **63**, 339–42.
SPIERS, P. S. (1973). Spina bifida, anencephaly and potato blight. *Lancet* **i**, 426–7.
—— (1973*a*). Multiple ovulation and risk of anencephaly and spina bifida. (letter). *Lancet* **ii**, 1149.

——, Pietrzyk, J. J., Piper, J. M., and Glebatis, D. M. (1974). Human potato consumption and neural tube malformation. *Teratology* **10**, 125–8.

Spoto, P. (1947). Alcuni dati clinico-statistici sulle malformazioni fetali. *Lattante (Parma)* **18**, 338–59.

Spreng, D. S. (1938). Fetal maldevelopment recurring in mother and four daughters. *Ohio State Med. J.* **34**, 520.

Stark, C. R. and Mantel, N. (1966). Effects of maternal age and birth order on the risk of mongolism and leukaemia. *J. Nat. Cancer Inst.* **37**, 687–98.

—— —— (1967). Lack of seasonal—or temporal—spatial clustering of Down's syndrome births in Michigan. *Am. J. Epidem.* **86**, 199–213.

Stark, G. D. (1977). *Spina bifida. Problems and management.* Blackwell, Oxford.

Steele, M. W. (1973). Screening for chromosomal abnormalities. *Lancet* **i**, 542.

Steffensen, J. (1956). Quoted by Penrose, L. S. (1957), p. 5.

Stein, Z. and Susser, M. (1976). Maternal starvation and birth defects. In *Birth defects: risks and consequences*, edited by Kelly, S., Hook, E. B., Janerich, D. T. and Porter, I. H. Academic Press Inc., New York, pp. 205–20.

—— ——, and Guterman, A. V. (1973). Screening program for prevention of Down's syndrome. *Lancet* **i**, 305–9.

—— ——, Saenger, G., and Marolla, F. (1975). *Famine and human development. The Dutch hunger winter of 1944–1945.* Oxford University Press, London.

Sternberg, H. (1929). Über Spaltbedingungen des Medullarohres bei jungen menschlichen embryonen, ein Beikrag zur entstehung der Anencephalie und der Rachischisis. *Virchows Arch. path. Anat.* **272**, 325–73.

Stevenson, A. C. (1959). The load of hereditary defects in human populations. *Radiat. Res., Suppl.* **1**, 306–25.

—— (1960). The relation of hydrammios with congenital malformations (with discussion). In *Ciba Foundation Symposium on congenital malformations*. Edited by Wolstenholme, G. E. W. and O'Connor, C. M. Little, Brown and Co., Boston, pp. 241–67.

—— and Warnock, H. A. (1959). Observations on the results of pregnancies in women resident in Belfast. I. Data relating to all pregnancies ending in 1957. *Ann. hum. Genet. Lond.* **23**, 382–94.

——, Johnson, H. A., Stewart, M. I. P., and Golding, D. R. (1966). Congenital malformations—a report of a study of series of consecutive births in 24 centres. *Bull. WHO* **34**(1), 1–125.

Stewart, A., Webb, J., Giles, D., and Hewitt, D. (1956). Malignant disease in childhood and diagnostic irradiation *in utero*. *Lancet* **ii**, 447.

Stewart, A. G. and Taylor, W. C. (1964). Amniotic fluid analysis as an aid to the ante-partum diagnosis of haemolytic disease. *J. Obstet. Gynecol. Br. Commonw.* **71**, 604–8.

Stewart, C. R., Ward, A. M., and Lorber, J. (1975). Amniotic fluid α-fetoprotein in the diagnosis of neural tract malformations. *Br. J. Obstet. Gynaec.* **82**, 257–61.

Stewart, M. A. (1946). Personal communication to Olmstead (1946), p. 194.

Stewart, T. D. (1931). Incidence of separate neural-arch in the lumbar vertebrae of Eskimos. *Am. J. Phys. Anthropol.* **16**, 51–62.

—— (1953). The age incidence of neural-arch defects in Alaskan natives, considered from the standpoint of etiology. *J. Bone Jt Surg.* **35A**, 937–50.

Stockard,, C. R. (1921). Developmental rate and structural expression: an experimental study of twins, 'double monsters' and single deformities, and the interaction among embryonic organs during their origin and development. *Am. J. Anat.* **28**, 115–277.

Stocks, P. (1970). Incidence of congenital malformations in the regions of England and Wales. *Br. J. prev. soc. Med.* **24**, 67–77.

Stoller, A. and Collman, R. D. (1965). Patterns of occurrence of births in Victoria, Australia, producing Down's syndrome (mongolism) and congenital anomalies of the central nervous system: a 21-year prospective and retrospective survey. *Med. J. Aust.* **1**, 1–4.

Streeter, G. L. (1942). Developmental horizons in human embryos, description of age group XI, 13 to 20 somites, and age group XII, 21 to 29 somites. *Contrib. Embryol.* **30**, 211–45.

—— (1945). Developmental horizons in human embryos, description of age group XIII embryos about 4 or 5 millimeters long, and age group XIV, period of indentation of lens vesicle. *Contrib. Embryol.* **31**, 27–63.

—— (1948). Developmental horizons in human embryos, description of age groups XV, XVI, XVII and XVIII, being the third issue of a survey of the Carnegie Collection. *Contrib. Embryol.* **32**, 133–203.

SUSSER, M. W. (1973). *Causal thinking in the health Sciences*. Oxford University Press, London.

SUTHERLAND, G. R., BROCK, D. J. H., AND SCRIMGEOUR, J. B. (1973). Amniotic-fluid macrophages and anencephaly. *Lancet* **ii**, 1098–9.

——, ——, ——, —— (1975). Amniotic fluid macrophages and the antenatal diagnosis of anencephaly and spina bifida. *J. med. Genet.* **12**, 135–7.

SWINYARD, C. A. AND CHAUBE, S. (1973). Are potatoes teratogenic for experimental animals? *Teratology* **8**, 349–58.

TARUFFI, C. (1881–94). *Storia della Teratologia*. Eight volumes. Regia Typographia, Bologna.

TAYLOR, A. I. (1968). Autosomal trisomy syndromes: A detailed study of 27 cases of Edwards' syndrome and 27 cases of Patau's syndrome. *J. med. Genet.* **5**, 227–52.

TEW, B. J., LAURENCE, K. M., PAYNE, H., AND RAWNSLEY. (1977). Marital stability following the birth of a child with spina bifida. *Br. J. Psychiat.* **131**, 79–82.

THIERSCH, J. B. (1952). Therapeutic abortions with folic acid antagonist, 4-aminopteroylglutamic acid (4-amino P.G.A.) administered by oral route. *Am. J. Obstet. Gynec.* **63**, 1298–1304.

—— (1956). The control of reproduction in rats with the aid of antimetabolites, and early experiences with antimetabolites as abortifacient agents in man. *Acta endocr., suppl.* **28**, 37–45.

THOMAS, W. D. S. (1977). The Badgley report on the Abortion Law. (letter). *Can. med. Ass. J.* **116**, 966.

THOMPSON, C. J. S. (1930). *The mystery and lore of monsters*. Williams and Norgate Ltd., London, p. 63.

THOMPSON, B. (1977). Problems of abortion in Britain—Aberdeen, a case study. *Pop. Stud.* **31**, 143–54.

THORBURN, M. J., WYNTER, H. H., AND BELL, R. (1969). Congenital malformations in Jamaica. An analysis of the perinatal populations of the University Hospital of the West Indies. *Trop. geogr. Med.* **21**, 147–56.

TIMONEN, S. AND CARPEN, E. (1968). Multiple pregnancies and photoperiodicity. *Ann. Chir. Gynaec. Fenn.* **57**, 135–8.

TOMLIN, P. J. (1978). Teratogenic effects of waste anaesthetic gases. (letter). *Br. med. J.* **1**, 300.

—— (1978*a*). Teratogenic effects of waste anesthetic gases. (letter). *Br. med. J.* **1**, 438.

TREXLER, R. C. (1973). Infanticide in Florence: new sources and first results. *Hist. Childhood Q.* **1**, 98–116.

TRICHOPOULOS, D., DESMOND, L., YEN, S., AND MACMAHON, B. (1971). A study of time-place clustering in anencephaly and spina bifida. *Am. J. Epidem.* **94**, 26–9.

TRIMBLE, B. K. AND DOUGHTY, J. H. (1974). The amount of hereditary disease in human populations. *Ann. hum. Genet. (Lond.)* **38**, 199–223.

—— AND BAIRD, P. A. (1978). Congenital anomalies of the central nervous system incidence in British Columbia 1952–72. *Teratology* **17**, 43–50.

TRUETT, J., CORNFIELD, J., AND KANNEL, W. (1967). A multivariate analysis of the risk of coronary heart disease in Framingham. *J. chron. Dis.* **20**, 511–24.

TSUCHIDA, Y., ENDO, Y., URANO, Y., AND ISHIDA, M. (1975). α-fetoprotein in yolk sac tumor. *Ann. N.Y. Acad. Sci.* **259**, 221–33.

TUCHMANN-DUPLESSIS, H. AND MERCIER-PAROT, L. (1957). Sur l'action tératogène de l'acide X-méthylfolique chez la souris. *C.R. Acad. Sci. (Paris)* **245**, 1963–5.

——, —— (1959*a*). Apropos of the teratogenic action of actinomycin. *C.R. Soc. Biol. (Paris)* **153**, 1697–1700.

——, —— (1959*b*). On the abortive and teratogenic action of 6-chloropurine. *C.R. Soc. Biol. (Paris)* **153**, 1133–6.

TULP, N. (1637). *Observations Medicae*. Amsterdam.

TÜNTE, W. (1965). *Verglechende Untersuchungen uber die Haufigheit angeborener menschlicher Missbildungen*. Gustav Fishcher, Stuttgart.

—— (1971). Fortpflanzungsfähigkeit, Heiratsh-aufigkeit und zahl und Beschaffenheit der Wachkommen bei Patienten init spina bifida aperta *Humangenetik* **13**, 43–8.

TYROLER, H. A. (1977). The Detroit project studies of blood pressure. A prologue and review of related studies and epidemiological issues. *J. Chron. Dis.* **30**, 613–24.

ULLRICH, O. (1951). Der status Bonnevie-Ullrich im Rahmen anderer 'Dyscranio-Dysphalangien'. *Ergebn. inn. Med. Kinderheilk.* **2**, 412–66.

UNITED KINGDOM COLLABORATIVE STUDY (1977). Maternal serum-alpha-fetoprotein measurement in antenatal screening for anencephaly and spina bifida in early pregnancy. Report of U.K. Collaborative Study on alpha-fetoprotein in relation to neural tube defects. *Lancet* **i**, 1323–32.

URIEL, J., DE NECHAND, B., STANISLAWSKI-BIRENWAJG, M., MASSEYEFF, R., LEBLANC, L., QUENUM, C. LOISILLIER, F. AND GRABAR, P. (1968). Le diagnostic du cancer primaire du foie par des méthodes immunologiques. *Presse Méd.* **76**, 1415–17.

USHER, R. H. (1977). Definition of perinatal mortality (letter). *Lancet* **ii**, 354.

VALENTI, C. (1978). Fetal blood sampling in early pregnancy. In *Towards the prevention of fetal malformation* edited by J. B. Scrimgeour, Edinburgh University Press, Edinburgh, pp. 273–86.

VAN DEN BOSCH, J. (1956). Personal communication, *see* Penrose, L. S. (1957).

VAN WENT, J. J., VAN WENT, G. F., DELLEMAN, J. W., AND BECKER, A. G. (1977). Spina bifida and so-called asplenia syndrome occurring separately in sibs. *Teratology* **15**, 195–8.

VAN DER VELDEN, W. H. M. (1957). *De betekenis van het hydramnion voor die ureogtijdige herkenning van zieten of afwijkingen bij moeder en kind*. Koch and Knuttel, Gouda.

VARIEND, S. AND EMERY, J. L. (1976). Cervical dislocation of the cerebellum in children with menignomyelocele. *Teratology* **13**, 281–90.

VERSLEGE, J. CH. W. (1971). *Anencephalie in Nederland 1951–1968*. Central Bureau voor de Statistiek, Staatsuitgeverij. (The Hague).

VIANNA, N. J. AND POLAN, A. K. (1976). Childhood lymphatic leukaemia: prenatal seasonality and possible association with congenital varicella. *Am. J. Epidem.* **103**, 321–32.

VOGEL, F. S. (1961). The anatomic character of the vascular anomalies associated with anencephaly: with consideration of the role of abnormal angiogenesis in the pathogenesis of the cerebral malformation. *Am. J. Path.* **39**, 163–9.

—— AND MACLENAHAN, J. L. (1952). Anomalies of major cerebral arteries associated with congenital malformations of the brain. *Am. J. Path.* **28**, 701–23.

VOGEL, H. P. AND KNOX, E. G. (1975). Reproductive patterns after stillbirth and early infant death. *J. biosoc. Sci.* **7**, 103–11.

WACKER, M. N. (1963). Congenital abnormalities. A survey of 296 cases occurring in a 10 year period. *Am. J. Obstet. Gynec.* **86**, 310–20.

WALD, N., BARKER, S., PETO, R., BROCK, D. J. H., AND BONNAR, J. (1975). Maternal serum α-fetoprotein levels in multiple pregnancy. *Br. med. J.* **1**, 651–2.

WALD, N. AND HAMBRIDGE, M. (1977). Maternal serum-copper concentration and neural tube defects (letter). *Lancet* **ii**, 560.

——, BARKER, S, PETO, R., BROCK, D. J. H., AND BONNAR, J. (1976). Maternal serum alpha-fetoprotein and previous neural tube defects. *Br. J. Obstet. Gynaec* **83**, 213–16.

——, ——, CUCKLE, H., BROCK, D. J. H., AND STIRRAT, G. M. (1977). Maternal serum alpha-fetoprotein and spontaneous abortion. *Br. J. Obstet. Gynaec.* **84**, 357–62.

——, CUCKLE, H., STIRRAT, G. M., BENNETT, M. J., AND TURNBULL, A. C. (1977). Maternal serum-alpha-fetoprotein and low birth-weight. *Lancet* **ii**, 268–70.

——, ——, AND STIRRAT, G. (1978). Maternal serum alpha-fetoprotein levels in triplet and quadruplet pregnancy. *Br. J. Obstet. and Gynaec.* **85**, 124–6.

——, ——, ——, AND TURNBULL, A. C. (1978). Maternal serum alpha-fetoprotein and birth weight in twin pregnancies. *Br. J. Obstet. Gynaec.* **85**, 582–4.

——, ——, ——, (1978*a*). Screening for neural-tube defects (letter). *Lancet,* **i**, 495.

——, ——, BROCK, D. J. H., AND POLANI, P. E. (1978). Screening for neural-tube defects (letter). *Lancet,* **ii**, 216–17.

WALDMANN, T. A. AND MCINTIRE, K. R. (1972). serum-alpha-fetoprotein levels in patients with ataxia-telengiectasia. *Lancet* **ii**, 1112–15.

WALKER, J. AND SMITH, A. (1961). Anencephaly in Dundee 1950–9. In *First International*

Conference on Congenital Malformations 1960. J. B. Lippincott and Co., Philadelphia, pp. 257–63.

WALKER, S. H. AND DUNCAN, D. B. (1967). Estimation of the probability of an event as a function of several independent variables. *Biometrika* **54**, 167–79.

WALKER, W. M. AND MCKEE, A. P. (1959). Asian influenza in pregnancy: relationship to fetal anomalies. *Obstet. Gynec.* **13**, 394–8.

WALLWORK, J. C., MCFARLANE, H., HINGLEY, S., AND WARD, A. M. (1975). Serum -fetoprotein in cystic fibrosis. (letter). *Br. med. J.* **1**, 392.

WALTER, S. D. (1977). Determination of significant relative risks and optimal sampling procedures in prospective and retrospective comparative studies of various sizes. *Am. J. Epidemiol.* **105**, 387–97.

—— (1977*a*). The power of a test for seasonality. *Br. J. prev. soc. Med.* **31**, 137–40.

—— AND ELWOOD, J. M. (1975). A test for seasonality of events with a variable population at risk. *Br. J. prev. soc. Med.* **29**, 18–21.

WARD, A. M. AND STEWART, C. R. (1974). False-positive results in antenatal diagnosis of neural-tube disorders. (letter) *Lancet* **ii**, 345–6.

WARD, I. V. AND IRVINE, E. D. (1961). The incidence of congenital abnormality in infants born to Exeter mothers, 1954–60 inclusive. *Med. Offr.* **106**, 381–3.

WARKANY, J. (1959). Congenital malformations in the past. *J. Chronic Dis.* **10**, 84–96.

—— (1971). *Congenital malformations*. Year Book Medical Publishers Inc., Chicago.

—— (1975). A warfarin embryopathy? *Am. J. Dis. Child* **129**, 287–8.

—— AND PETERING, H. G. (1972). Congenital malformations of the central nervous system in rats produced by maternal zinc deficiency. *Teratology* **5**, 319–34.

—— AND TAKACS, E. (1959). Experimental production of congenital malformations in rats by salicylate poisoning. *Am. J. Path.* **35**, 315–24.

——, —— (1965). Congenital malformations in rats from streptonigrin. *Arch. Pathol.* **79**, 65–79.

——, BEAUDRY, P. H., AND HORNSTEIN, S. (1959). Attempted abortion with aminopterin (4-amino-pteroylglutamic acid). *Am. J. Dis. Child* **97**, 274–81.

WARNER, W. L., MEEKER, M., AND EELIS, K. (1957). *Social class in America. A manual of procedure for the measurement of social status*. Peter Smith, Gloucester.

WEATHERALL, J. A. C. (1969). An assessment of the efficiency of notification of congenital malformations. *Med. Offr.* **121**, 65–8.

—— (1976). A follow-up study of children notified with spina bifida. In *Child health—a collection of studies*. Studies of Medical and Population Subjects No. 31. Office of Population Censuses and Surveys. HMSO, London, pp. 15–21.

—— AND HASKEY, J. C. (1976). Surveillance and malformations. *Br. med. Bull.* **32**, 39–44.

—— AND WHITE, G. C. (1976). A study of survival of children with spina bifida. In *Child health—a collection of studies*. Studies on Medical and Population Subjects No. 31. Office of Population Censuses and Surveys. HMSO, London, pp. 3–11.

WEHRUNG, D. A. AND HAY, S. (1970). A study of seasonal incidence of congenital malformations in the U.S. *Br. J. prev. soc. Med.* **24**, 24–32.

WEI, P. Y. AND CHEN, Y. P. (1965). Congenital malformations especially anencephalus in Taiwan. *Am. J. Obstet. Gynec.* **91**, 870–6.

WEINBERG, A. G. MILUNSKY, A. AND HARROD, M. J. (1975). Elevated amniotic fluid alphafetoprotein and duodenal atresia (letter). *Lancet* **ii**, 496.

WEINBERG, W. (1901). Beiträge zur Physiologie und Pathologie der Mehrlingsgeburten beim Menschen. *Pflügers Arch. ges. Physiol.* **88**, 346–430.

WELCH, J. P. (1976). Neural-tube defects (letter). *New Engl. J. med.* **294**, 1461–2.

WERTHEIMER, H. (1957). Relations des malformations congénitales avec l'age parental et l'ordre de Naissance et Répartition du sexe des enfants atteints. *J. Génet. Hum.* **6**, 49–63.

WHEELESS, C. R. (1976). Mortality from fetoscopy in mid trimester pregnancy. In *Intrauterine fetal visualization*. A *multidisciplinary approach*. Edited by Kaback, M. M. and Valenti, C. Excerpta Medica, Amsterdam, p. 184–90.

WHITFIELD, C. R., NEELEY, R. A., AND TELFORD, M. E. (1968). Amniotic fluid analysis in Rhesus iso-immunisation. *J. Obstet. Gynaec. Brit Common.* **75**, 121–7.

WHYLEY, G. A., WARD, R. H., AND HARDY, N. R. (1974). Alpha-fetoprotein levels in amniotic fluid in pregnancies complicated by rhesus immunisation. *J. Obstet. Gynaec. Brit. Common.* **81**, 459–65.

WILLIAMSON, A. P., BLATTNER, R. J., AND ROBERTSON, G. G. (1965). The relationship of viral antigen to virus-induced defects in chick embryos. Newcastle disease virus. *Dev. Biol.* **12**, 498–519.

WILLIAMSON, D. A. J. (1970). A syndrome of congenital malformations possibly due to maternal diabetes. *Develop. Med. Child. Neurol.* **12**, 145–52.

WILLIAMSON, E. M. (1965). Incidence and family aggregation of major congenital malformations of the central nervous system. *J. med. Genet.* **2**, 161–72.

WILLIS, R. A. (1962). *The borderland of embryology and pathology*. Second Edition. Butterworths, London, p. 460.

WILSON, J. G. (1955). Teratogenic activity of several Azo dyes chemically related to trypan blue. *Anat. Rec.* **123**, 313–33.

—— (1973). *Environment and birth defects*. Academic Press, London.

—— (1977). Current status of Teratology. General principles and mechanisms derived from animal studies. In *Handbook of teratology*. Vol. I. *General principles and etiology*, edited by Wilson, J. G. and Fraser, F. C. Plenum Press, New York, pp. 47–74.

—— (1977*a*). Embryotoxicity of Drugs in Man. In *Handbook of teratology*. Vol. I. *General principles and etiology*, edited by Wilson, J. G. and Fraser, F. C. Plenum Press, New York, pp. 309–55.

—— AND KARR, J. W. (1951). Effects of irradiation on embryonic development; X-rays on 10th day of gestation in rat. *Am. J. Anat.* **88**, 1–33.

——, JORDAN, H. C. AND BRENT, R. L. (1954). Effects of irradiation on embryonic development. *Am. J. Anat.* **92**, 153–87.

WILSON, J. K. (1955). Mono-amniotic multiple pregnancy. *J. Obstet. Gynaec. Brit. Eng.* **62**, 605–11.

WILSON, J. M. G. AND JUNGNER, G. (1968). *Principles and practice of screening for disease*. WHO, Geneva. Public Health Papers, **34**, p. 22.

WILSON, J. S. P. AND VALLENCE-OWEN, J. (1966). Congenital deformities and insulin antagonism. *Lancet* **ii**, 940–2.

WILSON, M. G., HEINS, H. L., IMAGAWA, D. T., AND ADAMS, J. M. (1959). Teratogenic effects of Asian influenza. *J. Am. med. Ass.* **171**, 638–41.

WILSON, T. S. (1971). A study of congenital malformations of the CNS among Glasgow births 1964–8. *Hlth. Bull. (Edinb.)* **29**, 79–87.

——, WATSON, R. S., AND RICHARDS, I. D. G. (1973). Anencephaly and water supply—a study of the problem in Glasgow. *Hlth. Bull. (Edinb.).* **31**, 76–8.

WILSON-DAVIS, K. (1974). The contraceptive situation in the Irish Republic. *J. biosoc. Sci.* **6**, 483–92.

WILSON-DAVIS, K. (1975). Some results of an Irish family planning survey. *J. biosoc. Sci.* **7**, 435–44.

WORLD HEALTH ORGANIZATION (1967). *International Classification of Diseases*. Eighth Revision, Volume I, Geneva, p. 271.

WRETE, M. (1959). Über die kenntnis des abnormen offenstehens des neuralrohres bei menschlichen Embryonen und jungen Feten. *Beitr. path. Anat. (Jena)* **121**, 329–46.

WRIGHT, Y. M., CLARK, W. E. AND BREG, W. R. (1974). Craniorachischisis in a partially trisomic 11 fetus in a family with reproductive failure and a reciprocal translocation, t(6p+; 11q−). *J. med. Genet.* **11**, 69–75.

WYSHAK, G. AND WHITE, C. (1969). Fertility of twins and parents of twins. *Hum. Biol.* **41**, 66–82.

YEN, S. (1975). Personal communication.

YEN, S. AND MACMAHON, B. (1968). Genetics of anencephaly and spina bifida? *Lancet* **ii**, 623–6.

YERUSHALMY, J., BIERMAN, J. M., KEMP, D. H., CONNOR, A., AND FRENCH, F. (1956). Longitudinal studies of pregnancy on the island of Kauai, Territory of Hawaii. *Am. J. Obstet. Gynec.* **71**, 80–96.

YORDAN, E. AND D'ESOPO, D. A., (1955). Hydramnios. A review of 204 cases at the Sloane Hospital for Women. *Am. J. Obstet. Gynec.* **70**, 266–73.

YOUNG, J. L., AND CRAWFORD, J. W. (1977). Omphalocoele and raised alpha-fetoprotein in maternal serum. Case Report. *Br. J. Obstet. Gynaec.* **84**, 578–9.

Younglai, E. V. and Lin, C. C. (1973). Fetal androgen and human chorionic gonadotrophin excretion in relation to genetic sex. *Am. J. Obstet. Gynec.* **117**, 291–2.

Zachary, R. B. (1977). Life with spina bifida. *Br. med. J.* **4**, 1460–2.

Zelen, M. (1971). The analysis of several 2 × 2 contingency tables. *Biometrika* **58**, 129–37.

Zimmermann, A. A. (1967). Embryologic and anatomic considerations of conjoined twins. *Birth Defects: Original Article Series* **3** (1), 18–27.

Index

Important page references are given in bold type